Global Challenges in Cardiovascular Prevention in Populations with Low Socioeconomic Status

Tomás Romero • Carolina Nazzal Nazal
Fernando Lanas
Editors

Global Challenges in Cardiovascular Prevention in Populations with Low Socioeconomic Status

Springer

Editors
Tomás Romero
Cardiovascular Medicine
University of California
San Diego, CA, USA

Carolina Nazzal Nazal
Epidemiology Programme
University of Chile
Santiago, Chile

Fernando Lanas
Internal Medicine
University of La Frontera
Temuco, Chile

ISBN 978-3-031-79053-9 ISBN 978-3-031-79051-5 (eBook)
https://doi.org/10.1007/978-3-031-79051-5

Fundacion Araucaria. This work was supported by Fundacion Araucaria.

This Springer imprint is published by the registered company Springer Nature Switzerland AG
The registered company address is: Gewerbestrasse 11, 6330 Cham, Switzerland

Foreword

> "Of all man's instruments, the most wondrous, no doubt, is the book. The other instruments are extensions of his body. The microscope, the telescope, are extensions of his sight; the telephone is the extension of his voice; then we have the plow and the sword, extensions of the arm. But the book is something else altogether: the book is an extension of memory and imagination."
>
> *Jorge Luis Borges (1899–1986)*

> "There is the joy of being healthy and fair, but there is overall the beauty, the immense joy of being useful."
>
> *Gabriela Mistral, 1945 Nobel Prize in Literature*

It is an honor, not without commitment, to write this foreword on *Global Challenges on Cardiovascular Prevention in Populations with Low Socioeconomic Status.*

Cardiovascular diseases (CVDs) are the leading cause of death in the world. At the end of the last century, there was a notable decrease in mortality rates from CVD associated with primary and secondary prevention strategies and with more effective treatments. However, in recent years, it has been observed that the total number of deaths and the global mortality rate related to CVD has increased**.** This highly worrying fact is related to the increase in the age of the population and, probably, to the increase in the prevalence of obesity, type 2 diabetes, dyslipoproteinemias, smoking, and high blood pressure. Lastly, evidence has accumulated pointing to socioeconomic and environmental factors as the fundamental causes of a wide range of health outcomes, and obviously CVD.

Global Challenges on Cardiovascular Prevention in Populations with Low Socioeconomic Status focuses on populations with limited or no access to basic health services, about half of the world population. The excellent textbooks published on current and updated resources on CVD prevention apply to populations with mostly unrestricted access to care. This textbook, as the Editors indicate, goes precisely in the opposite direction to define what is available or feasible to implement in CVD prevention in the still largest world population.

The book is published by Springer Nature Books and is available both in print and electronic formats plus an Open access option. The generous contribution of Tomás Romero, MD; Carolina Nazzal, PhD; and Fernando Lanas, MD as Editors of the book needs to be acknowledged. Fundación Araucaria Foundation, a nonprofit organization established in 1995 in San Diego California supporting research and educational activities in CVD prevention, is sponsoring this project and financially supporting it.

The experts and contributing authors of this edition are Cecilia Albala, MD; Mathew Allison, MD; L.F. Avendaño, MD; M. Canals, MD; Prabhakaran Dorairaj, MD; Tiny Jaarsma, PhD; Takeshi Kimura, MD; Fernando Lanas, MD; Kunihiro Matsushita, MD; Yubrine Moraa Gacchemba, MBChB; Cheryld Muttel, MSc; Carolina Nazzal, PhD; Elijah Ogola, MD; Neiko Ozasa, MD, PhD; Arun Pulikkottil, PhD; Barbara Riegel, PhD; Tomás Romero, MD; Pablo Ruiz, ScD; Doris Sau-Fa Yu, PhD; Maya Jean Salameh, MD; Pamela Serón, PhD; Sidney Smith Jr, MD; Kiyoaki Tanikawa, MD; Kathryn Taubert, PhD; Fernando Vio, MD; Karla Yohannessen, PhD; LiPolly Wai-Chi, PhD. All of them, with vast experience in CVD prevention from a wide range of the most populous world regions (Africa, the Americas, China, India, Japan) contribute a notable teaching capacity to their recognized academic hierarchy, covering not only the current state of knowledge but also the short- and long-term perspectives that the research envisions.

The book synthesizes contemporary concepts on the global challenges of cardiovascular prevention in populations with low socioeconomic status. The edition is extremely neat and well-cared-for, featuring a modern design, thoughtful layout and high- quality printing and binding.

I encourage everyone to take the time to read it and benefit from the insights it offers. Thank you again the authors for their hard work.

1. Albala Cecilia MD, MPH. Full Professor, Institute of Nutrition and Food Technology, Public Nutrition Unit, University of Chile.
2. Allison, Matthew. MD, MPH, FAHA. Professor and Chief. Division of Preventive Medicine. Department of Family Medicine. University of California San Diego
3. Alonso, Faustino, Ph.D. Assistant Professor, School of Public Health, Faculty of Medicine, University of Chile
4. Avendaño, Luis Fidel, MD. Pediatrician and Virologist. Professor. Faculty of Medicine, University of Chile. Honorary Member, Chilean Academy of Medicine
5. Canals, Mauricio MD, PhD. Full Professor, Department of Medicine and School of Public Health, Faculty of Medicine, University of Chile.
6. Dorairaj, Prabhakaran MBBS, MD, DM, MSc, Doctor of Science (Honoris Causa). Executive Director, Centre for Chronic Disease Control, New Delhi, India.
7. Gachemba Moraa, Yubrine. MBchB, MMed, PGD, MSc, Cardiology Fellow, Aberdeen Royal Infirmary, Aberdeen, United Kingdom. Honorary Associate Lecturer University of Aberdeen School of Medicine.
8. Gupta, Ishita. BDS, MPH, MSc. Assistant Director cum Research Scientist, Centre for Chronic Disease Control, New Delhi, India.
9. Jaarsma, Tiny. Ph.D, RN. Professor, Department of Health, Medicine and Caring Science, Linköping University.

10. Jose, Arun Pulikkottil. MBBS, MD. Head—BRIDGE Centre for Digital Health, Centre for Chronic Disease Control, New Delhi, India.
11. Lanas, Fernando. MD, PhD, Professor of Medicine, Universidad de La Frontera, Temuco, Chile
12. Li, Polly Wai-Chi. Ph.D. RN, MSc (Cardiology). School of Nursing, Faculty of Medicine, University of Hong Kong.
13. Matsushita, Kunihiro. MD, PhD, Professor, Department of Epidemiology, Johns Hopkins Bloomberg School of Public Health and Division of Cardiology, Johns Hopkins School of Medicine.
14. Muttel González, Cheryld. MD, Mg Clinical Epidemiology. Assistant Professor, Internal Medicine Department. Universidad de la Frontera.
15. Nazzal, Carolina. Ph.D. Associate Professor, Epidemiology Program, School of Public Health, Faculty of Medicine, University of Chile.
16. Ogola, Elijah N, MBChB, M.Med. Professor of Medicine and Cardiology, University of Nairobi.
17. Osokpo, Onome H. Ph.D, MSc, MSN, RN. Assistant Professor, Department of Population Health Nursing Science, University of Illinois.
18. Ozasa, Neiko MD, Ph.D. Associate Professor, Department of Cardiovascular Medicine, Kyoto University Graduate School of Medicine, Kyoto, Japan.
19. Riegel, Barbara. Ph.D, RN, FAHA, FAAN. Professor, School of Nursing, University of Pennsylvania and Senior Research Scientist, Center for Home Care Policy and Research at VNS Health.
20. Romero, Tomás. MD, FACC, FAHA, FSCAI, FACP. Associate Clinical Professor, Department of Medicine, Division of Cardiovascular Diseases, School of Medicine, University of California, San Diego. President, Fundacion Araucaria Foundation Board of Directors
21. Ruiz-Rudolph, Pablo Sc.D., Associate Professor, Epidemiology Program, Institute of Population Health, Faculty of Medicine, University of Chile.
22. Salameh, Maya. MD, FSVM. Assistant Professor of Medicine. Associate Director of the Johns Hopkins Center for Vascular Medicine. Division of Cardiology. Johns Hopkins University School of Medicine
23. Serón, Pamela Ph.D, MSc. Professor, Faculty of Medicine, Universidad de La Frontera.
24. Smith, Sidney C., Jr. MD, MACC, FAHA, FESC. Professor of Medicine and Cardiology, School of Medicine, Division of Cardiology, University of North Carolina.
25. Taubert, Kathryn, PhD. Department of Physiology, University of Texas Southwestern Medical Center, Dallas, Texas, USA.
26. Vio, Fernando MD, MPH. Full Professor, Institute of Nutrition and Food Technology, Public Nutrition Unit, University of Chile.
27. Westland, Heleen Ph.D. Department of General Practice and Nursing Science, University Medical Center Utrecht.
28. Ye, Fen. MN. Ph.D Candidate. School of Nursing, LKS Faculty of Medicine, The University of Hong Kong.

29. Yohannessen, Karla Ph.D., MPH. Assistant Professor, School of Public Health, Faculty of Medicine, University of Chile.
30. Yoshida, Toshiko RN, PHN, Ph.D. Dean, College of Nursing, Graduate School of Nursing Science, St. Luke's International University.
31. Yu, Doris Sau-fung. Ph.D., BSc in Nursing, RN, FAAN, FGSA, FHKAN. School of Nursing, Faculty of Medicine, University of Hong Kong.

Universidad de Buenos Aires
Buenos Aires, Argentina

Daniel José Piñeiro

Preface

This book addresses the reality of cardiovascular prevention (CVP) in more than half of the world's population with limited or no access to primary health care and thus, to CVP strategies.

Although there are excellent books on the established and recent advances in CVP, they are mostly applicable to populations with unlimited access to health care.

In this textbook, we want to go in the opposite direction: we are trying to define what is happening with the most basic and effective known CVP tools in the even larger segment of the world's population. A particular goal of the authors is to explore what effective and low-cost CVP resources can be applied to these populations, considering the social, economic, and cultural conditions of different regions of the world. To this end, we have been fortunate to have authors with expertise in cardiovascular prevention from the Americas, Africa, the Middle East, and Asia, as well as experts in environmental and public health issues who recognize the importance of social determinants in the development and control of cardiovascular disease. We believe that this book will appeal to a broad multinational readership, including primary care, cardiovascular, public health, and research professionals, as well as students of the medical professions.

San Diego, CA, USA — Tomás Romero
Santiago, Chile — Carolina Nazzal Nazal
Temuco, Chile — Fernando Lanas

Contents

Contributors

Cecilia Albala Public Health Nutrition Unit, Institute of Nutrition and Food Technology, Universidad de Chile, Santiago, Chile

Matthew Allison Division of Preventive Medicine, Department of Family Medicine, University of California San Diego, San Diego, CA, USA

Faustino Alonso Faculty of Medicine, School of Public Health, University of Chile, Santiago, Chile

Luis Fidel Avendaño Faculty of Medicine, University of Chile, Santiago, Chile

Mauricio Canals Faculty of Medicine, School of Public Health, University of Chile, Santiago, Chile

Yubrine M. Gachemba Aberdeen Royal Infirmary, University of Aberdeen School of Medicine, Aberdeen, UK

Ishita Gupta Centre for Chronic Disease Control, New Delhi, India

Tiny Jaarsma Department of Health, Medicine and Caring Sciences, Linkoping University, Linkoping, Sweden

Arun Pulikkottil Jose Centre for Chronic Disease Control, New Delhi, India

Fernando Lanas Facultad de Medicina, Universidad de La Frontera, Temuco, Chile

Polly Wai-Chi Li School of Nursing, Li Ka Shing Faculty of Medicine, The University of Hong Kong, Pok Fu Lam, Hong Kong

Kunihiro Matsushita Department of Epidemiology, Johns Hopkins Bloomberg School of Public Health, Johns Hopkins School of Medicine, Baltimore, MD, USA

Division of Cardiology, Johns Hopkins School of Medicine, Baltimore, MD, USA

Cheryld Muttel Facultad de Medicina, Universidad de La Frontera, Temuco, Chile

Carolina Nazzal Nazal Faculty of Medicine, School of Public Health, University of Chile, Santiago, Chile

Elijah N. Ogola University of Nairobi, Nairobi, Kenya

Onome H. Osokpo University of Illinois Chicago, Chicago, IL, USA

Neiko Ozasa Department of Cardiovascular Medicine, Kyoto University Graduate School of Medicine, Kyoto, Japan

Dorairaj Prabhakaran Centre for Chronic Disease Control, New Delhi, India

London School of Hygiene and Tropical Medicine, University of London, London, UK

Barbara Riegel University of Pennsylvania School of Nursing, Philadelphia, PA, USA

Center for Home Care Policy and Research at VNS Health, New York, NY, USA

Tomás Romero Department of Medicine, Division of Cardiovascular Diseases, School of Medicine, University of California, San Diego, San Diego, CA, USA

Fundacion Araucaria Foundation Board of Directors, San Diego, CA, USA

Pablo Ruiz-Rudolph Epidemiology Program, Faculty of Medicine, Institute of Population Health, University of Chile, Santiago, Chile

Maya Jean Salameh Division of Cardiology, Johns Hopkins School of Medicine, Baltimore, MD, USA

Pamela Serón Facultad de Medicina, Universidad de La Frontera, Temuco, Chile

Sidney C. Smith, Jr. Division of Cardiology, Department of Medicine and Cardiology, School of Medicine, University of North Carolina, Chapel Hill, NC, USA

Kathryn A. Taubert Department of Physiology, UT Southwestern Medical Center, Dallas, TX, USA

Fernando Vio Public Health Nutrition Unit, Institute of Nutrition and Food Technology, Universidad de Chile, Santiago, Chile

Heleen Westland Julius Center for Health Sciences and Primary Care, University Medical Center Utrecht, Utrecht, The Netherlands

Sophia Fen Ye School of Nursing, Li Ka Shing Faculty of Medicine, The University of Hong Kong, Pok Fu Lam, Hong Kong

Karla Yohannessen Faculty of Medicine, School of Public Health, University of Chile, Santiago, Chile

Toshiko Yoshida St. Luke's International University, College of Nursing, Graduate School of Nursing Science, Chuo City, Japan

Doris Sau-fung Yu School of Nursing, Li Ka Shing Faculty of Medicine, The University of Hong Kong, Pok Fu Lam, Hong Kong

Abbreviations

ABI	Ankle-brachial index
ACC	American College of Cardiology
ACE	Angiotensin-converting enzyme
ACEI	Angiotensin-converting enzyme inhibitor
ACS	Acute coronary syndrome
AHA	American Heart Association
AHWA	Amsterdam Healthy Weight Approach
AI	Artificial Intelligence
AIDS	Acquired immunodeficiency syndrome
AMI	Acute myocardial infarction
APPCAP	Air Pollution Prevention and Control Action Plan
ARB	Angiotensin-receptor blocker
ARIC	The Atherosclerosis Risk in Communities study
ARNI	Renin-angiotensin system inhibitors
ASCVD	Atherosclerotic cardiovascular disease
BCE	Before current age
BMI	Body mass index
BP	Blood pressure
CARRS	Cardiometabolic Risk Reduction in South Asia Study
CCB	Calcium channel blocker
CDC	US Centers for Disease Control and Prevention
CE	Current age
CH_4	Methane
CHA2DS2-VASc scores	Congestive heart failure, Hypertension, Age, Diabetes, previous Stroke/transient ischemic attack scores
CHD	Coronary heart disease
China CDC	Chinese Centre for Disease Control and Prevention
CHIP	Clonal hematopoiesis indeterminate potential
CI	Confidence interval
CLI	Critical limb ischemia
CMB	Centralized bed management

CMNN	Communicable, maternal, neonatal, and nutritional diseases
CO	Carbon monoxide
COVID 19	Coronavirus pandemic disease emerged in 2019
COVID-19	COronaVIrus Disease of 2019
CREOLE	Comparison of Dual Therapies for Lowering Blood Pressure Black Africans
CVD	Cardiovascular diseases
CVDP	Cardiovascular disease prevention
CVP	Cardiovascular prevention
DALY	Disability-Adjusted Life Years
DALYs	Disability Adjusted Life Years
DBP	Diastolic blood pressure
DLHS	District-Level Household Survey
DNA virus	Virus in which deoxyribonucleic acid strands set up their genomic code
DPSEEA	Driving Force-Pressure-State-Exposure-Effect-Action
ECLAC	Economic Commission for Latin America and the Caribbean
EHR	Electronic Health Record
ELSA	English Longitudinal Study of Ageing
EMF	Endomyocardial fibrosis
ENSANUT	Encuesta Nacional de Salud y Nutrición
EPIDEMCA	Epidemiology of Dementia in Central Africa study
ESC	European Society of Cardiology
FAD	Food for Agriculture Development
FAO	Food and Agriculture Organization
FCTC	Framework Convention on Tobacco Control
FLCMC	Free/Low-Cost Medical Care
G7	Group of Seven
GAP	Global action plan
GBD	Global Burden of Disease
GDP	Gross Domestic Product
GHGs	Greenhouse gases
HAP	Household air pollution
HDLc	High-density lipoprotein cholesterol
HER	Electronic Health Record
HFC	Hydrofluorocarbons
HFrEF	Heart failure with reduced ejection fraction
Hg	Mercury
HgA1c	Hemoglobin A1c
HIC	High-income country
HICs	High-income countries
HIV	Human immunodeficiency virus
HLM	High-level meeting

HR	Hazard ratio
HTN	hypertension
ICMR	Indian Council of Medical Research
ICU	Intensive care unit
IFAD	International Fund for Agricultural Development
IGT	Impaired glucose test
IHCI	India Hypertension Control Initiative
IHD	Ischemic heart disease
INDIAB	India Diabetes study
KCHF registry	Kyoto Congestive Heart Failure
KICKOFF registry	Kitakawachi Clinical Background and Outcome of Heart Failure
LA	Latin America
LDLc	Low-density lipoprotein cholesterol
LIC	Low-Income Country
LMIC	Low- and middle-income countries
LMICs	Low- and medium-income countries
MPOWER	Monitor, protect, offer, warn, enforce, raise
mRNA	Messenger RNA
N_2O	Nitrous oxide
NCD	Non-communicable diseases
NFHS	National Family Health Survey
NHANES	National Health and Nutrition Examination Survey
NO_X	Nitrogen oxides
NPHW	National Public Health Week
NPHW	Non-Physician Health Workers
NPI	Non-pharmaceutical interventions
O_3	Ozone
OECD	Organisation for Economic Co-operation and Development
OHCA	Out-of-hospital cardiorespiratory arrest events
OR	Odds ratio
PAD	Peripheral artery disease
PAHO	Pan American Health Organization
PASCAR	Pan-African Society of Cardiology
PFC	Perfluorocarbons
PHC	Primary health care
PM	Particulate matter
PM2.5	Particulate matter of size below 2.5 μm
PNS	Pesquisa Nacional de Saúde
PURE	Population Urban Rural Epidemiology
PURES	Prospective Urban Rural Epidemiology Study
PVR	Pulse volume recording
RCT	Randomized controlled trial
RHD	Rheumatic heart disease

RNA virus	Virus in which ribonucleic acid strands set up their genomic code
RT-PCR	Polymerase chain reaction test to detect an RNA virus
RTSL	Resolve to Save Lives
SALURBAL	Salud Urbana en América Latina
SARS	Severe acute respiratory syndrome
SARS-CoV-2	Coronavirus emerged in December 2019, responsible of COVID pandemic
SBP	Systolic blood pressure
SDG	Sustainable development goal
SDOH	Social determinants of health
SES	Socioeconomic status
SFE	Smoke-free environment
SMASH	Shandong Ministry of Health Action on Salt and Hypertension
SMS	Short messaging service
SO_2	Sulfur dioxide
ss	Single-stranded (nucleic acid)
SSA	Sub-Saharan Africa
SSB	Sugar-sweetened beverages
STEMI	ST-segment elevation myocardial infarction
TAVI	Transcatheter aortic valve implantation
TBI	Toe-brachial index
TTI	Trace-treat-isolate strategy
U.S.	United States
UFP	Ultrafine particles
UHC	Universal health coverage
UN	United Nations
UNGA	United Nations General Assembly
UNICEF	United Nations Children's Fund
US CDC	United States Centers for Disease Control and Prevention
VOCs	Volatile organic compounds
WFP	World Food Programme
WHA	World Health Assembly
WHF	World Heart Federation
WHO FCTC	WHO Framework Convention on Tobacco Control
WHO	World Health Organization
WISE	Women's Ischemia Syndrome Evaluation trial
YLDs	Years Lived with Disability
$\mu g/m^3$	Micrograms per cubic meter

Chapter 1
An Outlook of Cardiovascular Prevention (CVP): Cardiovascular Risk Factors, Current Resources, Future Promises, and Impact of Socioeconomic Factors

Tomás Romero

1.1 Historical Background

A healthy lifestyle that included diet and exercise were among the first recorded recommendations of what could be interpreted as the primordial steps in Cardiovascular Prevention. Sushruta in Benares, India, 600 BCE and later on Galen, a former physician of gladiators, developed programs based on those principles. Galen established himself at the Asklepion, originally a Greek health center in Pergamon, Turkey, then part of the Roman Empire, 150 CE [1]. The Asklepion may be seen as one of the first precursors of what is today an advanced hospital facility, with many of its activities focused on rehabilitation and prevention.

Cardiovascular Prevention (CVP) has evolved since then over similar stepping stones, identifying within the last 150 years other harmful factors and developing technical advances for additional support.

1.2 Textbook Objectives

The main objective of this textbook is the review and discussion of the socioeconomic factors associated with the implementation and outcomes of CVP in different world populations. From recent data published by the World Bank and Word Health Organization, approximately half of the world population have limited or no access

T. Romero (✉)
Department of Medicine, Division of Cardiovascular Diseases, School of Medicine, University of California, San Diego, San Diego, CA, USA

Fundacion Araucaria Foundation Board of Directors, San Diego, CA, USA

T. Romero et al. (eds.), *Global Challenges in Cardiovascular Prevention in Populations with Low Socioeconomic Status*,
https://doi.org/10.1007/978-3-031-79051-5_1

to basic primary health care services, the usual gate to CVP [2, 3]. The focus of our intent is precisely the assessment of what is the reality of CVP in these low socioeconomic status regions and populations, attempting an understanding of the social patterning involved and derived challenges in health care.

To further define this reality and for recommendations of potentially affordable improvements, we have compiled in our textbook reviews by authors with extensive work on cardiovascular prevention in different world regions and populations, most within the LIC or LMIC socioeconomic patterns.

1.3 Standard Approaches to Cardiovascular Prevention

CVP traditionally is analyzed in two phases interlocked to each other. Primary prevention starts identifying and managing the major risk factors (hypertension, obesity, diabetes mellitus, and smoking) that lead to the most common causes of cardiovascular diseases (CVDs) such as coronary heart disease, cerebrovascular and peripheral vascular disease, and congestive heart failure. Once the disease is manifest clinically, secondary prevention begins, continuing the management of risk factors with maximization of measures for control as needed, plus consideration of procedures to provide better blood supply to the coronary arteries and cerebrovascular and peripheral vascular territories or improve the mechanical/electrical heart function.

Since the 1900s, cardiovascular risk reduction began focused on the clinical management at the primary or secondary prevention level according to the progress in identifying the tools to manage the risk factors (lifestyle and dietary changes, pharmacological and interventional revascularization procedures). However, prevalence of CVD has globally increased steadily and doubled from 1990 to 2019 (271–523 million) as the number of CVD deaths raised from 12.1 to 19.7 millions attributed mostly to the increase in the aging population [4] although reduction of mortality in HMIC and HIC populations with less restricted access to health care resources has occurred [5].

A different approach aimed on population or community-oriented programs based on low-cost lifestyle modifications involving many subjects has been attempted. An example of such approach exceeding the improvements noted in the more restricted individual clinical management of risk factors is the North Karelia Project [6]. This region from Finland had the lowest socioeconomic status and the largest CVD mortality until the 1970s in comparison to the rest of the country. Preliminary observations in a cohort of 5817 subjects followed since 1972 through 1978 comparing the reduction of acute myocardial infarctions in North Karelia between clinical management of individuals with high risk for coronary heart disease (CHD, about 10% of the subjects) v/s a strategy to reduce cholesterol and blood pressure in the population at large projected clear advantages of the latter as shown in Table 1.1.

Table 1.1 North Karelia Project. Preliminary studies projections (5817 subjects, 1972–1978)

High risk strategy	Population strategy
33% AMI reduction	70% AMI reduction

Kottke et al. 1985 [7]

These estimates led to the largest CVD prevention (CVDP) community-population study done to our knowledge since 1972–1995 that included 433,000 subjects providing a solid justification for long-term community-oriented programs for CVDP. Finland in 1975 had the highest mortality for CHD in the world (673 males, 202 females/100,000), compared to most of HIC (USA 528, 168/100,000), Netherlands (363, 102/100,000), and Switzerland (226, 63/100,000). From 1969–1971 to 1995, the age-standardized CHD mortality (per 100, 000) decreased in North Karelia by 73% (from 672 to 185) and nationwide by 65% (from 465 to 165) with a similar reduction in CVD mortality. A community effort of volunteer leaders in every district in North Karelia (local housewives' groups such as Martha Association organized special festivities in local villages offering healthy food prepared and served by local villagers). Local TV involvement, newspaper publications, businesses, and available health professionals organized campaigns to cut down smoking, eating less saturated fats and salt, and continuing with the traditional regional high level of physical activities.

To what extent similar efforts may surge or already exist in low socioeconomic populations is unclear, and we expect that the information searched by our authors in the following chapters will fill some of these gaps.

1.4 Brief Review of Cardiovascular Risk Factor Status: Hypertension, Obesity, Diabetes, and Smoking

A case in point in CVDP within our objectives is hypertension, a primary risk factor that is discussed at length by Sidney Smith Jr., MD and Kathryn Taubert, PhD in Chap. 2. They will also address in Chap. 13, United Nation Sustainable Goals: Effective measures for CVP in LMIC and LIC populations. High blood pressure (HBP) is the leading risk factor for mortality, with attributable 10.8 million deaths in 2019. Alarming news are that HBP control currently around 50% in more affluent countries is near 10% in the poorest regions [8].

And this dependency of risk factor control and health outcomes from regional socioeconomic resources is a persistent global pattern discussed in detail in the following chapters.

Continuing with this brief outline, obesity has increased in all regions. Its prevalence in age-group 5–19 years was 6.8% in 2016, up from 2.9% in 2000. This increase has been noticed globally by WHO, but it has been highest in the Americas (12.4–16.6%). This trend has also occurred in adults >18 years old, with prevalence in 2016 of 13.1%, ranging from 4.7% in the South East Asia to 28.6% in the Americas [9].

As already noted, the influence of socioeconomic factors (income and education) in the global prevalence of hypertension, smoking, and diabetes mellitus is well documented. Obesity, however, follows a pattern determined mostly for limitations of access to a well-balanced diet in the lowest income and education groups, but with more readily access to cheaper ultra-processed high caloric food. The obesity prevalence still increasing in communities with higher income and education may be driven mostly by the middle-income groups, with less restrictions to food access as observed in the poorest, but still preferring high calorie ultra-processed foods instead of a healthier diet with a steady presence of vegetables and fruits.

Diabetes in 2021 affected approximately 537 million adults (20–79 years). The total number is projected to rise to 643 million by 2030 and 783 million by 2045, and three in four adults with diabetes live in low- and middle-income countries [9]. (Cecilia Albala, MD and Fernando Vio MD will address in detail Obesity and Diabetes in Chap. 3).

In 2020, smoking was estimated that 22.3% of the global population over age 15 were smokers, but down from 32.7% in 2000. This historical prevalence of smokers has been more prominent in men than in women (33% vs 7.7%). A study in 49 low- and middle-income countries conducted in 2010–2019 showed that smoking in men 19–49 years old was higher (25.6%) in individuals with no or low education vs 9.1% with higher education [10].

(Additional information on smoking will be addressed in Chaps. 4, 5, 8, 9, 10, 11, and 12)

1.5 Cardiovascular Prevention and Access to Drug Therapy

Information collected from the WHO and World Bank database and published in 2011 addressed the availability of antihypertensives and hypoglycemic agents among other medications for acute and chronic conditions in many low- and middle-income countries. The data was obtained from 2779 medical outlets (Africa, India, China, Eastern Mediterranean, Latin America, and Western Pacific). As an average, antihypertensive and antidiabetic medications were used in 42.1% at the public sector vs 62.5% at the private level, all of them below the WHO bench target of 80%. Factors included budget restrictions in stocking supplies in public facilities and reduced demand due to unaffordable expenses for higher drug prices in the private sector [11].

A PURE study published in 2016 reported that drugs frequently used in secondary prevention (ASA, beta blockers, angiotensin converting enzymes inhibitors, and statins) were all available in 90% of rural and in 95% of urban HIC, but only in 3% of rural and 25% of urban LIC [12].

The INTERHEART was a pioneer case-control study looking at the association of risk factors with Acute Myocardial Infarction (AMI). Included 52 countries with their population represented in both sex and age groups. Compared 15,152 AMI cases with 14,820 controls, showing an AMI positive association with history of hypertension and diabetes, ApoB/ApoA1 ratio, abdominal obesity and psychsocial factors. In contrast, daily consumption of fruits vegetables, and physical activities showed a protective effect [13].

A study published in 2022 done in 41 low- and middle-income populations that included a total of 116,649 subjects, 8% of subjects eligible for primary prevention and 21% of those for secondary prevention received statins, with a lower use in countries with lesser health spending. These findings were below the WHO threshold of 50% for statin use in eligible subjects [14]. More detailed information on the availability of pharmacological resources associated with socioeconomic status will be discussed further in the following chapters.

Data collected in the ALLHAT randomized control study of antihypertensive drugs in the USA which included 27,862 participants all of them provided with the assigned drug therapy showed that low-income subjects (2169) had poorer BP control and worse outcomes although no information on adherence was obtained other than less clinic visits by the low-income subjects [15].

A study published in 2019 done in 44 countries from Latin America, Caribe, Africa, and Bangladesh with a total of 1,100,507 participants, showed that 17.5% were hypertensive, 29.9% received antihypertensive treatment, and 10.3% achieved BP control which was higher in women, in subjects in the upper income and education levels, and in nonsmokers [16].

In a final analysis, the different aspects of access to drug therapy for cardiovascular prevention include a complex pattern of factors ranging from availability of drugs, their affordability, adherence to therapy, and the not well understood socioeconomic components.

1.6 Environment and Cardiovascular Health

Nature is shared by humans with all living and inert materials in the so-called biosphere, and from this interaction depends on some extent what we consider health and disease. A large number of environmental factors have been identified historically and more recently to influence cardiovascular health. Seasons and circadian rhythms have been associated with the timing and frequency of adverse cardiac events like myocardial infarction, heart rhythm disturbances, and strokes and so many other factors such as altitude, sunlight, social, built environment, and pollution (air, agriculture, and water) just to name a few (some of these factors are depicted in Table 1.2) [17].

Pablo Ruiz ScD and Karla Johannessen PhD will discuss at length this subject in Chap. 6.

L.F. Avendaño MD, M. Canals MD and C. Nazzal PhD will address the impact of the most recent pandemic (Covid-19) in the population access to health care providers (Chap. 7).

Table 1.2 Environmental domains

Natural environment	Personal environment	Social environment
Night and day cycles (circadian)	Physical activity	Built environment
Seasons (cold/heat)	Nutrition	Pollution
Sunlight	Smoking	Social networks
Altitude		Socioeconomic status
Latitude		
Greenspaces		

Content partially derived from figure in: Bhatnagar (2017) [17]; Illustration credit: Ben Smith

1.7 Future Expectations and New Steps in Cardiovascular Prevention

In a discussion presented by Eugene Braunwald MD at a Houston Methodist Grand rounds on January 16, 2022 [18], he pointed out six foreseeable steps in cardiovascular prevention:

Polygenic risk score (PRS) or how genetic risk profiling and risk factor interaction will help to identify susceptible populations to implement effective clinical risk assessment.

Primordial prevention of CHD focused on population-based healthy lifestyle choices to avoid the emergence or minimize coronary risk factors. Dietary adjustments, exercise, and abstention of smoking are part of this armamentarium common to many other cardiovascular risk factors.

More aggressive strategies that include new drugs to obtain maximal lipid control should go beyond statins. Once a year, injection of inclisiran (small interfering RNA that prevents PCSK synthesis) will reset the lipids levels by 40% and may prolong life in many.

More potent anti-inflammatory strategies are needed. Recurrence of coronary events in some subjects on statins with maximal reduction of LDL cholesterol suggests the need of stronger new anti-inflammatory drugs like canakinumab.

Clonal Hematopoiesis Indeterminate Potential (CHIP). Somatic mutations in leukocytes have been found independently associated with adverse outcomes in individuals with established atherosclerotic cardiovascular disease increasing risk from 25% to 85% and opening a potential new line for interventions.

Finally, artificial intelligence may become a guiding lead to integrate all the tools available in preventive cardiology.

The future of these developments in cardiovascular prevention seems promising but of uncertain usage. They will depend on increasing expenses that may go beyond affordability even in sectors of HMIC or HIC. However, as Braunwald and others have often remarked, the fundamental basic stepping stones in cardiovascular prevention are still the same, and we cannot do it without them. We just must find a way for half of the world population to walk on them.

Glossary

Primordial prevention Risk factor reduction targeted toward an entire population through modifications on social and environmental conditions.

Circadian Biological processes recurring naturally on a 24-hour cycle even in the absence of light fluctuations.

Built environment Human-made structures, features, and facilities interpreted as an environment in which people live and work.

Polygenic risk score (PRS) Genetic risk profiling and risk factor interaction to identify susceptible populations.

Artificial intelligence Computer systems able to perform human tasks that require human intelligence (visual, speech recognition, translations between languages, and decision-making).

CHIP Somatic mutations in leukocytes increase CHD risk.

PCSK Inhibits LDL cholesterol liver receptors, thus increasing LDL blood levels and CHD risk. Drugs like inclisiran inhibit PCSK synthesis.

References

1. Tipton CM. The history of "exercise is medicine" in ancient civilizations. Adv Physiol Educ. 2014;38(2):109–17. Available from: https://www.ncbi.nlm.nih.gov/pmc/articles/PMC4056176/
2. Tracking universal health coverage: 2017 global monitoring report (English). Washington, D.C.: World Bank Group. Available from: http://documents.worldbank.org/curated/en/640121513095868125/Tracking-universal-health-coverage-2017-global-monitoring-report
3. World Health Organization. World health statistics 2023. World Health Organization; 2023. Available from: https://www.who.int/publications/i/item/9789240074323
4. Roth GA, Mensah GA, Johnson CO, et al. Global burden of cardiovascular diseases and risk factors, 1990–2019: update from the GBD 2019 study. J Am Coll Cardiol. 2020;76(25):2982–3021. Available from: https://www.sciencedirect.com/science/article/pii/S0735109720377755
5. Ananth CV, Rutherford C, Rosenfeld EB, et al. Epidemiologic trends and risk factors associated with the decline in mortality from coronary heart disease in the United States, 1990–2019. Am Heart J. 2023;263:46–55. Available from: https://www.sciencedirect.com/science/article/pii/S0002870323001175?via%3Dihub
6. Puska P, Nissinen A, Tuomilehto J. The community-based strategy to prevent coronary heart disease: conclusions from the ten years of the North Karelia project. Annu Rev Public Health. 1985;6:147–93. https://doi.org/10.1146/annurev.pu.06.050185.001051.
7. Kottke TE, Puska P, Salonen JT, Tuomilehto J, Nissinen A. Projected effects of high-risk versus population-based prevention strategies in coronary heart disease. Am J Epidemiol. 1985;121(5):697–704. https://doi.org/10.1093/aje/121.5.697.
8. Schutte AE, Jafar TH, Poulter NR, et al. Addressing global disparities in blood pressure control: perspectives of the International Society of Hypertension. Cardiovasc Res. 2023;119(2):381–409. https://doi.org/10.1093/cvr/cvac130.
9. GBD results [Internet]. Institute for Health Metrics and Evaluation. Available from: https://vizhub.healthdata.org/gbd-results

10. WHO report on the global tobacco epidemic, 2023: protect people from tobacco smoke [Internet]. www.who.int. Available from: https://www.who.int/publications/i/item/9789240077164
11. Cameron A, Roubos I, Ewen M, Mantel-Teeuwisse AK, Leufkens HG, Laing RO. Differences in the availability of medicines for chronic and acute conditions in the public and private sectors of developing countries. Bull World Health Organ. 2011;89(6):412–21.
12. Khatib R, McKee M, Shannon H, et al. Availability and affordability of cardiovascular disease medicines and their effect on use in high-income, middle-income, and low-income countries: an analysis of the PURE study data. Lancet. 2016;387(10013):61–9.
13. Yusuf S, Hawken S, Ôunpuu S, et al. Effect of potentially modifiable risk factors associated with myocardial infarction in 52 countries (the INTERHEART study): case-control study. The Lancet. 2004;364(9438):937–52. Available from: https://pubmed.ncbi.nlm.nih.gov/15364185/
14. Marcus ME, Manne-Goehler J, Theilmann M, et al. Use of statins for the prevention of cardiovascular disease in 41 low-income and middle-income countries: a cross-sectional study of nationally representative, individual-level data. Lancet Glob Health. 2022;10(3):e369–79.
15. Shahu A, Herrin J, Dhruva SS, et al. Disparities in socioeconomic context and association with blood pressure control and cardiovascular outcomes in ALLHAT. J Am Heart Assoc. 2019;8(15):e012277.
16. Geldsetzer P, Manne-Goehler J, Marcus ME, et al. The state of hypertension care in 44 low-income and middle-income countries: a cross-sectional study of nationally representative individual-level data from 1·1 million adults. Lancet. 2019 Aug;394(10199):652–62.
17. Bhatnagar A. Environmental determinants of cardiovascular disease. Circ Res. 2017;121(2):162–80. Available from: https://www.ncbi.nlm.nih.gov/pmc/articles/PMC5777598/
18. Dr. S. Venkatesan MD. Dr Braunwald's Grand rounds on future of cardiology [Internet]. 2022 [cited 2023 Dec 6]. Available from: https://drsvenkatesan.com/2022/01/16/dr-braunwalds-grand-rounds-on-future-of-cardiology/

Chapter 2
Global Programs and Outcomes in Arterial Hypertension Management in Countries with Developing Economies

Sidney C. Smith, Jr. and Kathryn A. Taubert

2.1 Introduction

Noncommunicable diseases (NCDs) are the leading cause of death worldwide, being responsible for approximately three quarters of all deaths each year. Within the categories of NCDs, the leading cause of death is cardiovascular diseases (CVD; particularly ischemic heart disease and stroke) and within the category of CVD, a major risk factor for death (including premature death) and disability is hypertension (also known as high blood pressure). Recognizing the increasing global burden of hypertension, the World Health Organization (WHO) recently published a comprehensive report titled "Global report on hypertension - The race against a silent killer" [1]. The report highlights the devastating global impact of high blood pressure and acknowledges that the condition leads to stroke, heart attack, heart failure, kidney damage, and many other health problems. The report also notes that "High systolic blood pressure is the world's leading risk factor for mortality." In the Foreword to the document, WHO Director-General Dr. Tedros Adhanom Ghebreyesus states, "hypertension can be controlled effectively with simple, low-cost medication regimens, and yet only about one in five people with hypertension has controlled it." He continues saying that strengthening hypertension control must be part of every country's health system.

S. C. Smith, Jr. (✉)
Medicine and Cardiology, School of Medicine, Division of Cardiology, University of North Carolina, Chapel Hill, NC, USA
e-mail: scs@med.unc.edu

K. A. Taubert
Department of Physiology, UT Southwestern Medical Center, Dallas, TX, USA
e-mail: kathryn.taubert@utsouthwestern.edu

T. Romero et al. (eds.), *Global Challenges in Cardiovascular Prevention in Populations with Low Socioeconomic Status*,
https://doi.org/10.1007/978-3-031-79051-5_2

2.2 Global Burden of Hypertension

There are 1.3 billion adults in the world who have hypertension. The global distribution of hypertension as of 2015 is shown in Fig. 2.1 [2]. Hypertension is defined as a persistently raised arterial pressure above the normal range. While the determination of this normal range varies between countries/regions across the globe, the WHO states that hypertension is diagnosed if the systolic blood pressure readings on two different days are ≥140 mmHg and/or the diastolic blood pressure readings on both days are ≥90 mmHg [1]. Most of the population studies and databases use this definition, and unless otherwise stated, the data referred to in this chapter will use 140 systolic and/or 90 diastolic as the threshold for hypertension. In population studies, the total number of individuals considered to have hypertension is generally defined those having an elevated systolic or diastolic blood pressure as well as those taking medication for hypertension.

The global age-standardized prevalence of hypertension has remained relatively stable over the 3-decade 1990–2019-time interval at about 32–33% [3]. It was similar between genders (32% in women and 34% in men in 2019). However, there was a wide variation in these percentages between various parts of the world. Additionally, hypertension becomes progressively more common with advancing age, with one study showing that prevalence essentially doubled in the age-group older than 50 years compared to individuals of 50 years or younger [4].

The absolute number of people aged 30–79 with hypertension has increased markedly over the last few decades due to population growth and aging. In 1990, that number was reported to be 650 million adults while in 2019 the prevalence had

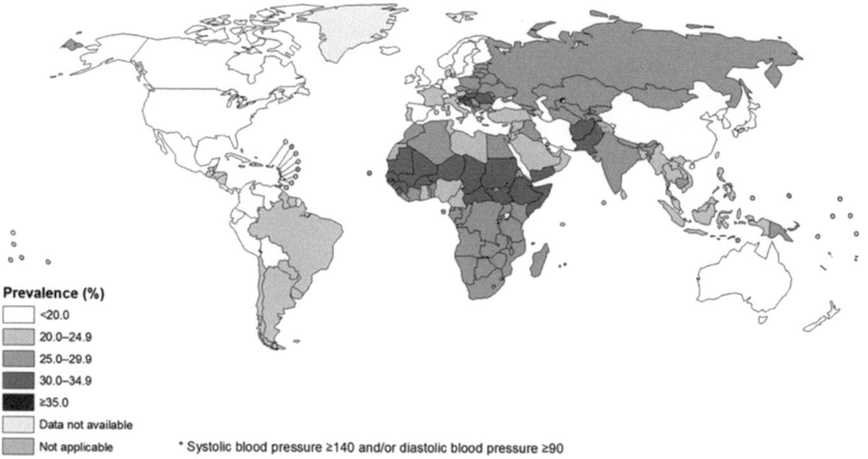

Fig. 2.1 Prevalence of raised blood pressure*, ages 18+, 2015 (age-standardized estimate). Both sexes. From Ref. [2]

jumped to 1.3 billion, doubling what it was in 1990 [3]. Worldwide, raised blood pressure is estimated to cause 10.8 million deaths per year [5].

Over the past few decades, the highest prevalence of hypertension has shifted from higher income countries to lower income countries [3, 6, 7]. Figure 2.2 illustrates these temporal global and regional changes in blood pressure during the 1990–2019 time period. As one can see, while the burden of hypertension is substantial globally, the number of undiagnosed cases tended to drop in the high-income countries while tending to increase in the less-rich ones. Furthermore, the steepest rise in the total number of cases over these three decades during these past few decades was seen in low- and middle-income countries (LMICs). In other words, hypertension is a huge global problem that puts a disproportionate burden on those who are least able to deal with it.

Although hypertension can be treated, controlled, and sometimes prevented, few countries currently do so effectively. Better hypertension management will save lives. According to the WHO's Global Health Observatory for adults ages 30–79 with hypertension, only 54% have been diagnosed, 42% are being treated, and 21% are considered to have their hypertension under control [1]. If one looks at only high-prevalence LMICs, the numbers are much worse—only one person in ten with hypertension has it under control.

Individual country profiles of hypertension burden and control are available to download from the WHO website [8]. Figure 2.3 is an example of one profile.

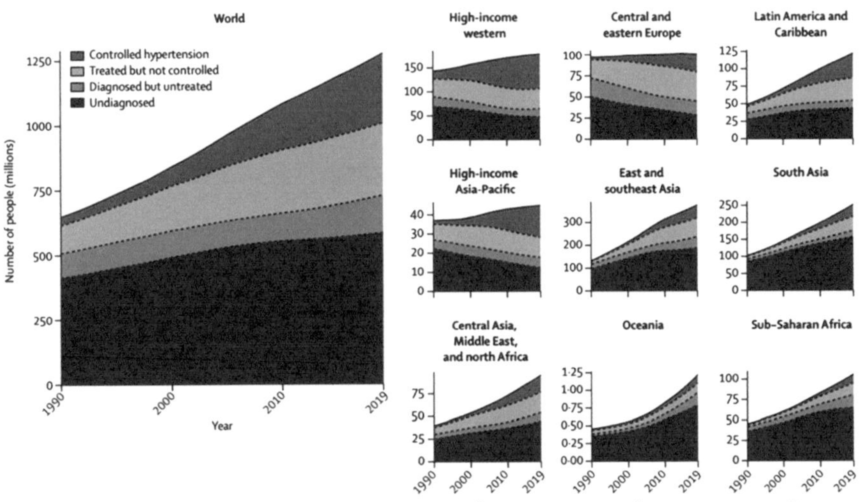

Fig. 2.2 Trends in the number of people with hypertension who reported a diagnosis, who used treatment, and whose blood pressure was effectively controlled, globally and by region. From Ref. [3]. Copyright © 2021 World Health Organization; licensee Elsevier. This is an Open Access article published under the CC BY 3.0 IGO license

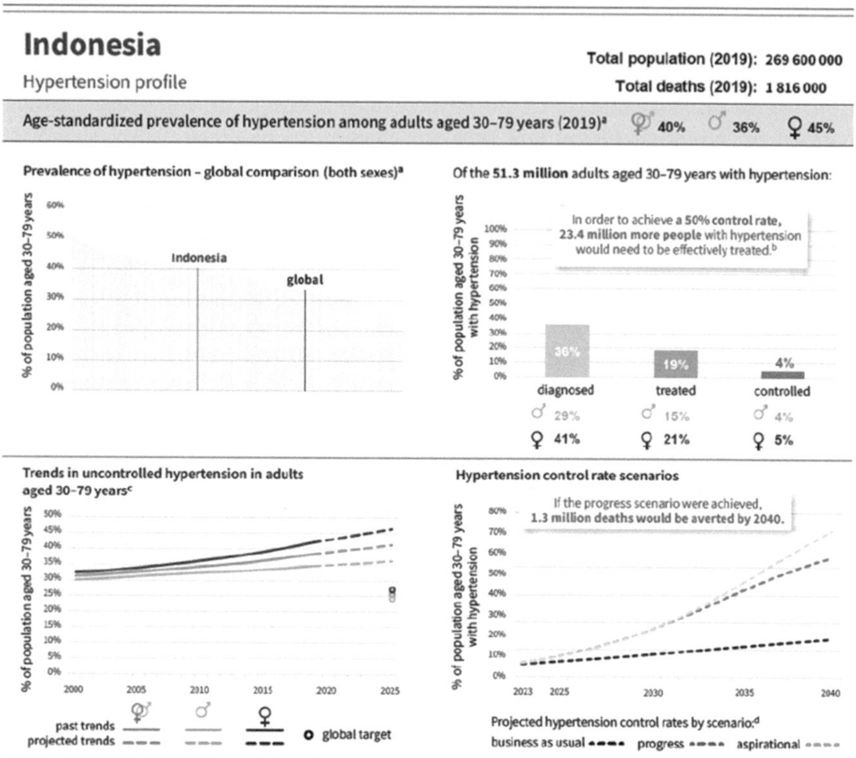

Mortality

	both sexes	males	females	year
Probability of premature mortality from NCDs (%)	25	28	21	2019
Cardiovascular disease deaths	697 000	355 000	342 000	2019
Cardiovascular disease deaths attributable to high systolic blood pressure (%)	69	67	71	2019

Risk factors[e]

	both sexes	males	females	year
Mean population salt intake, adults aged 25+ years (g/day)	10	11	10	2019
Current tobacco use, adults aged 15+ years (%)	37	71	4	2019
Obesity, adults aged 18+ years (%)	7	5	9	2016
Total alcohol per capita consumption, adults aged 15+ years (litres)	0	0	0	2019
Physical inactivity, adults aged 18+ years (%)	23	23	22	2016

National response

Targets
National target for blood pressure ✖
National target for salt consumption ✖
Surveillance
Conducted recent, national survey measuring raised blood pressure/hypertension ✔
Conducted recent, national survey on salt/sodium intake ✖
Functioning system for generating reliable cause-specific mortality data on a routine basis ✖

Treatment
Guidelines for management of hypertension ✔

Footnotes: a. SBP ≥140 mmHg or DBP ≥90 mmHg or taking medication for hypertension. b. Control rate: adults aged 30–79 years receiving treatment, with blood pressure SBP <140 mmHg and DBP <90 mmHg. c. SBP ≥140 mmHg or DBP ≥90 mmHg. d. Progress and aspirational scenarios reflect a theoretical scaling up of treatment and control. e. Age-standardized estimates are presented for all indicators except salt intake.

Fig. 2.3 Indonesia hypertension profile. From Ref. [8]

2.3 UN High Level Meeting on NCDs: Targets for Lowering Prevalence of Hypertension

As detailed in Chap. 13 in recognition of the rising global burden of NCDs, including CVD, over the past decades the United Nations (UN) held a High-Level Meeting on Prevention and Control of Noncommunicable Diseases in 2011 [9]. The WHO was tasked with developing goals and targets to reach those goals, and at the World Health Assembly (the governing body of the WHO) meeting in 2012, a global target of 25% reduction in premature mortality from noncommunicable diseases by 2025 was adopted (referred to as 25 by 25, or 25 x 25) [10]. To help reach the overarching 25% reduction in premature mortality from cardiovascular disease, a set of six goals targeting key CVD risk factors and two goals targeting health systems were developed (Fig. 2.4) [11, 12]. The hypertension control goal is to obtain a 25% reduction in raised blood pressure by 2025 (from a baseline of 2010). Building on the overarching NCD goal of 25% reduction in premature mortality by 2025, the Sustainable Development Goals (SDGs; specifically goal 3.4) include a target of a one-third reduction in premature mortality from NCDs noncommunicable diseases by 2030.

In recognition of the burden of high blood pressure, and mindful of the targets for lowering this burden in 25 by 25 and in Sustainable Development Goals, several organizations have developed or updated tools, guidelines, and roadmaps (Table 2.1). Some of these that are more focused on LMICs can be particularly helpful.

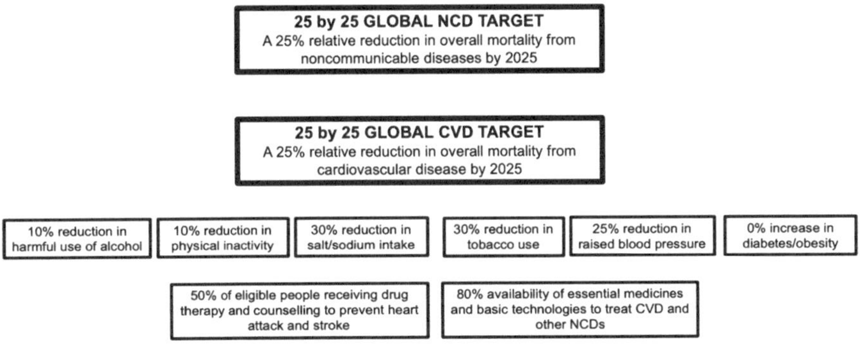

Fig. 2.4 The overall global target goal for noncommunicable disease mortality reduction (top line); the overall global target goal for cardiovascular disease mortality reduction (second line); the risk factors targeted to help reach the global goal (third line); health systems targeted to help reach the global goal (bottom line)

Table 2.1 Sample organizations with hypertension-focused programs, guidelines, or roadmaps

Guideline/program/roadmap	Brief description	Reference or website
WHO 2023 "Global report on hypertension: the race against a silent killer"	WHO, in partnership with Bloomberg Philanthropies and Resolve to Save Lives, issued this comprehensive publication which provides data on the global and national burden of HTN. It also provides targeted actions to manage HTN risk factors and gives recommendations for diagnosing and treating this preventable cause of death and disability.	Ref. [1], https://www.who.int/publications/i/item/9789240081062
WHO HEARTS technical package to improving CV health	The package provides a strategic approach to improving CV health in countries. It has six modules and an implementation guide. It supports ministries of health to strengthen CVD management in primary health care settings.	Ref. [13], https://www.who.int/publications/i/item/9789240001367
WHO 2021 Guideline for the pharmacological treatment of hypertension in adults	This guideline provides guidance on the initiation of pharmacological treatment for HTN in adults. The recommendations target adult patients who were diagnosed with HTN and counseled about lifestyle modifications. It also provides the basis for deciding whether to initiate treatment with monotherapy, dual therapy, or single-pill combinations.	Ref. [14], https://iris.who.int/bitstream/handle/10665/344424/9789240033986-eng.pdf
World Heart Federation (WHF) Hypertension Roadmap	This Roadmap goes through the continuum path of HTN, from preventive measures, screening and diagnosis, lifestyle modification, pharmacologic management, and long-term follow up. It also discusses roadblocks and solutions that can be met along the continuum.	Ref. [15], https://world-heart-federation.org/cvd-roadmaps/whf-global-roadmaps/hypertension/
Resolve to Save Lives	Resolve has a goal to increase global blood pressure control from 14% to 50%. They partner with global, national, and local partners to support their efforts to scale up proven blood pressure control strategies including the WHO's HEARTS technical package.	https://resolvetosavelives.org/cardiovascular-health/hypertension/
Pan-African Society of Cardiology (PASCAR) hypertension roadmap	PASCAR is an organization of physicians from across Africa involved in prevention and treatment of CVD. They have adapted the WHF roadmap at a national level.	Ref. [16]

2.4 Approach to Blood Pressure Management: Helpful Tools

2.4.1 HEARTS

In 2016, the WHO and the US Centers for Disease Control and Prevention (CDC) launched the new "Global Hearts Initiative." It was designed to support governments in strengthening the prevention and control of CVD in primary health care settings. As a part of this initiative, the HEARTS technical package (listed n Table 2.1) was developed [13]. The package contains six modules:

- **H**ealthy-lifestyle counseling
- **E**vidence-based treatment protocols
- **A**ccess to essential medicines and technology
- **R**isk-based CVD management
- **T**eam-based care
- **S**ystems for monitoring

There is also an implementation guide as well as a tool for the development of a consensus protocol for treatment of hypertension. The modules, which can be adapted to country-level needs, were designed to be most useful for Ministries of Health at the national level, Health/NCD program managers at the subnational level, and facility managers and primary health care trainers at the primary care level.

2.4.2 PAHO/HEARTS in the Americas

The Pan American Health Organization (PAHO) is the specialized international health agency for the Americas. It works with countries throughout the region to improve and protect people's health. PAHO wears two institutional hats: it is the specialized health agency of the Inter-American System, and it also serves as Regional Office for the Americas of the WHO. PAHO leads the implementation of HEARTS in the region of the Americas, ensuring that implementation actions are aligned with the strategic priorities of the region. The PAHO website homepage (www.PAHO.org) is available in English, Spanish, Portuguese, and French. All HEARTS materials are available Spanish as well as English.

2.4.3 Resolve to Save Lives (RTSL)

RTSL is a not-for-profit organization whose two-pronged mission is to (1) prevent 100 million deaths from cardiovascular disease and (2) make the world safer from epidemics. In 2017, WHO began a partnership with RTSL to support national governments in implementation of the Global Hearts Initiative. The RTSL website shows that by late 2023, approximately 17.4 million patients in 32 countries have been enrolled in RTSL-supported hypertension control programs [17].

RTSL, in a collaborative effort with the WHO and CDC, created an information-rich technical library called LINKS [18]. As part of this library, there is a section on "Tools and Guidance to Facilitate Scaling Up Effective Management of Hypertension—A six-step guide for program managers starting up national or sub-national hypertension control programs" [19].

2.4.4 World Heart Federation (WHF) Hypertension Roadmap

In 2015, the WHF published its first roadmap for hypertension [20]. This original roadmap was revised in 2021 to incorporate new information [15]. WHF states that their roadmaps "identify potential roadblocks and their solutions on the pathway to effective prevention, detection, and management of CVD and guide priority interventions on a global level." In addition to their roadmap on hypertension, they also have roadmaps focusing on other aspects of CV health and disease. All current roadmaps can be accessed on the WHF website [21]. The WHF Roadmaps are aimed to support 25 by 25 as well as goal 3.4 of the SDGs. They are designed to provide a generic global framework available for local adaptation and are intended to serve as a basis for developing region- or country-specific action plans.

Figure 2.5 illustrates the WHF Roadmap Continuum of Care. It covers screening, diagnosis, evidence-based treatments, monitoring adherence and BP control, and complications. This diagram and its supporting text can be quite helpful to staff in primary care facilities.

The paper has a large amount of information such as:

- A list of the newest (as of 2021) hypertension guidelines and key treatment recommendations in them
- A table containing the 2016 Lancet Commission on Hypertension 10 key global actions and a strategy across the life-course to address the global burden of hypertension
- Case studies on the implementation of the 2015 WHF Roadmap
- A table of roadblocks and possible solutions based on both WHF members' feedback and a review of the literature
- A diagram showing selected roadblocks on the way to the ideal patient journey
- Some prioritized solutions along the continuum of care for hypertension

2.4.5 Pan-African Society of Cardiology (PASCAR)

PASCAR is an organization of physicians from across Africa involved in prevention and treatment of CVD which is concerned by the lack of progress in the diagnosis and effective treatment of cardiovascular disease across Africa. Approximately

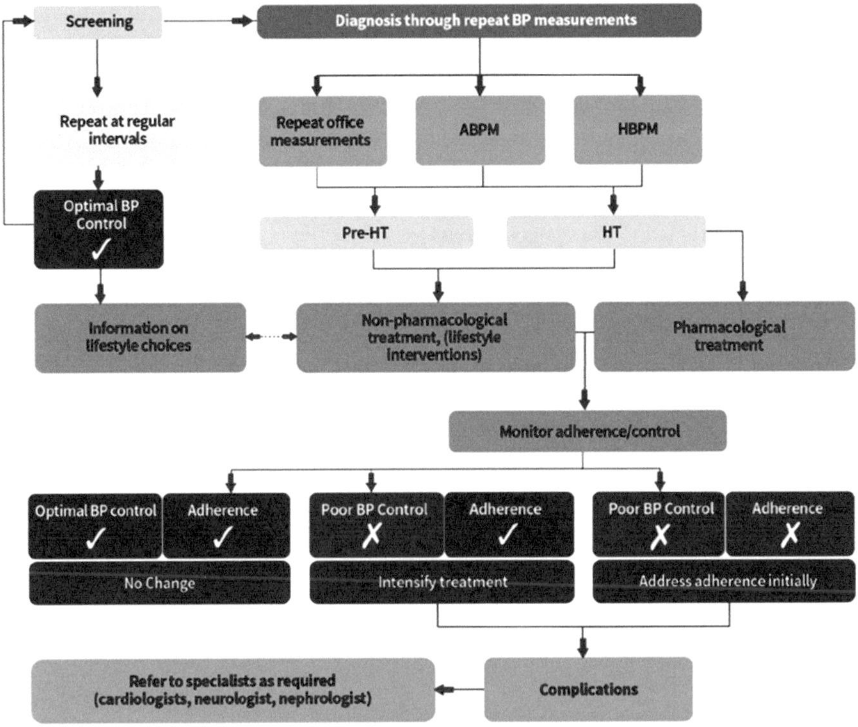

Fig. 2.5 The ideal patient pathway for hypertension, referred to as the Continuum of Care. From Ref. [15]. © World Heart Federation. *ABPM* 24-hour ambulatory BP monitoring, *HBPM* self-home BP monitoring, *HT* hypertension

10 years ago, recognizing that WHO estimated the global prevalence of hypertension was highest in the African region, PASCAR organized a task force of experts that met several times to identify key actions for a hypertension roadmap on the continent. Their ultimate goal was to develop a roadmap, modeled on the WHF roadmap but customized for the African continent to guide the nations to achieve 25% hypertension control in Africa by 2025. They identified roadblocks at the government and health-system level, healthcare professional level, and patient level. They then devised a 10-point action plan as well as a PASCAR roadmap to decrease the burden of hypertension in Africa [16]. These will be discussed later in this chapter.

2.5 Approach to Blood Pressure Management: Measuring Blood Pressure and Diagnosing Hypertension

To treat hypertension, one must first confirm a diagnosis. Because it usually has no symptoms and is referred to as the "silent killer," blood pressure must be measured. According to the WHO [1, 13], blood pressure in adults should be measured "opportunistically" during routine visits to primary health care facilities (including at first presentation to the facility). If it is normal, pressure should be measured periodically thereafter (e.g., every 1–5 years). Individuals with elevated blood pressure readings (≥140 mmHg systolic and/or ≥ 90 mmHg diastolic) require immediate follow-up to confirm a diagnosis. The type of follow-up depends on the initial reading. Generally, if the systolic pressure is 140–159 mmHg **OR** the diastolic is 90–99 mmHg, on the initial visit the confirmatory follow-up visit could be within a month; however, if the pressure is either ≥160 mmHg systolic **OR** ≥ 100 mmHg diastolic on two readings on a single day, medications to reduce blood pressure should begin as soon as possible (e.g., that day).

Unfortunately, many times blood pressure is not measured accurately. This can be due to mechanical reasons such as uncalibrated equipment or ill-fitting cuffs, or due to poor techniques used by the measurer. The staff member measuring blood pressure in clinics/offices should be trained in proper techniques. Equipment in working order (basic validated automated blood pressure measuring devices strongly preferred) should be available.

Blood pressure measurement and control are particularly important in adults who:

- Already have CVD or are at high risk for it
- Have diabetes
- Have chronic kidney disease
- Are obese
- Use tobacco
- Have a family history of heart attack or stroke

Table 2.2 is the HEARTS Module E instructions for measuring blood pressure [13]. A more detailed graphic from PAHO is seen in Fig. 2.6 [22].

Table 2.2 HEARTS: How to measure blood pressure. From Ref. [13]

Effective treatment algorithms for hypertension are dependent on accurate blood pressure measurement. The following advice should be followed for measuring blood pressure:
• Use the appropriate cuff size, noting the lines on the cuff to ensure that it is positioned correctly on the arm. (If the arm circumference is >32 cm, use large cuff.)
• Although at the initial evaluation it is preferable to measure blood pressure in both arms and use the arm with the higher reading thereafter, this may not be practical in a busy primary care environment.
• The patient should be sitting with back supported, legs uncrossed, empty bladder, relaxed for 5 min, and without talking.
• For persons who are getting their blood pressure measured for the first time, it is preferable to take at least two readings and to use the second reading.
Blood pressure can be measured either by a conventional sphygmomanometer, using a stethoscope, or by an automated electronic device. The electronic device, if available, is preferred because it provides more reproducible results and is not influenced by variations in technique or by the bias of the observers.
If the primary health care facility has electricity or regular access to batteries, then consider an automated validated blood pressure device with a digital reading. If the primary health care facility has no electricity or batteries, then a manual BP cuff will have to be used with a stethoscope.

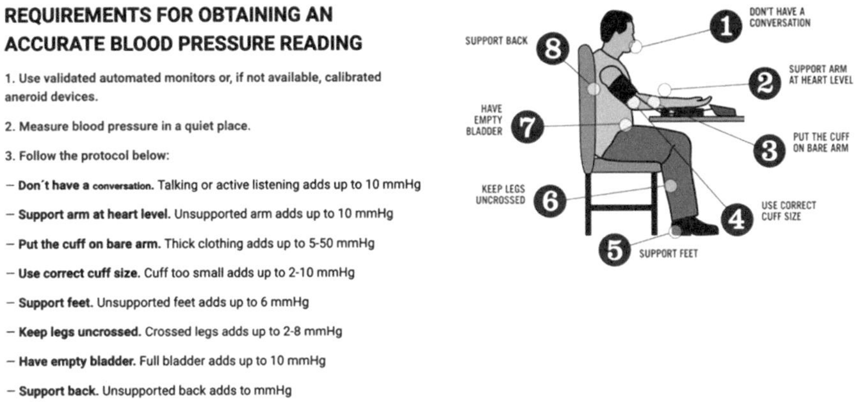

Fig. 2.6 PAHO illustrated guide for measuring blood pressure. From Ref. [22]

2.5.1 American Medical Association MAP™ Program

The AMA MAP™ Hypertension Quality Improvement (QI) Program (https://map.ama-assn.org) incorporates evidence-based strategies along with supporting tools, resources, performance metrics, and reports and coaching to help improve and sustain hypertension control rates. The program is based on the AMA MAP™ framework, which helps care teams organize their approach to providing evidence-based care by **M**easuring Accurately, that is obtaining actionable BP measurements to diagnose and assess BP control, **A**cting Rapidly by initiating and intensifying treatment when indicated and **P**artnering with Patients to support self-management activation, and improve adherence to treatment (**MAP**). The program is provided to health care organizations free of charge. Currently, the full quality improvement program is only available in the United States, but many of the supporting tools and resources are available through the program's website. A publication [23] laying the groundwork for the program shows the actions to take under each of the three pillars. For example, under the "Measure accurately" pillar, there is a screening checklist, a confirmatory checklist, and several evidence-based tips for correct positioning. Follow-up studies have shown a significant improvement in hypertension control in family medicine clinics whose staff had been trained compared to before the training began, even after coaching support was withdrawn [24].

2.6 Management of Hypertension

2.6.1 Lifestyle Modification

Various guidelines for management of blood pressure give recommendations for lifestyle modification [13–16, 25–27]). The essence of these recommendations is listed below. As pointed out in the various guidelines, these lifestyle modifications are beneficial for overall CV health.

1. Lose weight if needed/maintain an ideal body weight.
2. Stop all tobacco use, avoid second-hand tobacco smoke.
3. Increase physical activity to equivalent of brisk walk for 150 min per week.
4. Eat a healthy diet with several servings of fruits and vegetables (preferably fresh) a day. The DASH diet is often recommended [28].
5. Reduce salt intake—most guidelines recommend <5 g salt (2 g sodium) daily. Some recommend increasing potassium intake (see further comments below).
6. Alcohol consumption—limit intake to 1–2 drinks a day.

HEARTS Module "H" contains information on the four behavioral risk factors for CVD. Brief interventions are described as an approach to providing counseling on risk factors and encouraging people to have healthy lifestyles. The areas covered include tobacco use, unhealthy diet, insufficient physical activity, and harmful use of alcohol. Information on behavioral change, brief interventions for counseling, and key points for motivational interviewing is also included.

Sodium is an essential nutrient involved in many cellular processes. However, many studies have found that it is overconsumed compared to what the body physiologically needs. It has been reported that nearly two million people die each year from heart attacks and strokes caused by excess salt consumption [29]. WHO has pointed out that the average human consumption is more than 10 g of salt (4000 mg of sodium) a day, which is more than double the daily intake of <5 g of salt (<2000 mg sodium) for adults that is recommended by WHO.

In 2013, all 194 WHO Member States approved one of the 25 by 25 targets to focus on sodium—specifically, to commit to reducing population sodium intake by 30% by the year 2025. WHO has recommended several sodium-related "best buys" as actions that could be undertaken immediately to help prevent CVD and its associated costs. WHO recommendations included the following [30]:

- Reduce salt intake through the reformulation of food products to contain less salt and the setting of target levels for the amount of salt in foods and meals
- Reduce salt intake through the establishment of a supportive environment in public institutions such as hospitals, schools, workplaces, and nursing homes, to enable lower sodium options to be provided
- Reduce salt intake through a behavior change communication and mass media campaign
- Reduce salt intake through the implementation of front-of-pack labeling

Table 2.3 Estimated mean population dietary sodium intake in 2019 and projected mean population dietary sodium intake in 2025 and 2030 by WHO regions. From Ref. [32]

WHO region	2019		2025		2030	
	mg/day sodium	g/day salt	mg/day sodium	g/day salt	mg/day sodium	g/day salt
African	2687	6.72	2680	6.70	2674	6.69
Americas	3583	8.96	3574	8.94	3564	8.91
Eastern Mediterranean	2792	6.98	2800	7.00	2798	6.99
European	3445	8.61	3437	8.59	3430	8.57
South-East Asia	3921	9.80	3907	9.77	3896	9.74
Western Pacific[a]	6247	15.62	6189	15.47	6137	15.34
Global intake	4310	10.78	4230	10.58	4163	10.41
WHO's recommendation	<2000	<5.0	<2000	<5.0	<2000	<5.0

[a]The estimated intake for China is 6954 mg/day sodium, which is likely to be influencing the Western Pacific Region mean

A technical package for salt reduction, "SHAKE the salt habit" was developed by WHO under the auspices of the Global Hearts Initiative [31]. This package has a general framework of elements needed to create a successful salt reduction strategy and help reduce sodium consumption.

In 2023, the WHO issued a "Global Report on Sodium Intake Reduction" [32]. It contains helpful guidance on how countries might implement policies and measures to reduce salt consumption. It also shows sodium country score cards and contains overviews on mandatory and voluntary measures grouped by WHO region as well as by World Bank income groups. Progress has been slow with only a few countries reducing population sodium intake toward (but not yet reaching) the goal. Consideration is being given to extending the target to 2030.

Table 2.3, from the WHO Global Report on Sodium Intake Reduction, shows global sodium intake [32]. In 2019, the mean global sodium intake of adults was estimated at 4310 mg/day (10.78 g/day salt) which is more than double the WHO recommendation. Further breakout of countries by WHO regions is also shown in Table 2.3. Additionally, the Table includes projections, based on the trends 2010–2019, of what sodium intake could be in 2025 and 2030. Based on these 2010–2019 trends, sodium intake will reduce minimally and there is likely little chance for any/many countries to meet the 30% relative reduction. There have been some positive results, however. A study reported from a group of researchers in China was highlighted in the WHO report. The Shandong Ministry of Health Action on Salt and Hypertension (SMASH) program [33] was a government-led initiative aimed at curbing salt intake and reducing the prevalence of hypertension. Their program and results are highlighted in Box 2.1.

Box 2.1 Case study: The Shandong Ministry of Health Action on Salt Reduction and Hypertension (SMASH): Shandong, China. From Ref. [1]

The Shandong Ministry of Health Action on Salt and Hypertension (SMASH) programme was a government-led initiative aimed at curbing salt intake and reducing the prevalence of hypertension among adults. The programme employed various strategies, including a media campaign, distribution of scaled salt spoons, and public education activities.

The results of the programme were remarkable, with a significant 24.8% reduction in sodium intake observed over a 5-year period. This decrease was measured through 24-h urine sodium excretion, which dropped from 5338 mg/day to 4013 mg/day. Additionally, potassium excretion increased by 15.1%, and the sodium-to-potassium ratio decreased by 37.7%, indicating positive dietary changes. Beyond decreased sodium consumption, the SMASH programme demonstrated downstream improvement in blood pressure levels. The adjusted mean SBP decreased by 1.8 mmHg, and the adjusted mean DBP decreased by 3.1 mmHg, most likely due to decreased sodium intake.

Alongside these physiological changes, the programme positively impacted systematically assessed knowledge, attitudes, and behaviours related to sodium reduction and hypertension.

Participants showed increased awareness of the recommended salt intake, paid more attention to the labeling on processed foods, and took action to reduce sodium in their diets.

Resolve to Save Lives also has a focus on salt. RTSL's target, working with their partners, is to reduce the global intake by 30%, and their framework is based on WHO's "SHAKE" technical package. Their strategies target the areas where salt is most often found: (1) packaged food, (2) food prepared in the home, and (3) food prepared outside the home. Their strategies and action plans are on their website [34]. There is also further information in their technical LINKS library [35].

An often-mentioned drawback of lower sodium diets is that many people find them bland or distasteful compared to their "normal" diets. A 2022 study from China reported the results of the multicenter randomized DECIDE-Diet (Diet Exercise and Cardiovascular Health-Diet) [36]. Study participants (all with systolic BP between 130 and 159 mm Hg) were recruited from four major Chinese cities each of which has its own regional cuisine. Chinese heart-healthy diets were developed with study nutritionists, dietitians, and chefs in each area that conformed to the regional cuisines. Among other dietary ingredient modifications, these regional heart-healthy diets contained about half as much sodium and about 40% more potassium than the participants' regular diet and were palatable and affordable for Chinese adults. After a 1-month intervention period, individuals on the DECIDE-diet had significant lowering of blood pressure. The study authors listed three clinical implications of their study:

- The results support the idea that "food is medicine" and will give many patients with HBP the confidence to adopt a healthy diet as their lifestyle treatment.
- Clinicians should recommend that their Chinese patients with high blood pressure adopt a healthy diet with low sodium and high potassium, fiber, vegetables, and fruits as the first-line treatment.
- Restaurants and cafeterias should consider adopting the Chinese heart-healthy diet menu, particularly those providing services to institutional living populations.

The WHO 2023 Global Report on Hypertension discusses potassium in some detail [1]. The report states that blood pressure is reduced when dietary sodium intake is reduced and when potassium intake is increased, thus they support diets with lower dietary sodium and "...plenty of fruit and vegetables high in potassium...".

Several of the hypertension guidelines have included a potassium recommendation. For example, the ACC/AHA says: Potassium supplementation, preferably in dietary modification, is recommended for adults with elevated BP or hypertension unless contraindicated by the presence of chronic kidney disease or use of drugs that reduce potassium excretion [25]. The WHF recommends an enhanced intake of dietary potassium, aiming for 3500–5000 mg per day, preferably by a diet (such as locally available fruits and vegetables) rich in potassium [15]. Replacing high-sodium salt with potassium-rich salt is also recommended. The International Society of Hypertension has a healthy diets recommendation that states: Eating a diet that is rich in whole grains, fruits, vegetables, polyunsaturated fats, and dairy products and reducing food high in sugar, saturated fat, and trans fats, such as the DASH diet. Increase intake of vegetables high in nitrates known to reduce BP, such as leafy vegetables and beetroot. Other beneficial foods and nutrients include those high in magnesium, calcium, and potassium such as avocados, nuts, seeds, legumes, and tofu [37].

Lifestyle modification/lifestyle counseling is an important part of preventing/managing hypertension. Exactly what it entails, especially around dietary modifications, will vary in different regions of the world and in different cultures. Lifestyle modification may be recommended alone as a first step in blood pressure management, especially in individuals with borderline pressures of SBP 130–139 mmHg and/or DBP 80–89 mmHg. However, as has been pointed out in HEARTS materials, in settings where a person does not regularly visit the doctor, that person who is given *only* lifestyle modification may not return for re-evaluation and needed treatment, resulting in uncontrolled hypertension and associated complications. (See the HEARTS "H" module for more information on lifestyle counseling.)

2.6.2 Other Risks for Hypertension: Social Determinants of Health

The WHO recently released a document titled "Integrating the social determinants of health into health workforce education and training" [38]: In this publication, WHO states that "The social determinants of health are the social, economic and environmental conditions in which people are born, grow, live, work and age that impact health and well-being across the life course, and the inequities in access to power, decision-making, money and resources that give rise to these conditions."

The U.S. Centers for Disease Control and Prevention (CDC) states that social determinants of health "…encompasses economic and social conditions that influence the health of people and communities. These conditions are shaped by socioeconomic position, which is the amount of money, power, and resources that people have, all of which are influenced by socioeconomic and political factors (e.g., policies, culture, and societal values). An individual's socioeconomic position can be shaped by various factors such as their education, occupation, or income. All of these factors (social determinants) impact the health and well-being of people and the communities they interact with" [39].

The 2017 ACC/AHA hypertension guidelines [25]) list low socioeconomic/educational status among the CVD risk factors that are common in patients with hypertension. They point out that HTN control rates are higher for persons of higher socioeconomic status, for example. There also discuss accounting for age, race, ethnicity, sex, and special circumstances in antihypertensive treatment in their clinician's flow chart for HTN management.

The 2020 hypertension guidelines from the International Society of Hypertension [37] has a section on "Ethnicity, Race and Hypertension" which states that hypertension prevalence, treatment and control rates vary significantly according to ethnicity. Such differences are mainly attributed to genetic differences, but lifestyle and socioeconomic status possibly filters through into health behaviors such as diet—which appear to be major contributors." There are two subsections that discuss populations from African descent and populations from Asia.

Geldsetzer and colleagues [40] looked at HTN care in 44 LMICs and found that the performance of health systems in general was poor—less than half of those with hypertension were diagnosed, less than a third were taking antihypertensive medications, and only one in ten had their hypertension under control. They also observed that countries in Latin America and the Caribbean generally achieved the best performance relative to their predicted performance based on GDP per capita, whereas countries in sub-Saharan Africa performed worst.

A recently published study from 76 LMICs on the association of socioeconomic status with hypertension found that that hypertension affects countries across regions irrespective of their level of economic development and affects the full spectrum of socioeconomic groups within countries [41]. The data suggest, however, that hypertension may increasingly affect adults in the lowest socioeconomic groups as LMICs develop economically. They conclude that large-scale studies of hypertension disease burden in LMICs, and how this burden varies by socioeconomic groups, could better inform health policy in these settings than merely focusing on the prevalence of high BP.

2.6.3 Pharmacologic Treatment

When lifestyle intervention strategies alone are not sufficient to manage an individual's blood pressure, pharmacologic treatment is the next step. Pharmacologic therapy is not meant to take the place of lifestyle modifications; rather, these two management strategies should be used together.

In 2021, the WHO published new evidence-based global public health guideline for pharmacological treatment of hypertension in adults [14]. In order to produce the guidelines, WHO first organized a Guideline Development Group. As described in detail in the final document, the GDG then created an analytic framework linking hypertension treatment to important health outcomes, and 11 clinical questions were prioritized:

1. At what BP level should pharmacological therapy be initiated?
2. Are lab tests needed to start therapy?
3. Is risk assessment needed to start therapy?
4. Monotherapy vs no therapy?
5. Monotherapy vs another monotherapy?
6. Monotherapy vs combination therapy?
7. What choice of combination therapy?
8. Single-pill combination vs free combination?
9. Post-treatment target BP level?
10. When should BP be re-assessed after treatment initiation?
11. Management by physician vs non-physician provider?

Ultimately, these 11 questions led to eight areas of recommendations in the final guidelines, including guidance on BP threshold for initiating therapy, laboratory testing, CVD risk assessment, classes of medications to be used as first-line agents, combination therapy, target BP, frequency of assessment, and the role of non-physician health professionals. The eight recommendations are listed in detail in Table 2.4. Each recommendation has a "strength" associated with it. There were two strength categories: **A strong recommendation** is one for which the Guideline Development Group was confident that the desirable effects of adhering to the recommendation outweigh the undesirable effects.

A weak or conditional recommendation is one for which the Guideline Development Group concluded that the desirable effects of adhering to the recommendation probably outweigh the undesirable effects but was not confident about these trade-offs. Each recommendation has a certainty of evidence and its implications. The levels of certainty are defined as:

- Certainty Level **High**—WHO is very confident that the true effect lies close to that of the estimate of effect.
- Certainty Level **Moderate**—WHO is moderately confident in the effect estimate. (The true effect is likely to be close to the estimate of effect, but there is a possibility that it is substantially different.)

Table 2.4 WHO recommendations for pharmacological treatment of hypertension. From Ref. [14]

1. Recommendation on blood pressure threshold for initiation of pharmacological treatment
WHO recommends initiation of pharmacological antihypertensive treatment of individuals with a confirmed diagnosis of hypertension and systolic blood pressure of ≥140 mmHg or diastolic blood pressure of ≥90 mmHg.
Strong recommendation, moderate- to high-certainty evidence
WHO recommends pharmacological antihypertensive treatment of individuals with existing cardiovascular disease and systolic blood pressure of 130–139 mmHg.
Strong recommendation, moderate- to high-certainty evidence
WHO suggests pharmacological antihypertensive treatment of individuals without cardiovascular disease but with high cardiovascular risk, diabetes mellitus, or chronic kidney disease, and systolic blood pressure of 130–139 mmHg.
Conditional recommendation, moderate- to high-certainty evidence
2. Recommendation on laboratory testing
When starting pharmacological therapy for hypertension, WHO suggests obtaining tests to screen for comorbidities and secondary hypertension, but only when testing does not delay or impede starting treatment.
Conditional recommendation, low-certainty evidence
3. Recommendation on cardiovascular disease risk assessment
WHO suggests cardiovascular disease risk assessment at or after the initiation of pharmacological treatment for hypertension, but only where this is feasible and does not delay treatment.
Conditional recommendation, low-certainty evidence
4. Recommendation on drug classes to be used as first-line agents
For adults with hypertension requiring pharmacological treatment, WHO recommends the use of drugs from any of the following three classes of pharmacological antihypertensive medications as an initial treatment:
1. Thiazide and thiazide-like agents
2. Angiotensin-converting enzyme inhibitors (ACEis)/angiotensin-receptor blockers (ARBs)
3. Long-acting dihydropyridine calcium channel blockers (CCBs).
Strong recommendation, high-certainty evidence
5. Recommendation on combination therapy
For adults with hypertension requiring pharmacological treatment, WHO suggests combination therapy, preferably with a single-pill combination (to improve adherence and persistence), as an initial treatment. Antihypertensive medications used in combination therapy should be chosen from the following three drug classes: Diuretics (thiazide or thiazide-like), angiotensin-converting enzyme inhibitors (ACEis)/angiotensin-receptor blockers (ARBs), and long-acting dihydropyridine calcium channel blockers (CCBs).
Conditional recommendation, moderate-certainty evidence
6. Recommendations on target blood pressure
WHO recommends a target blood pressure treatment goal of <140/90 mmHg in all patients with hypertension without comorbidities.
Strong recommendation, moderate-certainty evidence
WHO recommends a target systolic blood pressure treatment goal of <130 mmHg in patients with hypertension and known cardiovascular disease (CVD).

(continued)

Table 2.4 (continued)

Strong recommendation, moderate-certainty evidence
WHO suggests a target systolic blood pressure treatment goal of <130 mmHg in high-risk patients with hypertension (those with high CVD risk, diabetes mellitus, chronic kidney disease).
Conditional recommendation, moderate-certainty evidence
7. Recommendations on frequency of assessment
WHO suggests a monthly follow-up after initiation or a change in antihypertensive medications until patients reach target.
Conditional recommendation, low-certainty evidence
WHO suggests a follow up every 3–6 months for patients whose blood pressure is under control.
Conditional recommendation, low-certainty evidence
8. Recommendation on treatment by nonphysician professionals
WHO suggests that pharmacological treatment of hypertension can be provided by nonphysician professionals such as pharmacists and nurses, as long as the following conditions are met: Proper training, prescribing authority, specific management protocols, and physician oversight.
Conditional recommendation, low-certainty evidence

- Certainty Level **Low**—WHO confidence in the effect estimate is limited. (The true effect may be substantially different from the estimate of the effect.)
- Certainty Level **Very Low**—WHO has very little confidence in the effect estimate. (The true effect is likely to be substantially different from the estimate of effect.)

It is noted in recommendation 1 of Table 2.4 that the threshold for initiation of pharmacological antihypertensive treatment is systolic blood pressure of ≥140 mmHg or diastolic blood pressure of ≥90 mmHg or systolic of ≥130 mmHg or in those with existing CVD, high CVD risk, diabetes mellitus, or chronic kidney disease. Nonpharmacologic therapy should be accompanying these treatment recommendations. However, some organizations/countries recommend initiating nonpharmacologic treatment for those with systolic BP of ≥120 mmHg or diastolic BP of ≥80 mmHg [25]. This is based on observational studies that have shown high blood pressure increases risk of death even when systolic blood pressure is in the 115–130 mmHg range, which is below the threshold for treatment of hypertension in most guidelines [1, 25].

2.6.4 *Specific Comments on Pharmacologic Agents*

1. Recommendation #4 indicates that any of three classes of antihypertensive medications are appropriate as an initial treatment: thiazide and thiazide-like agents, angiotensin-converting enzyme inhibitors (ACEIs)/angiotensin-receptor blockers (ARBs), and long-acting dihydropyridine calcium channel blockers (CCBs). This is a strong recommendation with high-level evidence. The Guideline Development Group explained that the anticipated benefits clearly outweighed

the potential harms these three classes of medications, and the adverse were infrequent, usually mild, and could be managed or another agent could be substituted. (NOTE—some WHO documents categorize ACEIs and ARBs as separate classes and therefore list 4 classes of first-line agents for initial treatment.)

2. Recommendation #5 suggests combination therapy, preferably with a single-pill combination (to improve adherence and persistence), be used as an initial treatment. The rationale for recommending a combination therapy, particularly in a single-pill approach, is based on the following considerations:

   - Most individuals with HTN will eventually require two or more antihypertensive agents to achieve BP control
   - The combination of two agents from complementary classes yields greater BP-reduction efficacy (at least equal to the sum of the efficacy of each chosen agent)
   - Lower doses of each agent are needed, which results in a reduction of side-effects and the fact that use of complementary classes of antihypertensive agents may mitigate the side-effects of each agent
   - Adherence and persistence are increased
   - Simplified logistics can lead to fewer stock-outs and a reduced pharmacy inventory

   The recommendation was classified conditional with moderate-certainty evidence. The Guideline Development Group explained that a comparison requires long-term data about hard clinical end points between monotherapy and combination therapy. Additionally, "real world" research studies are needed to determine if there is a difference in clinical outcomes and serious adverse events between single-pill combinations versus multiple-pill combinations.

3. Consider using diuretics or CCB in patients 65 years or older, or those of African or Afro-Caribbean descent; beta-blockers (BBs) post MI; and ACEIs/ARBs in those with diabetes mellitus, heart failure, or chronic kidney disease.
4. Hypertension in Pregnancy—There are clear contraindications to the use of some antihypertensive medications during pregnancy. The guidelines from WHO [14], ACC/AHA [25], and ESC [26] include all ACE inhibitors, ARBs, and direct renin inhibitors. WHO also includes the mineralocorticoid receptor antagonist spironolactone due to fetal anti-androgen effects. The use of the beta-blocker atenolol is also contraindicated due to the observation of intrauterine fetal growth inhibition. These three sets of guidelines all recommend that women with hypertension who become pregnant (or are planning to become pregnant) be treated with methyldopa, beta-blockers (particularly labetalol), CCBs (particularly nifedipine and, as an alternative, verapamil), and the direct-acting vasodilators (particularly hydralazine). WHO points out that there is evidence to suggest that among these agents, beta-blockers and CCBs appear to be more effective than methyldopa in decreasing the development of severe HTN later in the pregnancy. For further information on this topic, see the 2020 publication "WHO recommendations on drug treatment for non-severe hypertension in pregnancy" [42] as well as a recent scientific statement from the AHA [43].

2.6.5 WHO Essential Medicines List

WHO defines essential medicines as those that satisfy the priority health care needs of population. Medications on the list are chosen while considering: (a) disease prevalence and public health relevance, (b) evidence of efficacy and safety, and (c) comparative cost-effectiveness. These medicines, in appropriate dosage forms and affordable cost, should be always available in functioning health systems. Quality should be assured. The "antihypertensive medicines" section of the 2023 WHO Model List of Essential Medicines is shown in Table 2.5 [44].

In July 2019, the WHO added added single-pill combination (also referred to as fixed-dose combination or "polypill") antihypertensive medications to the WHO Essential Medicines List. Soon thereafter, a letter to the editor of Lancet from the American Heart Association, European Society of Hypertension, Lancet Commission on hypertension, International Society of Hypertension, Latin American Society of Hypertension, Resolve to Save Lives, World Heart Federation, World Hypertension League, and World Stroke Organization was published commending WHO for making single-pill combination antihypertensive medications more widely available by including them in the WHO Essential Medicines List [45]. Recognizing that the fixed dose combinations are safe, effective, and an emerging best practice, they cautioned that "…countries and health systems must ensure that everyone who needs treatments for hypertension can access them."

The complete 2021 WHO guidelines on pharmacological treatment of hypertension in adults and two annexes are available on the WHO website [14]. Annex A contains 104 tables with the summaries of evidence for each of the recommendations, and Annex B contains their evidence-to-decision frameworks.

A one-page summary of the WHO hypertension treatment guideline is shown in Fig. 2.7. It is also available in color on the WHO website [46].

Table 2.5 WHO essential antihypertensive medicines list. From Ref. [44]

Antihypertensive medicines	
Amlodipine (see footnote a) Therapeutic alternatives: – Fourth level of ATC chemical subgroup (C08CA dihydropyridine derivatives)	Tablet: 5 mg (as maleate, mesylate, or besylate).
Bisoprolol Therapeutic alternatives: – Atenolol* – Carvedilol – Metoprolol	Tablet: 1.25 mg; 5 mg. *Atenolol should not be used as a first-line agent in uncomplicated hypertension in patients >60 years
Enalapril (see footnote a) Therapeutic alternatives: – Fourth level of ATC chemical subgroup (C09AA ACE inhibitors, plain)	Oral liquid: 1 mg/mL (as hydrogen maleate) [note: There is a specific indication for restricting its use to children) Tablet: 2.5 mg; 5 mg; 10 mg (as hydrogen maleate).

(continued)

Table 2.5 (continued)

Antihypertensive medicines	
Hydralazine*	Powder for injection: 20 mg (hydrochloride) in ampoule. Tablet: 25 mg; 50 mg (hydrochloride). *Hydralazine is listed for use only in the acute management of severe pregnancy-induced hypertension. Its use in the treatment of essential hypertension is not recommended in view of the evidence of greater efficacy and safety of other medicines.
Hydrochlorothiazide (see footnote a) Therapeutic alternatives: – Chlorothiazide – Chlorthalidone – Indapamide	Oral liquid: 50 mg/5 mL. Solid oral dosage form: 12.5 mg; 25 mg.
Lisinopril + amlodipine (see footnote a) Therapeutic alternatives: – Fourth level of ATC chemical subgroup (C09AA ACE inhibitors, plain) (for lisinopril) – Fourth level of ATC chemical subgroup (C08CA dihydropyridine derivatives) (for amlodipine)	Tablet: 10 mg + 5 mg; 20 mg + 5 mg; 20 mg + 10 mg.
Lisinopril + hydrochlorothiazide (see footnote a) Therapeutic alternatives: – Fourth level of ATC chemical subgroup (C09AA ACE inhibitors, plain) (for lisinopril) – Chlorthalidone, chlorothiazide, and indapamide (for hydrochlorothiazide)	Tablet: 10 mg + 12.5 mg; 20 mg + 12.5 mg; 20 mg +25 mg.
Losartan (see footnote a) Therapeutic alternatives: – Fourth level of ATC chemical subgroup (C09CA Angiotensin II receptor blockers (ARBs), plain)	Tablet: 25 mg; 50 mg; 100 mg.
Methyldopa*	Tablet: 250 mg. *Methyldopa is listed for use only in the management of pregnancy-induced hypertension. Its use in the treatment of essential hypertension is not recommended in view of the evidence of greater efficacy and safety of other medicines.

(continued)

Table 2.5 (continued)

Antihypertensive medicines	
Telmisartan + amlodipine (see footnote a) Therapeutic alternatives: – Fourth level of ATC chemical subgroup (C09CA angiotensin II receptor blockers (ARBs), plain) (for telmisartan) – Fourth level of ATC chemical subgroup (C08CA dihydropyridine derivatives) (for amlodipine)	Tablet: 40 mg + 5 mg; 80 mg + 5 mg; 80 mg + 10 mg.
Telmisartan + hydrochlorothiazide (see footnote a) Therapeutic alternatives: – Fourth level of ATC chemical subgroup (C09CA angiotensin II receptor blockers (ARBs), plain) (for telmisartan) – Chlorthalidone, chlorothiazide, and indapamide (for hydrochlorothiazide)	Tablet: 40 mg + 12.5 mg; 80 mg + 12.5 mg; 80 mg +25 mg.
Complementary list (see footnote b)	
Sodium nitroprusside	*Power for infusion: 50 mg in ampoule.*

Footnote (a)—Intended to indicate therapeutic alternatives to the listed medicine that may be considered for selection in national essential medicines list
Footnote (b)—The complementary list presents essential medicines for priority diseases, for which specialized diagnostic or monitoring facilities, and/or specialist medical care, and/or specialist training are needed
For further explanation of the footnotes, please refer to the original document [44]

2.6.6 HEARTS Treatment Protocols

The HEARTS "E" module (Evidence-based treatment protocols) provides several sample hypertension treatment protocols using the medications discussed in the WHO treatment guidelines. As referenced in the module, it is intended for use by national governmental policymakers, subnational program managers, and primary health care facility managers who can adapt a protocol(s) and align to local context. This ensures that just one protocol is used at the national (or in some instances subnational) level. The protocols include:

- Hypertension protocol 1: Diuretic as first-line treatment
- Hypertension protocol 2: CCB as first-line treatment
- Hypertension protocol 3: ACE-I or ARB as first-line treatment
- Hypertension protocol 4: ACE-I or ARB + CCB as first-line treatment
- Hypertension protocol 5: CCB + diuretic as first-line of treatment
- Hypertension protocol 6: ACE-I or ARB + diuretic as first-line treatment
- Hypertension protocol 7: Use of BP-lowering drugs in patients with ischemic CVD
- Hypertension protocol 8: Adapted example: CCB as first-line treatment
- Hypertension protocol 9: Adapted example: telmisartan 40 mg/amlodipine 5 mg single-pill combination regimen

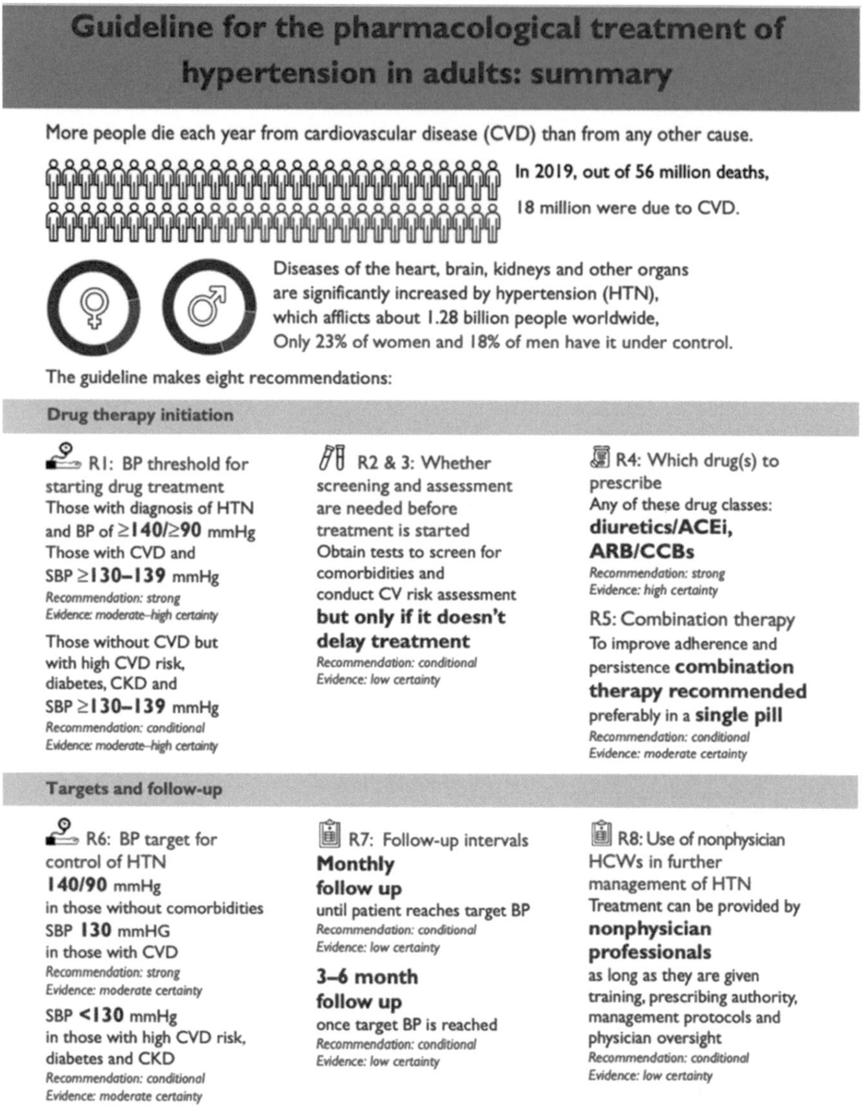

Fig. 2.7 Summary of guidelines for the pharmacological treatment of hypertension in adults. From Ref. [14]

Protocols 1–6 each have a different starting medication. Individual countries should choose and adapt the protocol(s) that best fits their local needs/preferences/resources. The seventh protocol is an example suited for individuals with hypertension and ischemic CVD (defined as ischemic stroke, TIA, or myocardial infarction >1 month ago). The eighth and ninth protocols are examples of adapted protocols based on two of the first six choices. It is noted that a non-comprehensive list of advantages and disadvantages is presented in a box relating to each protocol. These will help in the selection of the most suitable option for a given program/country. Selection of a single option greatly facilitates logistics, training, supervision, evaluation, and overall program implementation. **The simpler the protocol, the more likely it is to be followed and to achieve the program objective.**

2.6.7 *Other Components of HEARTS Package Relevant to Blood Pressure*

Module "A" (Access to essential medicines and technology) focuses on access to medicines and basic equipment for CVD management including:

- Information on the pharmaceutical management cycle and policies
- Selection of appropriate drugs and technologies
- Supply-chain management, including quantification, forecasting, distribution, storage, and handling
- Ensuring supply and accountability
- Rational use of medicines

Module "R" (Risk-based CV management) contains information on a total risk approach to the assessment and management of CVD, including country-specific risk charts.

Module "T" (Team-based care) describes team-based care and gives advantages and disadvantages of the approach. It also suggests steps on how to implement team-based care and contains case studies of team-based care in different countries and gives sample workflow charts and tables that can be customized to specific facilities.

Module "S" (Systems for monitoring) gives information on how to monitor and report on the prevention and management of CVD. It contains standardized indicators and data-collection tools.

In 2017, the WHO and RTSL partnered with country governments and other stakeholders to design, test, and scale up the WHO HEARTS hypertension services package to be implemented in primary care clinics. In 2020, WHO issued a report titled "Improving hypertension control in 3 million people: country experiences of programs development and implementation" [47]. In it, they reported on the programmatic experience of 18 countries that had adopted the HEARTS technical package for scaling up hypertension control. The included country case series described the development, implementation, and status (as of June 2020) of the hypertension control programs, based on information provided by each country.

In the same report, they listed five components that are necessary for a successful HEARTS hypertension control program:

- Drug- and dose-specific treatment protocols
- Access to quality-assured medications and blood pressure monitors

- Team-based care
- Patient-centered care delivered in the community
- Information systems to enable quality improvement

The 18 country cases measured the progress of each country against nine domains aligned to HEARTS technical package. In Fig. 2.8, these nine domains are numbered, and domains seven to nine show example data from Colombia and Vietnam. In the individual country reports in the 2020 report, all nine domains are populated with data for that particular country.

A more recent summary of the implementation of HEARTS in 32 countries through 2022 has been published [48] by 2022, HEARTS hypertension control programs treated 12.2 million patients in 165,000 primary care facilities. At the country level, median HTN control rate was 48% and ranged from 5% to 86%. The paper also contains a table showing the various HEARTS components, with advantages, barriers to implementation, and country examples for each of those components (Table 2.6). Additionally, there is information at the country or regional level regarding their partners, date the program was initiated, information system used, and program performance as of December 2022. The Global Hearts experience of implementing WHO HEARTS demonstrates the feasibility of controlling hypertension in low- and middle-income country primary care settings. A "central illustration" with an overview of the Global Hearts program at 5 years is shown in Fig. 2.9.

2.6.8 WHO Package of Essential Noncommunicable (PEN) Disease Interventions for Primary Health Care

Most primary health care clinics will be tasked with some management of other CV risk factors as well as CVD and other NCDs. The WHO **P**ackage of **E**ssential **N**oncommunicable (PEN) disease interventions for primary health care defines a minimum set of interventions to address major NCDs in primary care [49]. Components of WHO PEN include sections on cardiovascular diseases (including hypertension), diabetes mellitus, chronic respiratory diseases, cancer early diagnosis, healthy lifestyle counseling, self-care, palliative care, and adapting WHO PEN. Tools include a health facility assessment sample form, core list of medicines, essential technologies and tools list, sample clinical record, and table of indicators for hypertension, CVD, and diabetes. These components are feasible even in low resource settings and can be delivered by primary care physicians and non-physician health workers.

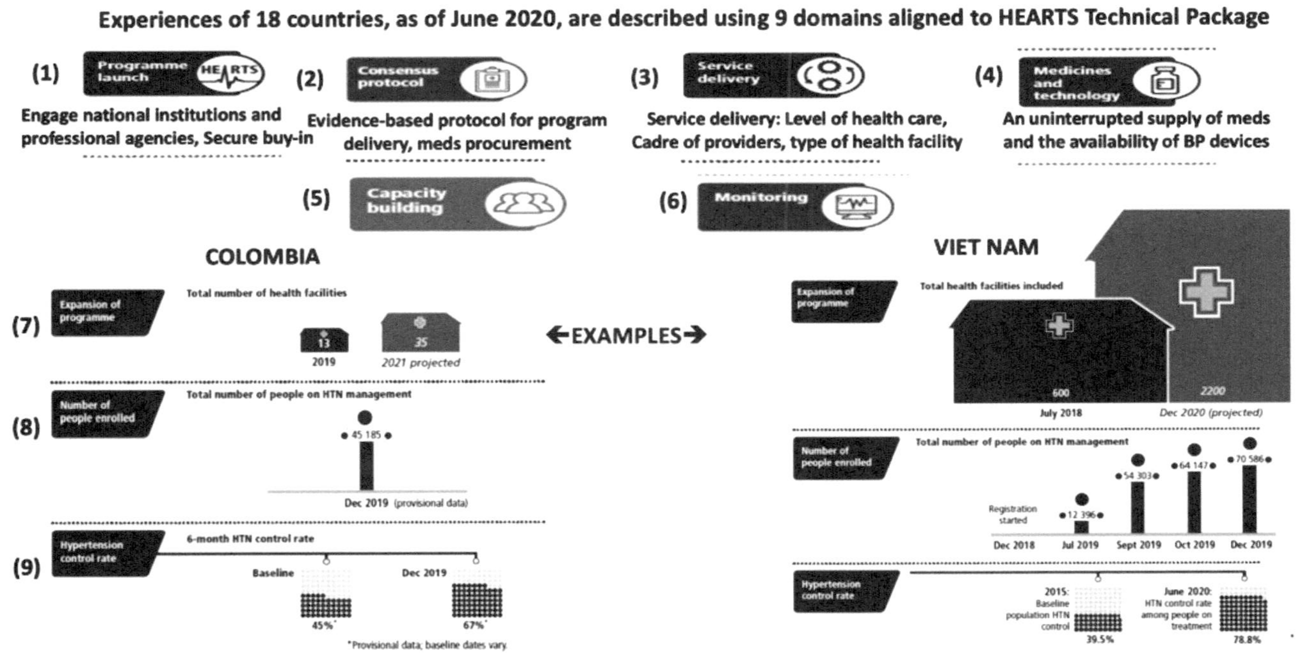

Source: Improving hypertension control in 3 million people: country experiences of programme development and implementation. Geneva: World Health Organization; 2020. Licence: CC BY-NC-SA 3.0 IGO.

Fig. 2.8 Improving hypertension control in three million people—Implementing WHO HEARTS. From Ref. [47]

Table 2.6 HEARTS components, advantages, barriers to implementation, and country examples. From Ref. [48]

HEARTS component	Advantages	Barriers to implementation	Solutions proven by global hearts program
H: Healthy lifestyle counseling	• Low cost	Education sessions are time-consuming for busy health workers	• Short lifestyle coaching modules delivered at the time of diagnosis by nonphysicians • Reinforcement by community health workers
E: Evidence-based treatment protocols	• Evidence-based medicines • Small number of HTN medicines in the treatment protocol consolidates demand and is relatively easy to implement	• Provider options constrained • Reluctance to adopt combination therapy • Unreliable drug supply	• Initial monotherapy (Fig. 2.1) • Initial dual therapy (Fig. 2.1)
A: Access to essential medicines and technology	• Improved patient retention • Fixed-dose medicines to accelerate control • Accurate hypertension diagnosis	• Incomplete inventory information • Inaccurate supply forecasting (based only on past consumption) • High prices • Price markups along supply chain • Low-quality medicines • Use of nonvalidated monitors • Broken blood pressure monitoring devices	• Medication quality assurance • Accurate inventory/forecasting/stock management • Pooled procurement • Streamlined supply chain • Regulations requiring validated blood pressure monitoring devices
R: Risk-based CVD management	• Benefits, without added risk, of intensive blood pressure lowering targeted to high-risk patients is established in major clinical trials • Allocates limited resources more efficiently by targeting treatment to highest benefit subgroups	• Lack of laboratory services at primary care level • Cognitive and time burden on health care workers working in facilities with high patient load/short visit time allocation • Potential for delayed HTN treatment or early loss-to-follow-up	• At the time of HTN diagnosis, defer risk assessment until after HTN treatment initiated • Offer intensive blood pressure lowering treatment to patients in high-risk categories defined by WHO 2021 treatment guideline • Offer lipid-lowering treatment (statin) to high risk, especially patients with diabetes complicated by HTN

(continued)

Table 2.6 (continued)

HEARTS component	Advantages	Barriers to implementation	Solutions proven by global hearts program
T: Team-based, patient-centered care			
1. Team-based care	• Increased system capacity • Highest trained spend time on complex cases • Empowers nonphysicians	• Doctors may be reluctant to share clinical tasks • Patient preference for hospital/ specialist care • Regulatory constraints on nonphysician scope of practice	• HTN effectively managed by nonphysician members of the health care team in India, Nepal, China, and other countries
2. Patient-centered care	• Retention in care • Cost-efficient	• Lack of infrastructure to deliver care in community • Regulations against visit spacing and multi-month prescription refills	• Delivery of HTN services in the community in HEARTS programs in India, Bangladesh Ethiopia, Vietnam, Philippines, and other countries
S: Systems for monitoring			
1. Hypertension indicators	• Standard across countries, good for tracking and comparing • Accurate monitoring	• Complexity	• WHO HEARTS HTN indicators
2. Digital health information systems	• Improve health worker satisfaction and performance • Timeliness • Eliminate duplicate data entry • QI driver	• Real-time data entry runs risk of complicating work routine • Lack of WIFI • Lack of smartphone • Lack of integration with national surveillance system	• Simple app • DHIS2 HTN tracker

HTN hypertension, *WHO* World Health Organization

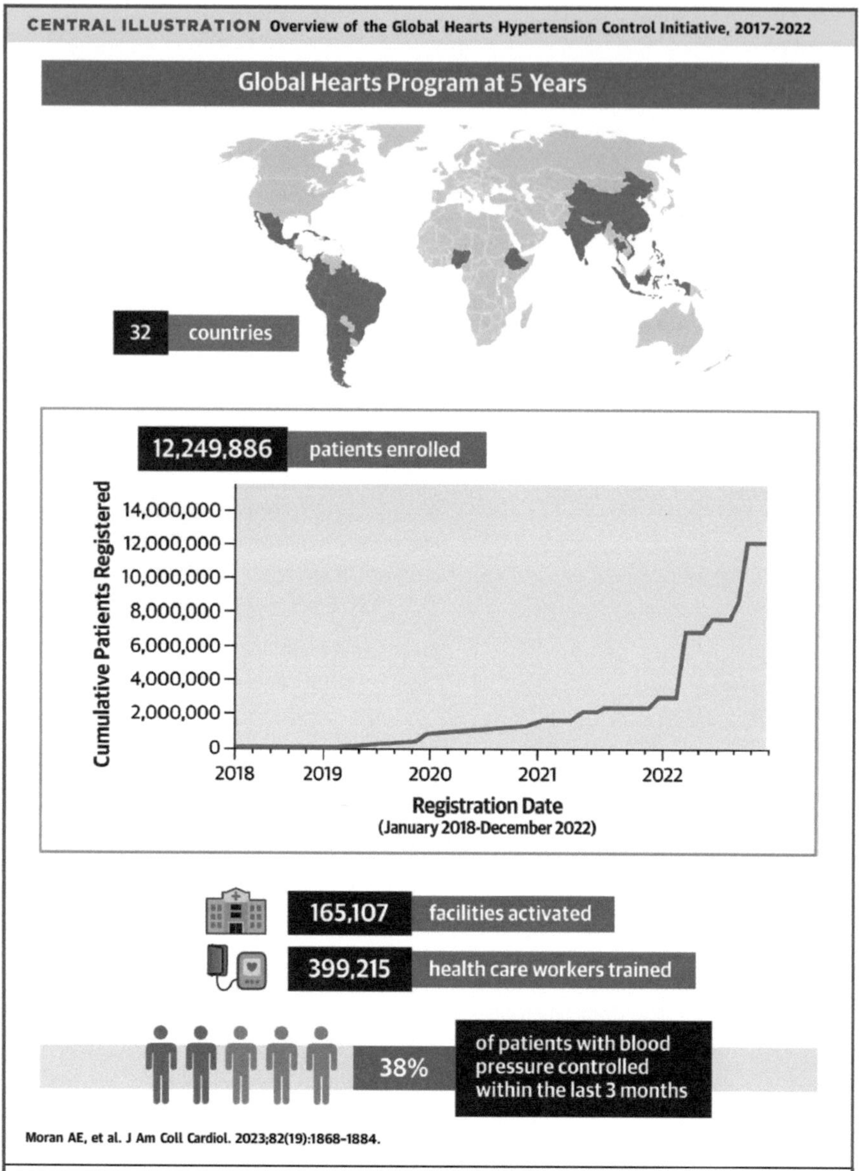

This dashboard includes a map of 32 Global Hearts countries as of December 2022, a trend plot of cumulative enrolled hypertension patients, counts of participating primary health care facilities activated and total health care workers trained in hypertension management, and health care facility-based crude proportion with blood pressure controlled (<140 mm Hg systolic and <90 mm Hg diastolic) in the 3 months before December 31, 2022.

Fig. 2.9 Overview of the global hearts hypertension control initiative, 2017–2022. From Ref. [48]

2.7 Lessons Learned: Resources That Can Help Along the Way

Successful control of blood pressure at the population level, especially in countries with limited resources, can be quite difficult. WHO's HEARTS technical package is a simple way to approach the problem, but trained staff, proper tools, and quality medications must be available. Patients must be willing and able to come to the clinic, be evaluated, receive lifestyle counseling and medications, and be adherent to the advice and medicines. Government officials must be willing to help where needed in adopting programs such as HEARTS at the regional or country level.

The implementation guide is a valuable tool for the HEARTS technical package. It discusses five steps for setting up the program: (1) engage stakeholders, (2) select demonstration site, (3) plan implementation, (4) implement and monitor, and (5) evaluate and scale up. There are also templates for rapid health system review as well as for baseline facility assessment. Additionally, there is an annex with a technical note regarding PAHO-HEARTS prerequisites and preparation for the implementation phase. The HEARTS module titled "Tool for the development of a consensus protocol for treatment of hypertension" is also quite useful. It discusses the need for a standardized protocol and gives the steps for the development of a consensus protocol. An annex contains examples of consensus protocols developed by states in India.

It may be necessary for multiple governmental and nongovernmental groups to work together to successfully initiate or sustain hypertension protocols. The India Hypertension Control Initiative (IHCI) is a collaborative initiative of several institutions including Ministry of Health and Family Welfare, national and state governments, Indian Council of Medical Research, WHO-India and Resolve to Save Lives as a technical partner. As detailed in the 2023 WHO hypertension report [1], the IHCI was started in 2018 to improve hypertension control in the community using the WHO HEARTS strategy and launched in selected districts of five states. Soon after initiation of the program, problems and setbacks related to procurement/availability of medicines emerged as the biggest challenge. However, WHO-recruited consultants, in conjunction with the Ministry of Health and Family Welfare and partners, provided technical and training support on strengthening the medicine supply chain, thus allowing for an adequate and uninterrupted availability of the needed drugs in Fig. 2.10. It was possible to decentralize the program to 18,000+ Ayushman Bharat Health and Wellness Centers (primary health care service providers) for improved access to care. By 2020, the IHCI had ensured that more than 70% of health care facilities had ensured 1 month's stock of the protocol medicines, and fewer than 10% had experienced stock-outs. As of mid-2023, IHCI had scaled up to 155 districts of 27 states with enrollment of 5.8 million hypertension patients. Figure 2.10 shows the incremental changes in procurement of amlodipine in five India states between 2017 and 2021. (Data and detailed description of this case study are from Ref. [1]).

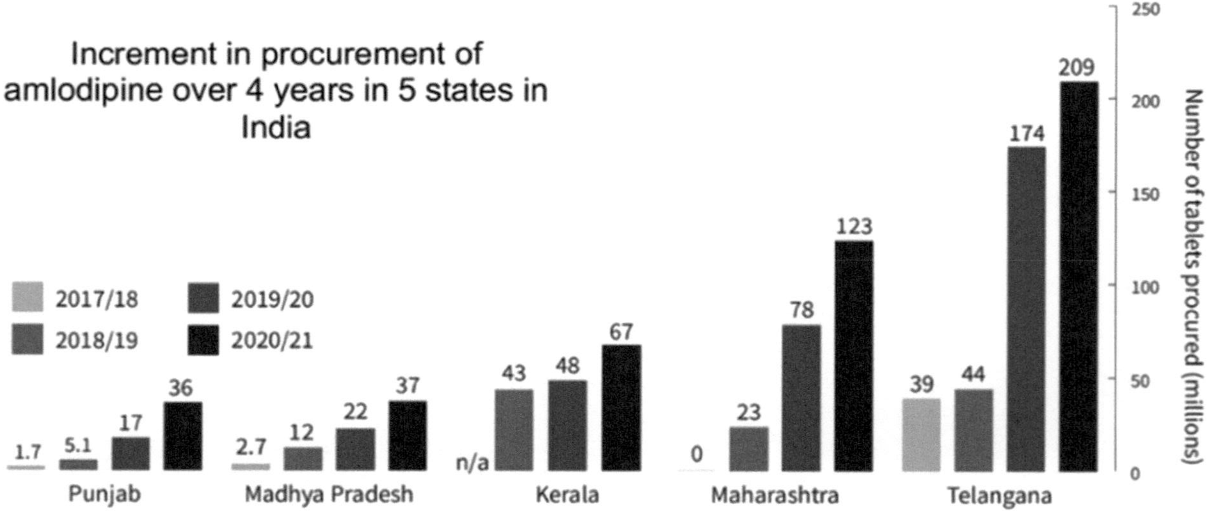

Fig. 2.10 India hypertension control initiative to strengthen the medical supply chain. From Ref. [1]

The HEARTS partner forum, led by WHO, with 11 partner organizations including the American Heart Association, Center for Chronic Disease Control, International Society of Hypertension, International Society of Nephrology, Pan American Health Organization, Resolve to Save Lives, US Centers for Disease Control, World Hypertension League, World Heart Federation, and World Stroke Organization is another useful resource. As described in a 2023 publication [50], the HEARTS partner forum supports countries in their implementation of the HEARTS technical package in various ways including technical expertise. According to this publication, forum members review the HEARTS strategic approach to improve CVD health, its advantages, feasibility, and progress of implementation and further outline future directions for HEARTS.

Several groups have addressed pitfalls, barriers, and roadblocks in achieving successful control of blood pressure. Examples of some of these are described below.

2.7.1 *Global Hearts Initiative*

As discussed earlier, a 2002 publication from the Global Hearts Collaborators summarized the implementation of HEARTS in 32 countries through 2022 [48]. For each of the six HEARTS components, the authors listed the advantages of the module as well as barriers to implementation, and solutions proven by the Global Hearts program (Table 2.6). These lessons learned can be quite helpful as more facilities adopt HEARTS.

2.7.2 *World Heart Federation Roadmap*

The WHF Roadmap (Fig. 2.11) points out selected roadblocks from both the demand side and the supply side in achieving their ideal pathway [15].

Their roadblocks and solutions are put into three general categories:

1. Pre-diagnosis and diagnosis
2. Start of treatment/drug therapy
3. Follow-up and retention

In a comprehensive table in their publication, within these three categories, WHF has listed dimensions as well as barriers and solutions for each dimension. For example, for the general category of pre-diagnosis/diagnosis, their dimensions, barriers, and solutions are shown in Table 2.7. The reader is referred to the full publication for the barriers and solutions in the categories of treatment/drug therapy and follow-up/retention [15].

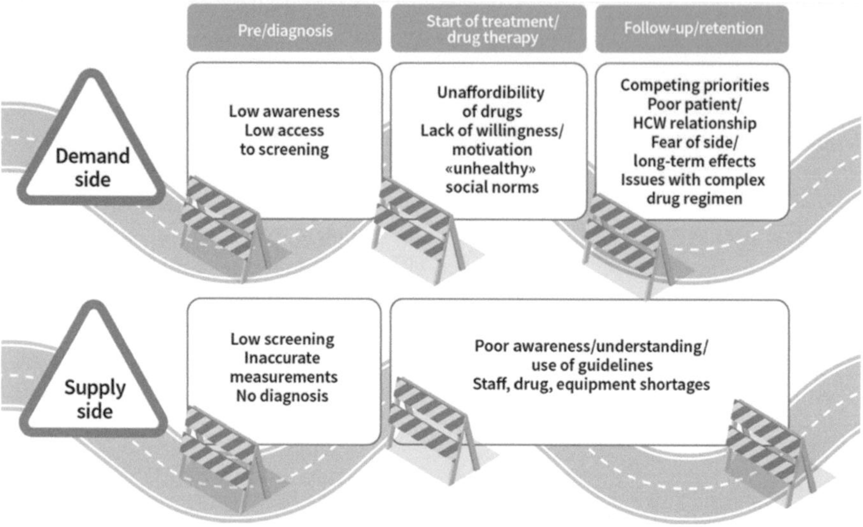

Fig. 2.11 Selected roadblocks on the way to the ideal patient journey © World Heart Federation. From Ref. [15]

2.7.3 Resolve to Save Lives Hypertension Management Program

In 2019, Frieden and colleagues published a summary of lessons learned in the first 2 years of the RTSL hypertension management program (operated in coordination with the WHO and other partners) [51]. They discussed hurdles encountered in hypertension control and noted that most of them were related to limitations in the healthcare system, not those related to patient behavior. The key lessons learned from this 2-year period were divided into categories of:

- Drug and dose-specific protocols
- Fixed dose combinations
- Drug supply
- Blood pressure measurement
- Team-based care
- Patient-centered services
- Monitoring
- Private sector
- Accountability.
- Prioritization

There is detailed discussion of each of these topics in the full open-access paper which is available online [51].

Table 2.7 Extracted from the WHF table on roadblocks and solutions. From Ref. [15]

Dimension	Barriers	Solutions
Demographic and socio-economic factors (individual level)	Lack of access to testing centres	Facilitate access to health centers where individuals can be diagnosed.
Knowledge and beliefs (individual level)	People are not aware that they are at risk of hypertension/have hypertension. Individuals have a poor understanding of the importance of detecting hypertension.	Implement community awareness campaigns. Roll out opportunistic screening (see case study 2). Implement community and worksite-based screening and education. Identify and engage local/national champions, including community health workers and volunteers and other non-traditional means to raise awareness. Encourage out-of-office BP measurement (see case study 3). Encourage involvement in and expansion of May Measurement Month.
Health systems resources and processes	Lack of health care professionals to screen/ prescribe priority interventions and to provide counseling	Promote task sharing/enhanced scope of practice for non-physician health workers for opportunistic screening and early diagnosis of HT (see case study 5). Provide clinical decision support systems and incentives for health care providers.
Social relations, norms, traditions		
Demographic and socio-economic factors (individual level)	Financial constraints Forgetfulness and poor motivation Competing family and work responsibilities	Support universal health care (UHC) for all and ensure hypertension is adequately covered in UHC coverage plans. Facilitate access to health centers where patients can be followed up free of charge. Provide financial and social support for patients (eliminate user fees and out-of-pocket medication costs). Choose low-cost alternatives in settings where there is idiosyncratic pricing.

RTSL also has developed an application known as "Simple" that is designed to support large-scale hypertension and diabetes management programs. As of December 2023, the app is actively used in 5465 public health facilities in India, Bangladesh, Ethiopia, and Sri Lanka to manage approximately 4.4 million patients with hypertension and diabetes. Healthcare workers record every patient's visit in an app, managers receive daily reports to monitor progress, and patients can chart their own BPs and blood sugars. The software is available on www.simple.org. A review of the implementation of Simple was published in 2023 [52].

Table 2.8 PASCAR 10-point action plan

1. All NCD national programs should additionally contain a plan for the detection of hypertension.
2. Allocate appropriate funding and resources for the early detection, efficient treatment, and control of hypertension.
3. Create or adopt simple and practical clinical evidence-based hypertension management guidelines.
4. Annually monitor and report the detection, treatment, and control rates of hypertension, with a clear target of improvement by 2025, using the WHO STEPwise[a] surveillance in all countries.
5. Integrate hypertension detection, treatment, and control within existing health services, such as vertical programs (e.g., HIV, TB).
6. Promote a task-sharing approach with adequately trained community health workers (shift-paradigm).
7. Ensure the availability of essential equipment and medicines for managing hypertension at all levels of care.
8. Provide universal access and coverage for detecting, treating, and controlling hypertension.
9. Support high-quality research to produce evidence that will guide interventions.
10. Invest in population-level interventions for preventing hypertension, such as reducing high levels of salt intake and obesity, increasing fruit and vegetable intake, and promoting physical activity.

Adapted from Ref. [16]

[a]The WHO STEPwise approach to surveillance (STEPS) is an internationally comparable, standardized and integrated surveillance tool through which countries can collect, analyze and disseminate core information on noncommunicable diseases. It allows country-level risk factor information to inform and improve public health policy. More information is available at https://www.who.int/teams/noncommunicable-diseases/surveillance/systems-tools/steps

2.7.4 Pan-African Society of Cardiology Roadmap

As mentioned earlier, PASCAR organized a task force of experts to identify targets and actions to lay the framework for developing a hypertension roadmap, modeled on the WHF roadmap but customized for the African continent. This document could then be used to guide the nations to achieve 25% hypertension control in Africa by 2025 [16]. They identified roadblocks at the government and health-system level, healthcare professional level, and patient level. PASCAR then identified a 10-point action plan which is summarized in Table 2.8. Their full plan includes an explanation of why and how each of these actions needs to be undertaken, as well as a discussion of steps that can be undertaken if there is a need to adapt the action plan at country level.

One of PASCAR's action plans was to integrate hypertension detection, treatment, and control within existing health services, such as vertical programs (e.g., HIV, TB). A case study in Box 2.2 describes a HIV-hypertension integrated care pilot in Uganda [1].

Box 2.2 Case Study: Human Immunodeficiency Virus (HIV) and Hypertension Integrated Care. From Ref. [1]

The integration of HIV and hypertension care, based on the WHO HEARTS technical package, has demonstrated that high levels of HIV viral suppression can be maintained while simultaneously achieving high blood pressure control.

A HIV-hypertension integration pilot in Uganda resulted in control of 73% at 24 months, up from 5.1% at baseline, while maintaining an HIV viral load suppression rate of 98%. Ninety-six percent of the patients were also retained in care while receiving integrated multi-month dispensing for both hypertension and HIV medications within a differentiated service delivery model *(155)*.

This arose from a 2-year grant awarded in 2019 by Resolve to Save Lives (RTSL) to Makerere University Joint AIDS Program (MJAP) to pilot HIV-hypertension care at Mulago ISS, the largest HIV clinic in Uganda. Uganda is home to about 1.4 million people living with HIV with an HIV prevalence of 5.1% among adults aged 15–49 years *(159; 160)*. Prior to the pilot, while more than 95% of the clinic's HIV patients were virally suppressed, of the 24.4% of patients diagnosed with hypertension, only 1% were initiated on treatment. Of those initiated on treatment, only 5.1% had achieved blood pressure control *(155; 156)*.

Note: Full citations for references 155, 156, 159 and 160 can be found in the 2023 WHO report [1].

2.7.5 WHO Regional Offices

In addition to WHO headquarters located in Geneva, Switzerland, WHO Member States are grouped into six regions: Africa, Americas, Eastern Mediterranean, Europe, South-East Asia, and Western Pacific. Each region has a regional office and has information tailored for that part of the world. For example, the South-East Asia Regional Office (SEARO), home to over a quarter of the world's population, has a SEAHEARTS Initiative adapting WHO HEARTS elements in the South-East Asia Region. As part of this, there are online courses to help adapt and implement HEARTS and PEN package. Regional website addresses can be found on the WHO at https://www.who.int/about/structure.

2.7.6 Universal Health Coverage (UHC)

In many documents concerning hypertension, CVD, and/or NCDs, it is acknowledged that achieving the 25 by 25 goals or the Sustainable Development Goals could be enhanced by governments enacting some form of UHC. WHO's work is aligned with SDG target 3.8, which focuses on achieving UHC. According to WHO, UHC means that all people have access to the full range of quality health services they need, when and where they need them, without financial hardship. It covers the full continuum of essential health services, from health promotion to prevention, treatment, rehabilitation, and palliative care [53].

WHO also acknowledges that progress toward UHC is a challenge. They state the progress in service coverage has stalled while the proportion of the population facing catastrophic out-of-pocket health spending increases continuously.

On 21 September 2023, the United Nations High-level Meeting (UN HLM) on UHC took place. It provided countries and stakeholders an opportunity to reinvigorate progress toward delivering health for all. At this meeting, world leaders recommitted to achieving UHC by 2030. The Political Declaration of the High-level Meeting on Universal Health Coverage, "Universal Health coverage: expanding our ambition for health and well-being in a post-COVID world" was subsequently adopted by the UN General Assembly on 5 October 2023 [54]. A summary of this UN HLM on Universal Health Coverage can be accessed on the UN website [55].

2.8 Take Home Message

It has been shown that, even if difficult, countries can lower blood pressure with programs such as HEARTS described in this chapter. WHO, in a September 2023 press release accompanying the launch of their first-ever global hypertension report, stated: An increase in the number of patients effectively treated for hypertension to levels observed in high-performing countries could prevent 76 million deaths, 120 million strokes, 79 million heart attacks, and 17 million cases of heart failure between now and 2050 [56].

Glossary

DECIDE Diet Diet, ExerCIse and CarDiovascular hEalth (DECIDE)-Diet is a multicenter randomized controlled feeding trial to evaluate Chinese heart healthy diets tailored to participants' own regional cuisine.

HEARTS The WHO HEARTS technical package for CVD management in primary health care supports policymakers and program managers at different levels within the Ministry of Health, primarily in LMICs, who can influence CVD primary care delivery.

Social determinants of health The social, economic, and environmental conditions in which people are born, grow, live, work, and age that impact health and well-being across the life course, and the inequities in access to power, decision-making, money, and resources that give rise to these conditions.

PEN Package The WHO **P**ackage of **E**ssential **N**oncommunicable (PEN) disease interventions for primary health care defines a minimum set of interventions to address major NCDs, including CVD, in primary care. The components are feasible even in low resource settings and can be delivered by primary care physicians and non-physician health workers.

SHAKE WHO technical package for salt reduction strategies to enable to achieve a reduction in population salt intake.

References

1. World Health Organization. Global report on hypertension: the race against a silent killer. Geneva: World Health Organization; 2023 [cited 2023 Nov 27]. License: CC BY-NC-SA 3.0 IGO. Available from: https://www.who.int/publications/i/item/9789240081062
2. WHO Global Health Observatory Map Gallery [cited 2023 Nov 27]. Available from: https://www.who.int/data/gho/map-gallery-search-results?&maptopics=1a7eb31d-4803-42d1-9c92-2890bf9b2c48
3. NCD Risk Factor Collaboration (NCD-RisC). Worldwide trends in hypertension prevalence and progress in treatment and control from 1990 to 2019: a pooled analysis of 1201 population-representative studies with 104 million participants. Lancet. 2021;398:957–80.
4. Chow CK, Teo KK, Rangarajan S, et al. PURE Study Investigators. Prevalence, awareness, treatment, and control of hypertension in rural and urban communities in high-, middle-, and low-income countries. JAMA. 2013;310:959–68.
5. GBD 2019 Risk Factors Collaborators. Global burden of 87 risk factors in 204 countries and territories, 1990–2019: a systematic analysis for the global burden of disease study 2019. Lancet. 2020;396(10258):1223–49. https://doi.org/10.1016/S0140-6736(20)30752-2.
6. NCD Risk Factor Collaboration (NCD-RisC). Worldwide trends in blood pressure from 1975 to 2015: a pooled analysis of 1479 population-based measurement studies with 19·1 million participants. Lancet. 2017;389:37–55.
7. Zhou B, Pablo P, Mensah GA, Ezzati M. Global epidemiology, health burden and effective interventions for elevated blood pressure and hypertension. Nat Rev Cardiol. 2021;18:785–802.
8. World Health Organization [cited 2024 Jan 3]. Available from: https://www.who.int/teams/noncommunicable-diseases/hypertension-report
9. United Nations. Political declaration of the high-level meeting of the general assembly on the prevention and control of non-communicable diseases: draft resolution/submitted by the President of the General Assembly. United Nations Digital Library [cited 2023 Nov 25]. Available from: https://digitallibrary.un.org/record/710899?ln=en
10. World Health Assembly. Sixty-Fifth World Health Assembly, Geneva, 21–26 May 2012. Resolutions and decisions, Annexes [cited 2023 Nov 25]. Available from: https://apps.who.int/gb/DGNP/pdf_files/A65_REC1-en.pdf
11. World Health Organization. Global action plan for the prevention and control of noncommunicable diseases 2013–2020. World Health Organization [cited 2023 Nov 26]. Available from: https://iris.who.int/handle/10665/94384
12. Sacco RL, Roth GA, Reddy KS, Arnett DK, Bonita R, Gaziano TA. The heart of 25 by 25: achieving the goal of reducing global and regional premature deaths from cardiovascular diseases and stroke: a modeling study from the American Heart Association and World Heart Federation. Circulation. 2016;133:e674–90. https://doi.org/10.1161/CIR.0000000000000395.
13. World Health Organization. HEARTS technical package for cardiovascular disease management in primary health care: risk based CVD management. Geneva: World Health Organization;

2020. Licence: CC BY-NC-SA 3.0 IGO. Available from: https://www.who.int/publications/i/item/hearts-technical-package
14. World Health Organization. Guideline for the pharmacological treatment of hypertension in adults. Geneva: World Health Organization; 2021. License: CC BY-NC-SA 3.0 IGO. Available from: https://www.who.int/publications/i/item/9789240033986
15. Jeemon P, Séverin T, Amodeo C, Balabanova D, Campbell NRC, Gaita D. World Heart Federation roadmap for hypertension—a 2021 update. Glob Heart. 2021;16(1):63. https://doi.org/10.5334/gh.1066.
16. Dzudie A, Rayner B, Ojji D, et al. Roadmap to achieve 25% hypertension control in Africa by 2025. Glob Heart. 2018;13(1):45–59. https://doi.org/10.1016/j.gheart.2017.06.001. Copublished in Cardiovasc J Afr. 2017;28(4):261–72. https://doi.org/10.5830/CVJA-2017-040.
17. Resolve to Save Lives [cited 2024 Jan 01]. Available from: https://resolvetosavelives.org/cardiovascular-health/hypertension/
18. Resolve to Save Lives [cited 2024 Jan 03]. Available from: https://linkscommunity.org/about
19. Resolve to Save Lives [cited 2024 Jan 03]. Available from: https://linkscommunity.org/toolkit/hypertension-six-steps/
20. Adler AJ, Prabhakaran D, Bovet P, et al. Reducing cardiovascular mortality through prevention and management of raised blood pressure: a World Heart Federation roadmap. Glob Heart. 2015;10(2):111–22. https://doi.org/10.1016/j.gheart.2015.04.006.
21. World Heart Federation [cited 2024 Jan 06]. Available from: https://world-heart-federation.org/cvd-roadmaps/
22. Pan American Health Organization [cited 2024 Jan 06]. Available from: https://www.paho.org/pt/hearts-nas-americas/hearts-americas-blood-pressure-measurement
23. Boonyasai RT, Rakotz MK, Lubomski LH, et al. Measure accurately, act rapidly, and partner with patients: an intuitive and practical three-part framework to guide efforts to improve hypertension control. J Clin Hypertens. 2017;19:684–94. https://doi.org/10.1111/jch.12995.
24. Egan BM, Sutherland SE, Rakotz M, et al. Improving hypertension control in primary care with the measure accurately, act rapidly, and partner with patients protocol - results at 6 and 12 months. Hypertension. 2018;72:1320–7. https://doi.org/10.1161/HYPERTENSIONAHA.118.11558.).
25. Whelton PK, Carey RM, Aronow WS, et al. 2017 ACC/AHA/AAPA/ABC/ACPM/AGS/APhA/ASH/ASPC/NMA/PCNA guideline for the prevention, detection, evaluation, and management of high blood pressure in adults: a report of the American College of Cardiology/American Heart Association Task Force on clinical practice guidelines. Hypertension. 2018;71(6):e13–e115. https://doi.org/10.1161/HYP.0000000000000065.
26. Williams B, Mancia G, Spiering W, et al. 2018 ESC/ESH guidelines for the management of arterial hypertension: the Task Force for the management of arterial hypertension of the European Society of Cardiology (ESC) and the European Society of Hypertension (ESH). Eur Heart J. 2018;39:3021–104. https://doi.org/10.1093/eurheartj/ehy339.
27. Weber MA, Schiffrin EL, White WB, et al. Clinical practice guidelines for the management of hypertension in the community: a statement by the American Society of Hypertension and the International Society of Hypertension. J Clin Hypertens (Greenwich). 2014;16(1):14–26. https://doi.org/10.1111/jch.12237.
28. National Heart, Lung, and Blood Institute [cited 2024 Jan 26]. Available from: https://www.nhlbi.nih.gov/education/dash-eating-plan
29. Global burden of disease (GBD) results tool. Institute for Health Metrics and Evaluation; 2019. Available from: http://ghdx.healthdata.org/gbd-results-tool
30. World Health Organization. Tackling NCDs 'best buys' and other recommended interventions for the prevention and control of noncommunicable diseases. World Health Organization. Licence: CC BY-NC-SA 3.0 IGO. Available from: https://iris.who.int/handle/10665/259232
31. World Health Organization [cited 2024 Jan 08]. Available from: https://iris.who.int/bitstream/handle/10665/250135/9789241511346-eng.pdf
32. World Health Organization. WHO global report on sodium intake reduction. Geneva: World Health Organization; 2023. Licence: CC BY-NC-SA 3.0 IGO. Available from: https://iris.who.int/bitstream/handle/10665/366393/9789240069985-eng.pdf?sequence=1

33. Neal B, Wu Y, Feng X, et al. Effect of salt substitution on cardiovascular events and death. N Engl J Med. 2021;385:1067–77. https://doi.org/10.1056/NEJMoa2105675.
34. Resolve to Save Lives [cited 2024 Jan 26]. Available from: https://resolvetosavelives.org/wp-content/uploads/2023/08/Salt-Reduction-Strategies.pdf
35. Resolve to Save Lives [cited 2024 Jan 26]. Available from: https://linkscommunity.org/toolkit
36. Wang Y, Feng L, Zeng G, et al. Effects of cuisine-based Chinese heart-healthy diet in lowering blood pressure among adults in China: multicenter, single-blind, randomized, parallel controlled feeding trial. Circulation. 2022;146:303–15. https://doi.org/10.1161/CIRCULATIONAHA.122.05904537.
37. Unger T, Borghi C, Charchar F, et al. International Society of Hypertension global hypertension practice guidelines. Hypertension. 2020;75:1334–57. https://doi.org/10.1161/HYPERTENSIONAHA.120.15026.
38. World Health Organization. Integrating the social determinants of health into health workforce education and training. Geneva: World Health Organization; 2023. Licence: CC BY-NC-SA 3.0 IGO.
39. Centers for Disease Control and Prevention [cited 2024 Jan 07]. Available from: https://www.cdc.gov/nchhstp/socialdeterminants/faq.html#what-are-social-determinants
40. Geldserzer P, Manne-Goehler J, Marcus M-E, et al. The state of hypertension care in 44 low-income and middle-income countries: a cross-sectional study of nationally representative individual-level data from 1·1 million adults. Lancet. 2019;394:6452–662.
41. Kirschbaum TK, Sudharsanan N, Manne-Goehler J, et al. The association of socioeconomic status with hypertension in 76 low- and middle-income countries. J Am Coll Cardiol. 2022;80:804–17.
42. World Health Organization. Available from: https://www.who.int/publications/i/item/9789240008793
43. Garovic VD, Dechend R, Easterling T, et al. on behalf of the American Heart Association Council on Hypertension, Council on the Kidney in Cardiovascular Disease, Kidney in Heart Disease Science Committee, Council on Arteriosclerosis, Thrombosis and Vascular Biology, Council on Lifestyle and Cardiometabolic Health, Council on Peripheral Vascular Disease, Stroke Council. Hypertension in pregnancy: diagnosis, blood pressure goals, and pharmacotherapy: a scientific statement from the American Heart Association. Hypertension. 2022;79:e21–41. https://doi.org/10.1161/HYP.0000000000000208.
44. World Health Organization. Web Annex A. World Health Organization model list of essential medicines – 23rd list, 2023. In: The selection and use of essential medicines 2023: executive summary of the report of the 24th WHO Expert Committee on the Selection and Use of Essential Medicines, 24–28 April 2023. Geneva: World Health Organization; 2023 (WHO/MHP/HPS/EML/2023.02). Licence: CC BYNC-SA 3.0 IGO.
45. Benjamin IJ, Kreutz R, Olsen MH, et al. Fixed-dose combination antihypertensive medications. Lancet. 2019;394:637–8. https://doi.org/10.1016/S0140-6736(19)31629-0.
46. World Health Organization. Available from: https://www.who.int/publications/i/item/9789240050969
47. World Health Organization. Improving hypertension control in 3 million people: country experiences of programme development and implementation. Geneva: World Health Organization; 2020. Licence: CC BY-NC-SA 3.0 IGO.
48. Moran AE, Gupta R, Global Hearts Initiative Collaborators. Implementation of global hearts hypertension control programs in 32 low- and middle-income countries. J Am Coll Cardiol. 2023;82:1868–84.
49. WHO package of essential noncommunicable (PEN) disease interventions for primary health care. Geneva: World Health Organization; 2020. Licence: CC BY-NC-SA 3.0 IGO. Available from: https://iris.who.int/bitstream/handle/10665/334186/9789240009226-eng.pdf?sequence=1
50. Khan T, Moran AE, Perel P, et al. The HEARTS partner forum—supporting implementation of HEARTS to treat and control hypertension. Front Public Health. 2023;11:1146441. https://doi.org/10.3389/fpubh.2023.1146441.

51. Frieden TR, Varghese CV, Kishore SP, et al. Scaling up effective treatment of hypertension-a pathfinder for universal health coverage. J Clin Hypertens (Greenwich). 2019;21(10):1442–9. https://doi.org/10.1111/jch.13655.
52. Burka D, Gupta R, Moran AE, et al. Keep it simple: designing a user-centred digital information system to support chronic disease management in low/middle-income countries. BMJ Health Care Inform. 2023;30:e100641. https://doi.org/10.1136/bmjhci-2022-100641.
53. World Health Organization. Available from: https://www.who.int/health-topics/universal-health-coverage#tab=tab_1
54. [cited 2024 Jan 03]. Available from: https://documents-dds-ny.un.org/doc/UNDOC/GEN/N23/306/84/PDF/N2330684.pdf?OpenElement (English version); for other available languages go to https://www.undocs.org/Home/Mobile?FinalSymbol=A%2FRES%2F78%2F4&Language=E&DeviceType=Desktop&LangRequested=False
55. UHC2020 [cited 2024 Jan 26]. Available from: https://www.uhc2030.org/news-and-events/news/the-2023-un-hlm-on-uhc-was-a-moment-to-renew-commitment-to-uhc-and-set-the-path-for-action-and-investment/
56. World Health Organization. First WHO report details devastating impact of hypertension and ways to stop it. 2023 Sep 19 [cited 2024 Jan 26]. News release New York. Available from: https://www.who.int/news/item/19-09-2023-first-who-report-details-devastating-impact-of-hypertension-and-ways-to-stop-it

Chapter 3
Obesity and Diabetes in Latin America: The Impact of Socioeconomic Status on Programs and Outcomes

Cecilia Albala and Fernando Vio

3.1 Introduction

Important changes in socioeconomic and environmental conditions and the rapid aging of the population in the last decades in Latin American countries have led to profound changes in health conditions [1]. The aging of the population leads to an accumulation of chronic diseases at the end of life, and on the other hand, the socioeconomic and environmental conditions have led to an accelerated increase in obesity, the most important risk factor for chronic diseases. At global level, cardiovascular diseases are the most frequent chronic diseases; however, their evolution has not been the same throughout the world. In middle- and low-income countries, such as most Latin Americans, an increase in frequency has been observed, while in high-income countries, the prevalence has decreased [2, 3]. This is fundamentally attributed to the accelerated increase in obesity in all age-groups, affecting mainly low-income people. The related increase in diabetes 2 poses both obesity and diabetes among the main five modifiable risks for cardiovascular disease [3].

In this chapter, we analyze the impact of both diseases, obesity and diabetes 2, in Latin America (LA), the associated risk of chronic diseases, and the main causes, outcomes, and interventions.

C. Albala (✉) · F. Vio
Public Health Nutrition Unit, Institute of Nutrition and Food Technology, Universidad de Chile, Santiago, Chile
e-mail: calbala@uchile.cl; fvio@inta.uchile.cl

T. Romero et al. (eds.), *Global Challenges in Cardiovascular Prevention in Populations with Low Socioeconomic Status*,
https://doi.org/10.1007/978-3-031-79051-5_3

3.2 The Increase of Obesity in Latin America (LA)

3.2.1 Obesity in Adults

Obesity is a serious public health problem globally. With 62.5% of overweight in adults (Body Mass Index or BMI >25) from which 28% are obese (BMI ≥30), nowadays the Region of the Americas has the higher prevalence of overweight or obesity in adults from all regions of the World Health Organization (WHO) [4]. In LA about 64% of adults are overweight, from which 30.5% are obese, with numbers on the rise and affecting the entire population from early childhood. According to the United Nations Children's Fund (UNICEF) data [5], between 2000 and 2016, the prevalence of obesity doubled in Latin America (LA), and figures that tripled in Haiti and Costa Rica. Likewise, deaths associated with obesity have also increased, exceeding 8.5% in 2019. The main determinants of this phenomenon have been energy-dense fast-food exposition, adverse environments, and sedentary lifestyle [6].

Table 3.1 describes the last available data on the prevalence of overweight and obesity in adults in LA, where most of the countries have more than half of the population with overweight or obesity. Mexico, Chile, and Argentina have the higher rates of obesity, surpassing one-third of the adult population. The lowest rate in the Region corresponds to Cuba and Dominican Republic with figures of 15.8% and 16.6%, respectively, although the last one Dominican Republic has one of the highest prevalence of infant obesity in the Region (Table 3.2). Obesity prevalence in adults is higher in women than men in all the countries with the single exception of Colombia where men have twice the prevalence of obesity than women (29.4% vs. 12.6%, respectively). The countries with the highest prevalence of obesity in men are Mexico, Argentina, and Chile, with a prevalence over 30% (Table 3.1).

3.2.2 Children's Obesity

The most concerning problem is the accelerated increase in obesity and overweight in childhood that has affected all countries in Latin America. According to UNICEF data [5], between 2000 and 2016, an accelerated increase in childhood obesity and overweight was observed throughout the Region, with great inequalities to the detriment of low socioeconomic levels.

Table 3.2 describes the prevalence of children obesity (5–19 years) according to UNICEF report 2023 [5], with data from 2016. The higher rates are observed in Mexico, Argentina, Dominican Rep., Chile, Venezuela, and Uruguay, with rates of obesity about 15% and overweight of 25% or higher. In this group of age, the prevalence of obesity is higher in boys than girls in all South American countries and Mexico, Dominican Rep., Costa Rica, and Cuba. According to FAO and UNICEF, overweight in Latin America affects 7.3% of children under 5 years, rate over the global rate of 5.6% [5, 8].

Table 3.1 Prevalence of overweight and obesity in adults in Latin America

	Males		Females		Total	
Region/country	Overweight	Obesity	Overweight	Obesity	Overweight	Obesity
Mexico, Central America, and Caribbean						
Mexico (2021) ≥20 years	37.8	31.8	33.9	41.1	35.7	36.9
Dominican Rep (2013) 15–49 years	27.8	13.0	29.7	20.8	28.1	16.6
Costa Rica (2008/2009) 20–64 years	43.5	18.9	35.3	31.3	39.4	25.1
Cuba (2010) ≥18 years	32.7	12.8	30.8	18.8	31.7	15.8
El Salvador (2014/2015) ≥20 years	39.5	19.5				
Nicaragua (2007/2009) 20–60 years	30.9	11.9	34.7	29.8	33.1	22.0
South America						
Argentina (2018) ≥18 years	38.7	31.4	29.1	33.4	33.7	32.4
Bolivia (2019) 18–69 years	39.1	20.8	35.10	31.8	37.1	26.2
Brazil (2019) ≥18 years	35.7	21.8	33.1	29.5	34.4	25.9
Chile (2016/2017) ≥15 years	43.3	30.3	36.4	38.4	39.8	34.4
Colombia (2018) 18–75 years	36.4	29.4	36.0	12.6	36.2	21.3
Ecuador (2018) 19–59 years	43.1	18.3	39.7	27.9	41.3	23.4
Paraguay (2011) 15–74 years	35.3	19.9	34.4	26.6	34.8	23.2
Peru (2017/2018) 18–59 years	39.1	21.3	38.3	29.4	38.7	26.0
Uruguay (2013/2014) 15–64 years	38.6	22.1	31.3	25.0	34.8	23.7
Venezuela (2014/2017) ≥20 years	38.2	22.2	31.2	26.7	34.5	24.6

Source [7]: Global obesity observatory https://data.worldobesity.org/region/who-americas-region-3/#data_prevalence

3.2.3 *Obesity and Non-communicable Diseases*

A high BMI is a major risk factor for non-communicable diseases, such as heart disease, stroke, diabetes, musculoskeletal disorders, and some cancers. The consequences of obesity are observed throughout the entire life cycle and increase with increasing BMI. Childhood obesity is associated with a higher likelihood of diabetes, premature death, and disability in adulthood. In addition to these increased future risks, obese children suffer from breathing difficulties, increased risk of fractures and hypertension, and present early markers of cardiovascular disease, insulin resistance, and psychological effects. All these problems produce a high burden of disease associated with obesity.

Table 3.2 Children obesity (5–19 years) prevalence in Latin America (data from 2016)

Region/ country	Boys		Girls		Total	
	Overweight (%)	Obesity (%)	Overweight (%)	Obesity (%)	Overweight (%)	Obesity (%)
Mexico, Central America, and Caribbean						
Mexico	35.7	16.7	35.1	12.8	35.4	14.8
Dominican Rep	33.1	15.8	32.6	14.2	32.8	15.0
Costa Rica	30.1	12.6	33.0	11.9	31.5	12.3
Cuba	31.0	12.4	29.0	10.3	30.6	11.4
El Salvador	27.7	11.0	33.1	12.5	30.4	11.7
Guatemala	26.7	10.0	30.7	9.8	28.6	9.9
Honduras	25.0	9.3	29.6	9.8	27.3	9.6
Nicaragua	26.7	10.3	32.0	11.4	29.3	10.8
Panama	26.9	9.6	32.0	11.4	28.6	9.9
South America						
Argentina	36.5	20.7	31.8	12.9	36.5	16.9
Bolivia	28.1	9.8	30.0	8.5	28.1	9.1
Brazil	28.0	12.4	26.3	9.2	28.0	10.8
Chile	35.4	17.5	33.5	12.9	35.4	15.2
Colombia	24.3	7.5	26.2	6.4	24.3	7.0
Ecuador	28.3	10.5	29.1	8.3	28.3	9.4
Paraguay	27.9	11.7	26.9	9.3	27.9	10.5
Peru	27.0	8.8	27.9	6.8	27.0	7.8
Uruguay	33.4	16.1	31.0	11.4	33.4	13.8
Venezuela	34.1	14.9	33.4	13.2	34.1	14.1

Source [5]: United Nations Children's Fund, Childhood overweight on the rise. Is it too late to turn the tide in Latin America and the Caribbean? 2023 Report, UNICEF, Panama City, August 2023

According to the Global Burden of Disease (GBD) study 2015, the increasing obesity has been faster than the related disease burden but with a wide range of variation between countries. Among the obesity related deaths, more than 60% were related to cardiovascular diseases, the first problem of Disability Adjusted Life Years (DALY) lost, followed by chronic kidney disease, diabetes, cancer, and musculoskeletal disorders [4].

The other growing problem, associated with population aging are neurodegenerative disorders as dementia, a disease that could be decreased in 40% by controlling modifiable risk factors, such as obesity, diabetes, and physical inactivity [9].

3.3 Diabetes 2 in Latin America

Children and adult obesity are increasing in Latin America. The accelerated increase in obesity has also meant an increase in diabetes 2. It is estimated that between 2021 and 2045 [10], there will be a 50% increase in cases of diabetes 2 in Latin America. Andean LA and Southern LA are among the six regions of the world that increased diabetes 2 by more than 100% between 1990 and 2021 [11].

According to the Global Burden of Diseases study [10], in 2021 diabetes 2 accounted for 96.0% of diabetes cases and 95.4% of diabetes DALYs worldwide, from which 52.2% of global diabetes 2 DALYs were attributable to high BMI. By 2050, the same study estimates total diabetes 2 prevalence of 11.3% in LA, second after North Africa and the Middle East, with estimates of 16.8%.

Table 3.3 shows the age adjusted prevalence of diabetes estimates (according to WHO population), for people 20–79 years. Although some countries show a decrease between 2011 and 2021, it is estimated that all the countries in the Region will increase the prevalence of diabetes in 2030. By 2021, four countries on the Region surpass 10%: Mexico, Dominican Republic, Guatemala, and Chile, but in 2030, the same situation will be observed also in Brazil, Venezuela, Uruguay, Costa Rica, and Guatemala. The higher rate in the Region is exhibited by Mexico with 16.8% in 2021 and an estimated 18.3% in 2030. A high rate of undiagnosed diabetes is observed in all the Region where the rates are over 30%, with the sole exception of Venezuela and Ecuador with estimates of 20% of undiagnosed diabetes 2.

The mortality attributed to diabetes 2 in 2021 in South American Countries fluctuates between 1.35% and 2.8%, but in Mexico, Central America, and Caribbean, the rates are higher, fluctuating between 1.7% in Cuba and 9.9% in Mexico. Impaired glucose test (IGT) is about 10% in all the countries, fluctuating from 7.3% in Bolivia to 16.1% in Honduras [12].

The main risk factors for diabetes 2 are obesity, the most important driver; dietary risks, physical inactivity, tobacco use, and air pollution are also well documented, most of them increasing in LA [13].

The high rates of under diagnoses, the knowledge about the natural history of disease, and the identification of obesity as the main risk factor for diabetes reinforce the need of population-based interventional strategies to address the avoidable risk factors, and early screening for detection from IGT to diabetes 2 [14]. In China, a 6-year lifestyle intervention program among people with impaired glucose tolerance demonstrated a significant decrease in cumulative incidence of cardiovascular disease mortality, all-cause mortality, and incidence of diabetes 2 [15].

Table 3.3 Age adjusted prevalence of diabetes 2 in Latin America by 2011, 2021, and 2030

	Age adjusted prevalence % (WHO pop) 20–79 years estimates				% people with diabetes 2 undiagnosed	Mortality attributable to diabetes 2 <60 year %
	Diabetes 2011 (%)	Diabetes 2021 (%)	Diabetes 2030 (%)	IGT 2021 (%)	2021 (%)	2021 (%)
Mexico, Central America, and Caribbean						
Mexico	15.6	16.9	18.3	8.7	47.5	9.9
Dominican Rep.	8.1	10.5	12.5	10.8	37.3	4.4
Costa Rica	9.6	8.8	10.1	10.3	37.3	2.6
Cuba	9.4	7.6	7.8	9.9	37.3	1.7
El Salvador	9.4	6.3	6.9	10.8	37.3	2.8
Guatemala	9.5	13.1	14.1	9.9	48.8	6.1
Honduras	6.7	5.1	5.6	16.1	50.0	2.2
Nicaragua	11.0	9.3	10.2	12.1	44.8	3.2
Panama	9.4	8.2	8.9	11.8	31.2	2.7
Venezuela	10.2	9.6	11.9	9.9	20.0	4.0
South America						
Argentina	5.5	5.4	6.1	11.8	31.2	1.3
Bolivia	6.6	5.5	6.1	7.3	39.6	1.5
Brazil	10.1	8.8	10.2	9.9	31.9	2.8
Chile	9.5	10.8	10.9	11.8	31.2	2.5
Colombia	9.8	8.3	8.9	10.8	36.0	2.8
Ecuador	6.6	4.4	4.6	9.9	20.0	1.8
Paraguay	6.5	7.5	8.3	9.9	37.3	2.3
Peru	6.0	4.8	5.3	9.9	37.3	2.0
Uruguay	5.7	9.0	10	11.8	31.2	1.3

Source [12]: https://diabetesatlas.org/data/en/country/ IDF Diabetes Atlas 10th Ed. 2021

In 2019, premature death accounts for most of the diabetes 2 burden in the Americas; by 2019, 5.9% of all deaths in adults 20 year and older in the Region were due to diabetes 2 [13]. The fraction of the diabetes 2 burden attributed to disability increased from 1990 to 2019 reaching figures near 50% in all Regions [13]. Central America and the Caribbean have the higher DALY lost in Latin America. On the other side, Southern America exhibits the lower DALYs in the Region. The diabetes 2 burden increases according to increasing prevalence, but better access to health care and higher income decreased it. Among the main attributable risk for the diabetes 2 burden is the high BMI accounting for 63.2% attributable population fraction of the diabetes 2 burden, seconded by dietary pattern with 27.5% [10].

3.4 Obesity and Diabetes and Determinants of Health

Among all the countries, obesity affects mainly low-income people, where children's obesity coexists with important problems of undernutrition. The FAO report (2018) indicates that hunger, malnutrition, micronutrient deficiencies, overweight, and obesity mostly affect people with lower incomes, women, indigenous people, and people of African descent and rural families [8]. Although important improvements in the fight against undernutrition, childhood obesity is on the rise [5]. One of the main causes of the rise in malnutrition among the most vulnerable is the change that the region's food systems have undergone, from production to consumption.

Until a couple of decades ago, the fight against obesity and chronic diseases associated with poor diet was focused on individual behavior change and education. However, these strategies proved to be very little cost-effective in non-experimental conditions, along with increasing the gap between people with greater income and education, and those who are more disadvantaged. For this reason, since the 2000s it has been proposed that people's behaviors are also influenced by their environments and that we could achieve greater advances in food and nutrition if we intervene in these environments. Food environments refer to all the social, political, and cultural characteristics that influence people's eating decisions and include prices, forms of promotion, and availability and quality of food, among a series of other factors. Examples of such policy are tax on sugar-sweetened beverages and the food warning labeling. The food industry can play a significant role in promoting healthy diets by reducing the fat, sugar, and salt content of processed foods, ensuring that healthy and nutritious choices are available and affordable to all consumers; restricting marketing of foods high in sugars, salt, and fats, especially those foods aimed at children and teenagers; and ensuring the availability of healthy food choices and supporting regular physical activity practice in the workplace [16, 17].

However, the problem of obesity is multifactorial. It must be approached comprehensively, with structural, environmental, and cultural policies, considering critical issues such as food and physical activity, but also the effect of urban and school environments, screens, personal image and self-esteem, the family environment with the model of parents and the habits they transmit, attachment and their love expressed through food, the regularity, and timing of eating and sleeping. The findings make emphasis in the long-term clinical benefits of lifestyle intervention for patients with impaired glucose tolerance and provide further justification for adoption of lifestyle interventions as public health measures to control the consequences of diabetes.

3.5 Interventions

The most important interventions to address the problem with tax on sugar-sweetened beverages and the food warning labeling policies in the Region have been led by Mexico and Chile.

Since June 2014, a tax on sugary drinks and ultra-processed sugary foods was implemented in Mexico. The evaluation of results shows a decrease in purchases and a decrease in dental cavities [18]. These results are very encouraging considering that Mexico is the country with the highest prevalence of diabetes 2 in Latin America and one of the countries with the highest sugar consumption through soft drinks beverages.

The first food warning labeling worldwide (black octagon) was designed in Chile and has been replicated in countries in the region such as Mexico, Uruguay, Peru, and Argentina and was also being discussed in countries in other regions, such as South Africa, India, Canada, among others. The design process was carried out by a multidisciplinary team that included experts in public health and nutrition, but also experts in food marketing and behavioral economics, exporting techniques and designs from those areas. The proposed labeling was finally implemented in June 2016 through a Food Labeling Law, which also considered advertising restrictions for foods with warning labels and protection of school environments regarding the sale, promotion, and delivery of foods with seals, becoming a pioneering law in the promotion of better food environments [19].

The first partial evaluations show that in general terms, the sale of labeled foods has decreased, especially sodium, sugars, and saturated fats, which are nutrients that have been related to the appearance of diabetes, cardiovascular disease, and hypertension among others. The marketing restrictions have worked. Today Chilean children are exposed to almost half of the advertising of unhealthy foods compared to what occurred before the implementation of the law. At the school level, feeding program was reformulated, the entire supply of these unhealthy foods was reduced, and significant reductions in calories and the consumption of sodium, saturated fats, and sugars have been observed [20].

Despite the initial evaluations showing positive results although insufficient, children obesity continued increasing in Chile which must be complemented with other actions in the coming years. Although these are very valuables policies, the addition of more initiatives related to the environment, such as improving urban and school environments, controlling time in front of screens, the family environment, sleep time, and other factors are needed to address the whole problem [21, 22].

A recent systematic review of label interventions provides evidence for supporting nutrition labels with interactive digital interventions, such as basket feedback, or financial incentives is promising. Overall, the findings indicate that more intrusive interventions are required to give cause to act on nutrition labels [23].

3.6 Discussion

The fast increase in overweight and obesity and its consequent higher risk of diabetes 2 and chronic diseases since earlier ages poses a serious challenge over to healthy aging, quality of life, and health care systems [6]. Obesity and diabetes 2 are among five modifiable risks for cardiovascular disease [3] as well as other diseases. The data in this article demonstrate that obesity is a growing problem in Latin America, whose consequences impact the entire life cycle, especially healthy aging, and therefore, policy measures need to be taken urgently.

To date, no public policy has been able to stop the advance of obesity, despite the efforts made by international organizations such as the WHO and many governments. These policies have been based on addressing structural issues, such as taxes, advertising, and stamps on processed foods high in critical nutrients such as saturated fats, sugar, and salt.

Some interesting examples of public policy related to prevent obesity in the world are The Amsterdam Healthy Weight Approach (AHWA) and the Shuku (food) Iku (intellectual, moral, and physical education) program in Japan. The AHWA is a long-term program run by the municipality of Amsterdam to improve the physical activity and diet of children from the poorest sectors where obesity is concentrated, through school, home, neighborhood, and the city, with a comprehensive personalized support program for each child. Since 2013, the program has reached more than 15,000 children. During this period, the prevalence of overweight and obesity among 2–18 years of age decreased from 21% in 2012 to 18.7% in 2017 [24].

In Japan, the Shuku Iku program has existed since 2005. The objective is to increase student information about the food chain, the origin and production of food, and food education from the beginning of the early years to secondary school. The program establishes: (a) healthy menus in schools and specific classes on nutrition; (b) hiring professional nutritionists who also have teaching degrees; (c) promotion of a social culture around food, in which children help prepare and distribute food in schools, and at mealtime they transform the dining room into a kind of restaurant, where they help set the table, the tablecloth, they serve each other and eat together in class. The idea is "eating is a social act" and in schools there are no shops or food machines, which makes the environment healthy, without access to chips, soft drinks, and snacks [25, 26].

Additional research and research capacity are needed to address the growing epidemic of obesity and diabetes 2, particularly with respect to designing, implementing, and evaluating the impact of evidence-based obesity prevention interventions [6].

Considering that although overweight and obesity are preventable, no country has reversed the epidemic, WHO is providing new recommendations to accelerate and urgently confront this worrying panorama that is the fight against obesity [27, 28].

References

1. Albala C. El envejecimiento de la población chilena y los desafíos para la salud y el bienestar de las personas mayores. Rev Med Clin Condes. 2020;31(1):7–12.
2. Abarca-Gomez L, Abdeen Z, Abdul Hamid Z, Abu-Rmeileh NM, Acosta Cazares B, et al. Worldwide trends in body-mass index, underweight, overweight, and obesity from 1975 to 2016: a pooled analysis of 2416 population-based measurement studies in 128.9 million children, adolescents, and adults. Lancet. 2017;390(10113):2627–42.
3. Global Cardiovascular Risk Consortium, Magnussen C, Ojeda FM, Leong DP, Alegre-Diaz J, Amouyel P, et al. Global effect of modifiable risk factors on cardiovascular disease and mortality. N Engl J Med. 2023;389(14):1273–85.
4. GBD 2015 Obesity Collaborators, Afshin A, Forouzanfar MH, Reitsma MB, Sur P, Estep K, et al. Health effects of overweight and obesity in 195 countries over 25 years. N Engl J Med. 2017;377(1):13–27. https://doi.org/10.1056/NEJMoa1614362. Epub 2017 Jun 12.
5. United Nations Children's Fund. Childhood overweight on the rise. Is it too late to turn the tide in Latin America and the Caribbean? 2023 Report. Panama City: UNICEF; 2023.
6. Popkin BM, Corvalan C, Grummer-Strawn LM. Dynamics of the double burden of malnutrition and the changing nutrition reality. Lancet. 2020;395(10217):65–74. https://doi.org/10.1016/S0140-6736(19)32497-3. Epub 2019 Dec 15.
7. Global Obesity Observatory. https://data.worldobesity.org/tables/prevalence-of-adult-overweight-obesity-2/. https://data.worldobesity.org/region/who-americas-region-3/#data_prevalence.
8. FAO, IFAD, UNICEF, WFP and WHO. The state of food security and nutrition in the world 2018. Building climate resilience for food security and nutrition. Rome: FAO; 2018. Licence: CC BY-NC-SA 3.0 IGO.
9. Nichols E, Szoeke CEI, Vollset SE, Abbasi N, Abd-Allah F, Abdela J, et al. Global, regional, and national burden of Alzheimer's disease and other dementias, a systematic analysis for the Global Burden of Disease Study 2016. Lancet Neurol. 2019;18:88–106. https://doi.org/10.1016/S1474-4422(18)30403-4.
10. GBD 2021 Diabetes Collaborators. Global, regional, and national burden of diabetes from 1990 to 2021, with projections of prevalence to 2050: a systematic analysis for the global burden of disease study 2021. Lancet. 2023;402(10397):203–34. https://doi.org/10.1016/S0140-6736(23)01301-6.
11. Avilés-Santa ML, Monroig-Rivera A, Soto-Soto A, Lindberg NM. Current state of diabetes mellitus prevalence, awareness, treatment, and control in Latin America: challenges and innovative solutions to improve health outcomes across the continent. Curr Diab Rep. 2020;20(11):62. https://doi.org/10.1007/s11892-020-01341-9.
12. International Diabetes Federation. IDF diabetes atlas. 10th ed. Brussels, Belgium: IDF; 2021. https://www.diabetesatlas.org.
13. Diabetes in the Americas Collaborators. Burden of diabetes and hyperglycaemia in adults in the Americas, 1990–2019: a systematic analysis for the Global Burden of Disease Study 2019 GBD 2019. Lancet Diabetes Endocrinol. 2022;10:655–67.
14. Mechanick J, Garber AJ, Grunberger G, Handelsman Y, Garvey WT. Dysglycemia-based chronic disease: an American Association of Clinical Endocrinologists Position Statement. Endocr Pract. 2018;24:995–1011.
15. Li G, Zhang P, Wang J, et al. Cardiovascular mortality, all-cause mortality, and diabetes incidence after lifestyle intervention for people with impaired glucose tolerance in the Da Qing Diabetes Prevention Study: a 23-year follow-up study. Lancet Diabetes Endocrinol. 2014;2:474–80.
16. Corvalán C, Garmendia ML, Jones-Smith J, Lutter CK, Miranda JJ, et al. Nutrition status of children in Latin America. Obes Rev. 2017;18(Suppl 2):7–18. https://doi.org/10.1111/obr.12571.

17. Miranda JJ, Barrientos-Gutiérrez T, Corvalan C, Hyder AA, Lazo-Porras M, Oni T, Wells JCK. Understanding the rise of cardiometabolic diseases in low- and middle-income countries. Nat Med. 2019;25(11):1667–79. https://doi.org/10.1038/s41591-019-0644-7. Epub 2019 Nov 7.
18. Hernández-Fa MK, Cantorala MA, Colcherob A. Taxes to unhealthy food and beverages and oral health in Mexico: an observational study. Caries Res. 2021;55:183–92.
19. Corvalán C, Reyes M, Garmendia ML, Uauy R. Structural responses to the obesity and non-communicable diseases epidemic: update on the Chilean law of food labelling and advertising. Obes Rev. 2019;20:367–74. https://doi.org/10.1111/obr.12802. Epub 2018 Dec 13.
20. Taillie LS, Bercholz M, Popkin B, Reyes M, Colchero MA, Corvalán C. Changes in food purchases after the Chilean policies on food labelling, marketing, and sales in schools: a before and after study. Lancet Planet Health. 2021;5:526–33. https://doi.org/10.1016/S2542-5196(21)00172-8.
21. Olafsdottir S, Berg C, Eiben G, et al. Young children's screen activities, sweet drink consumption and anthropometry: results from a prospective European study. Eur J Clin Nutr. 2014;68:223–8.
22. Hense S, Pohlabeln H, De Henauw S, et al. Sleep duration and overweight in European children: is the association modified by geographic region. Sleep. 2011;34:885–90.
23. Schruff-Lim EM, van Loo EJ, van Kleef E, van Trijp HCM. Turning FOP nutrition labels into action: a systematic review of label+ interventions. Food Policy. 2023;120:102479. https://doi.org/10.1016/j.foodpol.2023.102479.
24. Sawyer A, den Hertog K, Verhoeff AP, et al. Developing the logic framework underpinning a whole-systems approach to childhood overweight and obesity prevention: Amsterdam Healthy Weight Approach. Obes Sci Pract. 2021;7:591–605.
25. Miyoshi M, Tsuboyama-Kasaoka N, Nishi N. School-based "Shokuiku" program in Japan: application to nutrition education in Asian countries. Asia Pac J Clin Nutr. 2012;21:159–62.
26. Tanaka N, Miyoshi M. School lunch program for health promotion among children in Japan. Asia Pac J Clin Nutr. 2012;21:155–8.
27. World Health Organization. Global action plan on physical activity 2018–2030: more active people for a healthier world. World Health Organization; 2018. https://iris.who.int/handle/10665/272722.
28. World Health Organization. Acceleration plan to stop obesity. World Health Organization; 2023. ISBN: 978-92-4-007563-4. https://www.who.int/publications/i/item/9789240075634.

Chapter 4
Peripheral Artery Disease in Regions with Limited Socioeconomic Resources

Kunihiro Matsushita, Maya Jean Salameh, and Matthew Allison

4.1 Background

Lower extremity peripheral artery disease (PAD) is an occlusive arterial disease that is associated with significant cardiovascular and limb complications. Despite representing a significant public health problem, PAD continues to be underdiagnosed and undertreated [1], receiving substantially less public attention compared to coronary heart disease (CHD) and stroke [2]. A large percentage of individuals with PAD have concomitant atherosclerotic disease in other vascular beds [3] and, when compared to the general population, are at significantly higher risk for myocardial infarction, stroke, and cardiovascular disease mortality [4, 5]. Furthermore, patients with PAD are at higher risk of major adverse cardiovascular events compared to patients with CHD or stroke [6], while those with concomitant PAD and CHD/stroke have the worst prognosis with a reported 12-year survival of only 26% [7]. Patients with PAD are also at risk for claudication and/or loss of mobility, with over 50% of patients with PAD exhibiting some degree of walking impairment [8], as well as more severe limb outcomes including ischemic rest pain, ischemic

K. Matsushita (✉)
Department of Epidemiology, Johns Hopkins Bloomberg School of Public Health, Johns Hopkins School of Medicine, Baltimore, MD, USA

Division of Cardiology, Johns Hopkins School of Medicine, Baltimore, MD, USA
e-mail: kmatsus5@jhmi.edu

M. J. Salameh
Division of Cardiology, Johns Hopkins School of Medicine, Baltimore, MD, USA
e-mail: msalame1@jhmi.edu

M. Allison
Division of Preventive Medicine, Department of Family Medicine, University of California San Diego, San Diego, CA, USA

T. Romero et al. (eds.), *Global Challenges in Cardiovascular Prevention in Populations with Low Socioeconomic Status*,
https://doi.org/10.1007/978-3-031-79051-5_4

ulceration, and limb loss. These complications can be associated with poor quality of life [9, 10]. As such, PAD imposes a significant economic burden on health systems [11], with the additional morbidity associated with PAD also contributing to an increase in indirect costs due to loss of productivity.

While the burden of PAD in high-income countries (HICs) has been well documented [12], its impact on low- and middle-income countries (LMICs) has been largely overlooked [13]. In recent years, LMICs have been undergoing an epidemiological transition whereby the burden of cardiovascular disease (CVD) has been growing exponentially with the World Health Report of 1999 estimating that 85% of the CVD burden worldwide arose from LMICs [14]. Indeed, a pattern of premature CVD mortality has been observed in LMICs, with about half the deaths attributable to CVD occurring in people aged below 70 years, compared to about 25% in HICs [15].

The increasing burden of CVD in LMICs can be attributed to the increased prevalence of atherosclerotic diseases due to the aging of the population, as well as industrialization, urbanization, and changing lifestyles with an increase in risk factors such as obesity, smoking, diabetes, hyperlipidemia, and hypertension. Urbanization represents one of the most significant environmental changes associated with the observed increase in CVD burden worldwide [16]. Rates of urbanization continue to increase globally, with approximately 60% of the global population projected to be living in urban areas by 2025 [16]. Urbanization is associated with an increase in consumption of energy-rich foods accompanied by a decrease in physical activity and a loss of traditional social support mechanisms [15].

4.2 Prevalence

The clinical spectrum of PAD is wide. Specifically, individuals with PAD may be asymptomatic or present with a variety of symptoms including intermittent claudication, atypical leg pain, critical limb ischemia (CLI), or acute limb ischemia. The reported prevalence of PAD in any given population depends on the characteristics and risk factors of the assessed population and the methods used for diagnosis [17]. Around 20–40 million people with PAD worldwide are likely to suffer from intermittent claudication while an even larger number of PAD patients likely experience atypical leg symptoms resulting in significant limitations in mobility and reduced quality of life. Even asymptomatic patients with PAD experience impaired lower function and loss of mobility, as well as functional decline, compared to individuals without PAD [18–20]. These effects are of even more concern in LMICs where significant walking distances may be required to obtain daily life necessities.

PAD (defined as ankle-brachial index [ABI] ≤0.9) is estimated to affect more than 230 million people worldwide or 5.6% of the global population [21] with about 73% of people with PAD living in LMICs [21]. The overall prevalence of PAD in 2015 represented a relative increase of approximately 17% from 2010. There was a notable disparity in the increasing prevalence between HICs and LMICs over the

5-year period. Specifically, the increase in prevalence was higher in LMICs (22.6%) versus HICs (4.5%), with the Western Pacific Region having the largest share of global PAD cases at approximately 75 million. The largest share of cases in LMICs was observed in people aged 45–49 years, versus those aged 65–69 years in HICs. More specifically, the age group with the largest number of cases in the Southeast Asia and the Western Pacific Region was 45–54 years, and in the African and Eastern Mediterranean region the largest number of cases occurred in people aged 25–34 years. Approximately 52.2% of people living with PAD worldwide were women. The age- and sex-specific prevalence of PAD worldwide is summarized in Fig. 4.1.

Literature from LMICs Although the global and regional estimates of PAD prevalence are available, there are a limited number of studies quantifying the prevalence of PAD in LMICs, especially South Asia, Middle East, Africa, and Latin America.

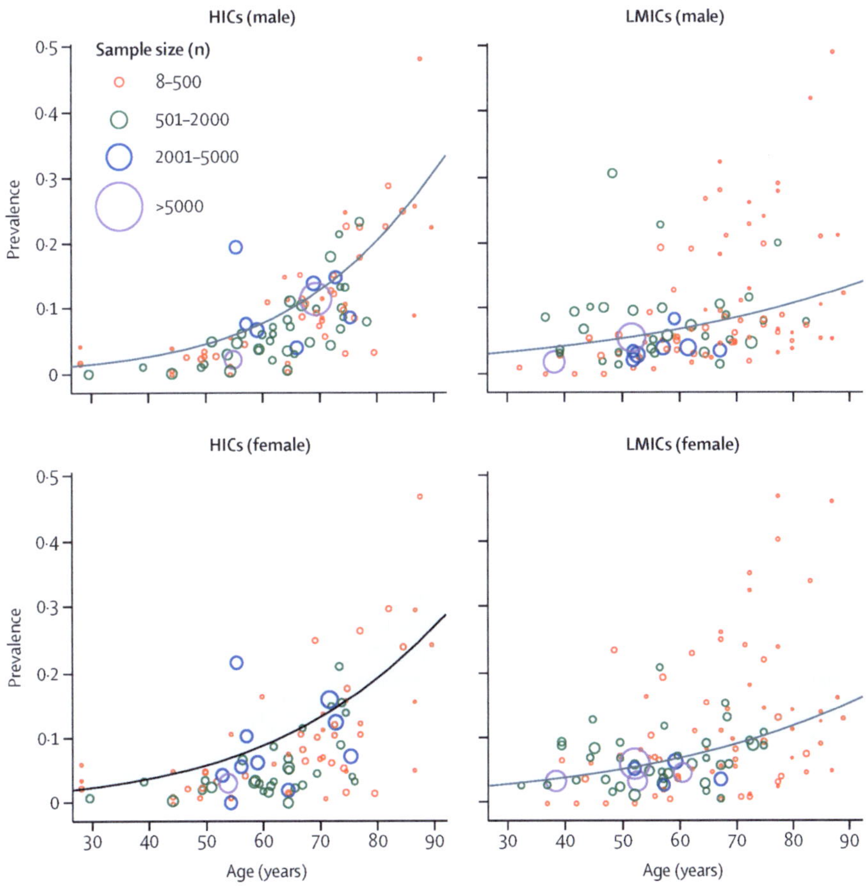

Fig. 4.1 Prevalence of peripheral artery disease by age in men and women in high-income and low-income or middle-income countries. (Song et al. [21])

Also, differences in reported prevalence may be variable based on the population selected for testing and variations in measurement technique [13]. For example, in China, the prevalence of PAD in men aged 60–70 years varied between 2.5% and 6.9% and in women aged 60–70 years the prevalence varied between 1.7% and 10.4% in several different population surveys [22–25]. The Epidemiology of Dementia in Central Africa (EPIDEMCA) study, a cross-sectional population-based study in rural and urban areas of two countries of Central Africa, including the Central African Republic and the Republic of Congo, reported an overall prevalence of PAD of 14.8% based on ABI ≤0.9 [26]. The prevalence of PAD was significantly higher in the Republic of Congo compared to the Central African Republic (17.4% vs. 12.2%, $p = 0.007$). There was a significant difference in the urban vs. rural prevalence of PAD in the Republic of Congo (urban 20.7% vs. rural 14.4%, $p = 0.011$) but not in the Central African Republic (11.5% vs. 12.9%).

4.3 Factors Associated with the Risk of PAD

4.3.1 Age

Song et al. conducted a review of 118 studies from 61 HICs and 57 LMICs and reported that the prevalence of PAD increased consistently with increasing age. Specifically, the prevalence of PAD was 4.3% in LMICs and 3.5% in HICs at 40–44 years, compared to a prevalence of 12.0% in LMICs and 21.2% in HICs at 80–84 years [21]. The study noted a modestly higher prevalence of PAD in LMICs vs. HICs at younger ages, whereas the prevalence was higher at older ages in HICs vs. LMICs [21]. Fowkes et al. reported that the increase in the prevalence of PAD was particularly striking in the older age groups. The increase was also more pronounced in all age categories in LMICs vs. HICs [17].

Literature from LMICs As urbanization in regions like sub-Saharan Africa increases, life expectancy is expected to also increase [27]. This will likely lead to an increase in the PAD burden at a rate proportional to increases in life expectancy, particularly in urban populations, due to greater exposure to risk factors such as smoking and obesity [28]. Indeed, the fastest-growing population around the world is the one above the age of 80 years, projected to increase 5.5-fold from 2000 to 2050 globally and 8.3-fold in less developed countries [29]. By 2050, countries such as Colombia, Malaysia, Kenya, Thailand, and Ghana are expected to see an increase of 200–300% in their elderly population [30].

4.3.2 Gender

Globally, Fowkes et al. reported higher prevalence of PAD in men in HICs whereas a higher prevalence in women was observed in LMICs, with more pronounced relative differences at younger ages [17]. A subsequent analysis by Song et al. reported similar prevalence between women and men in LMICs (e.g., ~6.4% in both sexes at age 55–59 years), whereas in HICs, the prevalence was slightly higher in women than in men, up to age 75 years (e.g., 7.8% vs. 6.6%, at 55–59 years). Overall, 52.2% of people living with PAD worldwide were women [21].

4.3.3 Race/Ethnicity

In epidemiological studies, race-ethnicity has also been associated with the presence of PAD. The National Health and Nutrition Examination Survey (NHANES) reported that the prevalence of PAD in non-Hispanic Blacks was as high as 7.8%, compared to 4.4% in Whites [31]. Data from seven community-based studies in the United States revealed the prevalence of PAD in Blacks was twice that of non-Hispanic Whites at any given age [9, 12]. The highest prevalence of PAD was reported in Black men ≥50 years of age. Specifically, the prevalence of PAD in Black men was approximately 5% at ages 50–59%; 13% at ages 60–69 years; and 59% ages >80 years (compared to approximately 2%, 5%, and 23% in non-Hispanic Whites at similar ages) [9, 12]. The Atherosclerosis Risk in Communities (ARIC) study also reported a higher prevalence of PAD in Black males compared to White males (3.3% vs. 2.3%) as well as in Black females compared to White females (4.0% vs. 3.3%) [10, 32]. A study using data from six US community-based cohorts estimated approximately 30% of Black men and women would develop PAD during their lifetime, compared to approximately 20% of Whites and Hispanics [31]. Studies have also shown that Black patients present at more advanced stages of PAD than White patients, with the former having a 37% higher risk of amputation [33]. Other studies have also revealed that Black patients experience higher risk of major adverse limb events (hazard ratio [HR] 1.15 [95% CI 1.06–1.25], $p < 0.001$) and amputation (HR 1.33 [1.18–1.51], $p < 0.001$), irrespective of the region in the United States [34].

Community-based studies have shown a similar prevalence of PAD in Hispanics compared to non-Hispanic Whites [35, 36] though differences in PAD prevalence have been noted among Hispanic subgroups. One study of an ethnically diverse Hispanic population in the United States revealed that Cuban Americans had the highest risk of PAD (odds ratio [OR] 2.9 [95% CI, 1.9–4.4]) compared with Mexican Americans, after adjusting for multiple cardiovascular risk factors [37]. Another study reported that Hispanics present with more advanced stages of disease, with higher rates of limb-threatening ischemia, failed lower extremity revascularization, and amputations compared to non-Hispanic Whites [38]. The racial-ethnic difference in the prevalence of PAD may be largely explained by social determinants of health. See Sect. 3.3.4 (below) for more details.

Literature from LMICs A study conducted at Mthatha General Hospital, a district hospital in a rural and low socioeconomic area of South Africa, enrolled 542 mostly Black patients age >50 with no prior diagnosis of PAD. Overall, 159 patients were identified as having PAD by an ABI ≤0.9, resulting in a prevalence of 29%. Similarly, a study by Krishan et al. conducted in Kerala, India revealed an age-adjusted prevalence of PAD of 26.7% and asymptomatic PAD was more prevalent among women (25.35% vs. 20.37%, $p = 0.0485$). The high prevalence of PAD in that study population was attributed to the high frequency of risk factors, most notably smoking [39].

4.3.4 Socioeconomic Status

Among HICs, studies have shown that the prevalence of PAD is higher in poorer socioeconomic groups. For example, the NHANES study demonstrated a strong relationship between indicators of lower socioeconomic status (SES) such as income or education level, and the presence of PAD, even after multivariate adjustment [40]. The Edinburgh Artery Study reported that a lower ABI was associated with lower SES, less education achievement, and a higher deprivation score [41]. A study based on nationwide ambulatory claims data covering approximately 87% of the German population revealed an increase in the prevalence of PAD of a 10-year period, with a higher prevalence in patients living in low-income areas (4.8%) compared to high-income areas (2.8%) by 2018 [41]. The ARIC Study examined the association between PAD and SES in the United States and reported that the risk of hospitalization due to PAD was more than twice as high in a cohort with low median household income (<$12,000) compared with a cohort with a household income >$25,000, after adjusting for age, sex, and race [42]. PAD-associated hospitalization risk was also twice as high in those with a lower education level (less than high school) compared to those with a higher level of education (more than high school) [42].

4.3.5 Smoking

Cigarette smoking is one of the strongest modifiable risk factors for PAD, increasing the risk of PAD by two- to sixfold [43]. Smokers are twice as likely to develop PAD compared to CHD [44]. The ARIC study reported that individuals who smoked >40 pack years had an HR of ~4 for PAD, compared to an HR of ~2 for CHD and stroke [45]. Further, the elevated risk of PAD persisted for up to 30 years after smoking cessation vs. less than 20 years for CHD and stroke [45]. Current smokers with PAD have lower survival rates, reduced bypass graft patency rates, and increased likelihood of progression to CLI and amputation [46]. Conversely, patients with PAD who quit smoking have improved prognosis and are less likely to develop CLI [47]. The global effect of smoking is likely to continue increasing. Recent projections indicate that the number of smokers will increase from 794 million in 2010 to 872 million by 2030 [48]. In contrast to an overall decline in HICs, tobacco consumption in LMICs continues to rise [29]. In fact, more than 80% of smokers worldwide reside in LMICs [49]. The Global Adult Tobacco Survey revealed that in 14 LMICs, 48.6% of men and 11.3% of women were tobacco users [50].

Literature from LMICs A national population-based survey conducted in China reported that cigarette smoking is highly prevalent among Chinese males (over 60%) and increasing [51]. A study by Krishan et al. revealed a high age-adjusted prevalence of PAD (26.7%) in Kerala, India. The high prevalence of PAD was attributed to the high frequency of risk factors, especially smoking [39]. Among rural South Africans aged 50 or older, the prevalence of PAD was 29% based on ABI <0.9 with smokers being 4.5 times more likely to have PAD compared to non-smokers [52].

4.3.6 Obesity/Diabetes

The presence of diabetes in turn increases the risk of developing both symptomatic and asymptomatic PAD by up to fourfold [53, 54]. Patients with diabetes and PAD usually display a more distal distribution of disease with more calcified, longer occlusions and fewer collaterals compared to non-diabetic patients with PAD [55]. Patients with diabetes and PAD are also at increased risk for complications, including major limb amputations and higher mortality. The prevalence of diabetes is increasing at an alarming rate worldwide, with a projected 330 million living with diabetes by 2030, over 75% of them in developing countries [56]. In addition, while older age groups are most affected by diabetes in HICs, the most frequently affected age group in LMICs is 35–64 years old, resulting in a heavier burden of Disability Adjusted Life Years (DALYs) and Years Lived with Disability (YLDs) in those countries [57]. Studies have shown that diabetes is a costly disease in many countries, accounting for up to 15% of healthcare expenditure [58].

Literature from LMICs Urbanization rates are growing significantly worldwide, with over 60% of the world population expected to live in urban areas by 2025 [59]. As populations become more urban, a nutrition transition is expected to occur, whereby dietary patterns will change to include a higher proportion of saturated fat, sugar, and refined foods, accompanied by a sedentary lifestyle [60]. In addition, advances in mechanization and expansion in modes of transport can lead to a more sedentary lifestyle and reduced levels of exercise [13]. As an example, a population-based study in Curacao revealed that 37% of the population did not eat vegetables daily, 50% did not eat fruit daily, and 75% did not exercise regularly [61]. This expected transition in diet and lifestyle will likely lead to a higher prevalence of obesity and diabetes [29].

4.3.7 Hypertension

Several epidemiologic studies have demonstrated a strong association between hypertension and PAD. Population growth and aging is leading to an increase in the number of individuals with uncontrolled hypertension worldwide [62] and given its high prevalence in the elderly population, hypertension is considered a significant contributor to the burden of PAD in the global population. For example, the Heart Professionals Follow-up Study revealed that the population-attributable risk of PAD due to hypertension exceeds 40% [63].

Literature from LMICs The World Health Organization (WHO) Study on Global Aging and Adult Health revealed strikingly high rates of hypertension in LMICs. The prevalence of hypertension among individuals 50 years of age or older was 53%, ranging from 32% in India to 78% in South Africa, with consistently higher levels for women [64]. By 2025, the global prevalence of hypertension is estimated to increase by 60% to a total of 1.56 billion cases, with a rise of more than 80% predicted for developing countries from 639 million to 1.15 billion [65]. Hypertension is also an emerging risk factor in LMICs, particularly in west Africa [66], where it may have a significant effect in the development of PAD. In this regard, a community-based survey of two districts in Central African Republic reported a prevalence of PAD of up to 32% in those aged >65 based on an ABI < 0.9. Notably, subjects with hypertension were approximately two to four times more likely to have PAD [67].

4.3.8 Dyslipidemia

Several studies have reported a significant association between total cholesterol and PAD. The NHANES study reported that the prevalence of PAD was 5.8% in US adults (age ≥40 years) with hyperlipidemia vs. 3.2% in those without [8]. One study demonstrated that the likelihood of developing PAD increased by 10% for every 10 mg/dL increase in total cholesterol [68]. In addition, a recent study using data from the ARIC study showed that triglyceride-related and high-density lipoprotein-related lipids were particularly robustly associated with future risk of PAD [69]. In the Physicians' Health Study of incident PAD, the ratio of total to high-density lipoprotein cholesterol had the strongest association with PAD compared to other lipid measures [70].

Literature from LMICs A prospective observational study of over 9000 Chinese men and women between ages 35 and 64 showed a low mean serum cholesterol in the overall study population (mean 4.2 mmol/L at baseline); however, serum cholesterol was found to be directly related to mortality from CHD [71]. A systematic review and meta-analysis from ten different African countries revealed a prevalence of dyslipidemia of 52.8% [72]. Individuals with a body mass index >25.0 kg/m^2 and waist circumference >94 cm were approximately 2.4 times more likely to develop dyslipidemia compared to those with lower values [72].

4.3.9 Environmental Factors

Long-term air pollution exposure has been associated with an increased risk of atherosclerotic diseases, including PAD [73]. In Germany, pollution from road traffic was associated with increased risk of low ABI in exposed individuals. Specifically, individuals living within 50 m of a major road had an OR of 1.8 for PAD compared with those living more than 200 m away [74].

Toxic metals such as lead and cadmium, by-products of industry that can be found in ambient air near industrial or combustion sources, have also been associated with an increased risk of PAD [75]. In one study analyzing data from 2125 participants ≥40 years of age in the 1999 to 2000 NHANES, individuals with PAD had 13.8% (95% CI, 5.9–12.9) higher mean levels of lead and 16.1% (95% CI, 4.7–28.7) higher mean levels of cadmium than those without PAD, after adjustment for demographic and cardiovascular risk factors [76]. The Strong Heart Study revealed that cadmium exposure, measured by urine cadmium concentrations, was prospectively associated with increased risk of new-onset PAD in Native American individuals followed for up to 10 years, independent of smoking [75].

Literature from LMICs In a study conducted using data on 18,000 individuals in China, those living in urban areas with high levels of air pollution had a two- to threefold increased risk of PAD compared with individuals living in rural areas, independent of traditional cardiovascular risk factors [25]. In LMICs, the risk of PAD may be increased by the consequences of industrialization. Potential mechanisms are shown in Fig. 4.2.

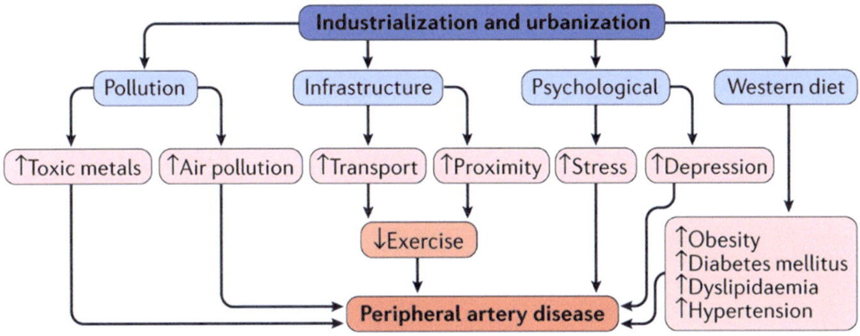

Fig. 4.2 Possible effects of industrialization and urbanization in LMICs on risk of peripheral artery disease. (Fowkes et al. [13])

4.3.10 Summary of Risk Factors

Globally, cigarette smoking and diabetes are the strongest modifiable risk factors for PAD [77]. Risk factors for PAD reported in HICs are similar to those observed in LMICs, except for an increased risk in women compared with men in LMICs and conversely, an increased risk in men in HICs (Fig. 4.3).

4.4 Diagnostic Tests of PAD

Ankle-Brachial Index The ABI (the ratio of ankle systolic blood pressure to brachial systolic blood pressure) is typically used as the first-line diagnostic test for PAD [78]. An ABI ≤0.9 is diagnostic of PAD. The ABI can be measured using an oscillometric device, but guidelines recommend using a Doppler probe to measure brachial and ankle blood pressure [78]. Using the Doppler technique, a low ABI has consistently shown high specificity (e.g., >85–90%), whereas the sensitivity has been variable probably reflecting the different populations studied. For instance, studies with a combination of patients with PAD and healthy subjects showed high sensitivity (e.g., >90%), while other studies that included people without diagnosis of PAD reported a low sensitivity ~20% [79, 80]. This means that a number of individuals with PAD may not be captured by a single test of low ABI ≤0.9. Another caveat of the ABI is that ABI can be falsely high (e.g., >1.4) when there is medial calcification in ankle arteries.

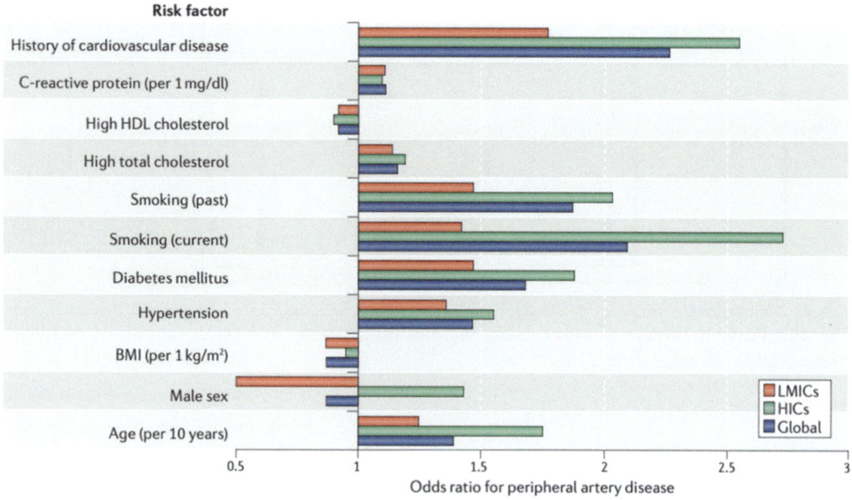

Fig. 4.3 Risk factors for peripheral artery disease in high-income and low- to middle-income countries. (Criqui and Aboyans [77])

Other Tests Supplementing ABI There are a few tests to supplement ABI: toe-brachial index (TBI, the ratio of great toe systolic blood pressure to brachial systolic blood pressure), Doppler waveforms, pulse volume recording (PVR), and post-exercise ABI (Table 4.1). Since digital arteries are less likely to be calcified, the TBI can be particularly useful among patients suspected of having stiff ankle arteries potentially due to medial calcification (e.g., diabetes). Clinical guidelines recommend TBI <0.7 as a threshold to diagnose PAD, but a few studies suggest that a TBI <0.6 may be preferable [81, 82]. Doppler waveforms can be recorded using a Doppler probe and provide information on blood flow in each ankle artery (i.e., dorsalis pedis and popliteal tibial). Normal waveforms are defined as triphasic or biphasic with good acceleration and deceleration, while abnormal waveforms include biphasic (without the aforementioned qualifiers) and monophasic. PVR is measured by a sphygmomanometer with a defined volume of air (usually ~60 mmHg) and provides comprehensive information on blood flow in ankle arteries (not each ankle artery). Normal PVRs have a systolic upstroke with sharp systolic peak and downstroke with dicrotic notch. Loss of the dicrotic notch, flat peak, and low amplitude constitute abnormal PVRs. Finally, the ABI can be measured after a defined period of exercise (typically using treadmill, but heel raises are a validated alternative approach). A post-exercise ABI ≤0.9, drop of ABI >20%, or drop of ankle blood pressure >30 mmHg are considered diagnostic of PAD [78].

Table 4.1 Representative non-invasive diagnostic tests for PAD

Measure	Methodology	Clinical implication
Ankle-brachial index (ABI) at rest	Ratio of ankle and brachial systolic blood pressures at rest	Peripheral artery disease, defined by ABI ≤0.9 (ABI 0.9–1.0 is "borderline low"). ABI >1.4 indicates medial calcification
Post-exercise ABI	Ratio of ankle and brachial systolic blood pressures after exercise (usually treadmill but can be heel raise)	Following findings after exercise: ABI ≤0.9 or drop of ABI >20% or drop of ankle blood pressure >30 mmHg
Toe-brachial index (TBI)	Ratio of toe and brachial systolic blood pressures	PAD defined by TBI <0.7. TBI useful particularly when ABI >1.4
Doppler waveforms	Waveforms of the ankle arteries are collected using a Doppler probe	Normal waveforms are defined as triphasic or biphasic with good acceleration and deceleration, while abnormal waveforms include biphasic (without the aforementioned qualifiers) and monophasic
Pulse volume recordings (PVR)	PVR measured by cuffs inflated with a certain volume of air (usually ~60 mmHg)	Normal PVRs have a systolic upstroke with sharp systolic peak and downstroke with dicrotic notch, and loss of dicrotic notch, flat peak, and low amplitude constitute abnormal PVRs
Lower extremity Duplex	The presence of significant stenosis is recorded for distal aorta, femoral, and popliteal arteries	Presence of atherosclerotic plaque and peak systolic velocities in the conduit arteries of the lower extremities. The latter can be used to classify obstructive disease

Duplex Ultrasound Although angiography using computed tomography or magnetic resonance imaging can be used to identify significant stenosis in the leg arteries, Duplex ultrasound has several important advantages over those approaches such as being non-invasive, lack of a contrast agent, and usually lower price; all of which are relevant to resource-limited settings. A few limitations include the need of trained technicians and potential difficulty visualizing the abdominal aorta, iliac arteries, and calcified arteries. A US guideline recommends imaging tests only for strategize revascularization in patients with PAD and ischemic symptoms [83].

Literature in LMICs A Nigerian study explored an oscillometric device to measure ABI and reported the sensitivity of 61% and specificity of 90%, compared with ABI measured using Doppler method. A study from Pakistan compared the palpatory method vs. Doppler method for detecting PAD and reported Pearson's correlation coefficient of 0.73 between ABI measured by the two methods [84]. Although Doppler method should be the preferable option, these alternative methods can be considered in resource-limited settings.

4.5 Outcomes

Other Cardiovascular Outcomes Since PAD is an atherosclerotic disease, it is intuitive that patients with PAD demonstrate elevated risk of other atherosclerotic diseases (e.g., myocardial infarction and stroke). For example, a study using data from the ARIC study showed a significant association of ABI ≤0.9 vs. 1.1–1.2 with the composite outcome of myocardial infarction and stroke, independent of major CVD risk factors such as smoking, diabetes, blood pressure, and lipids (adjusted hazard ratio 2.40 [95% CI 1.55–3.71]) [85]. Interestingly, a few studies consistently reported a robust association of PAD with an increased risk of heart failure (HF) [85, 86]. In addition, a high prevalence of abdominal aortic aneurysm (AAA) is recognized in patients with PAD [87], and thus clinical guidelines recommend screening for AAA in this clinical population [83].

Leg Outcomes Not surprisingly, individuals with PAD are at high risk of leg outcomes such as acute limb ischemia (ALI) and chronic limb-threatening ischemia. Some people require leg amputation to improve limb and life survival. For example, a study using data from a clinical trial of patients with symptomatic PAD showed that 1.3% of patients developed ALI within 1 year and 1.2% required leg amputation [88]. In the general population, ABI was independently associated with elevated risk of leg amputation over a follow-up of ~30 years (adjusted HR of leg amputation 2.72 [95% CI 1.25–5.91] in ABI ≤0.9 vs. 1.1–1.2) (Fig. 4.4) [89].

Literature in LMICs Studies have confirmed the prognostic impact of PAD for all-cause mortality in Congo [90] and China [91] as well as major cardiovascular events in an international registry with data from 17 LMICs [92]. Although cross-

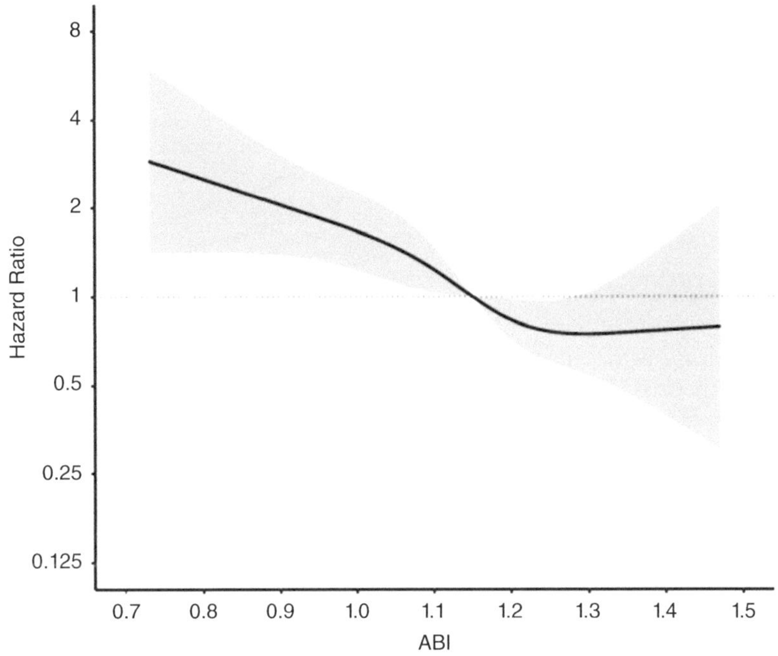

Fig. 4.4 Adjusted* hazard ratio of leg amputation according to ABI in the ARIC study. *Adjusted for age, sex, race, study site, education level, adiposity, total cholesterol, high-density lipoprotein cholesterol, cholesterol-lowering drugs, systolic blood pressure, antihypertensive drugs, smoking status, drinking status, diabetes, kidney function, prevalent coronary heart disease, prevalent heart failure, and prevalent stroke. (Paskiewicz et al. [89])

sectional, a study with data from Central African Republic and Republic of Congo showed the association between PAD and dementia [93].

Depression Major depression is a common comorbidity among patients with PAD, particularly in women. In one cohort study of 1635 participants with PAD, women were found to have an almost twofold greater prevalence of comorbid depression than men (46% vs. 26%) [94]. The higher rates of comorbid depression in female patients with PAD are of particular concern because depressive symptoms are associated with more significant physical disability and functional decline over time [95]. The Heart and Soul study [96] revealed that patients with depression had a twofold increased risk of developing PAD after adjustment for sex and age. Patients with both PAD and depression demonstrate worse functional outcomes and reduced quality of life [97, 98]. In addition, one Veterans Affairs study found that PAD patients with depression have a higher long-term risk of limb loss, especially if their depression is untreated [HR 1.42; 95% CI, 1.27–1.58] [99]. In LMICs, industrialization and urbanization may lead to changes in environment and lifestyle that can result in adverse psychological effects, such as stress and depression. These effects may in turn contribute to an increased risk of developing PAD [9]. Studies are needed to test these hypotheses.

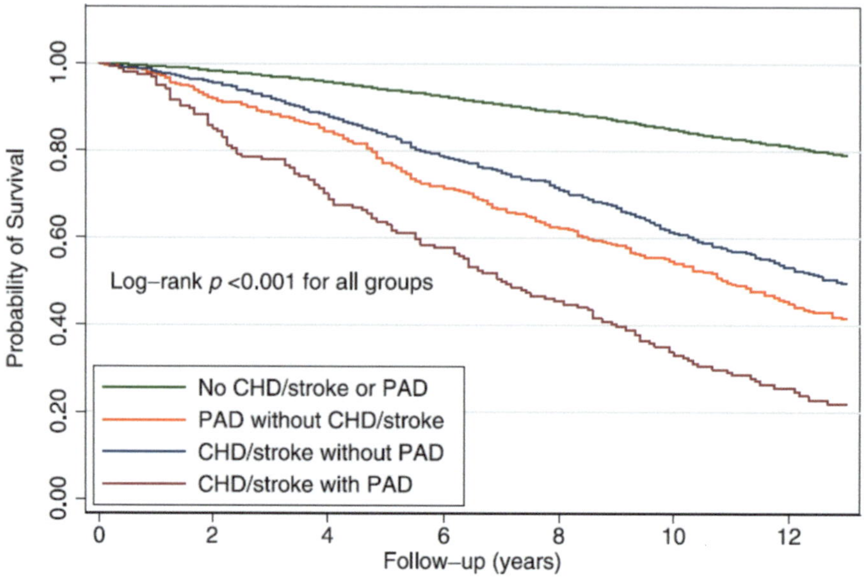

Fig. 4.5 Survival estimates by the status of PAD, coronary heart disease, and stroke in the 1999–2004 National Health and Nutrition Examination Survey. (Matsushita et al. [7])

Other Outcomes A US study showed that the prognostic impact of PAD is similar or may be even greater than that of CHD or stroke [7]. More specifically, individuals with PAD without CHD/stroke had worse overall survival than those with CHD/stroke without PAD (47.7% vs. 53.2% over 12 years, respectively) (Fig. 4.5). The combination of PAD plus CHD/stroke had the worst prognosis (25.5% over 12 years). The patterns were similar even after accounting for potential confounders like age, smoking status, and diabetes. This impact of PAD on all-cause mortality is consistent with several studies showing that individuals with PAD at elevated risk of adverse outcomes beyond CVD, such as cancer [100] and infectious diseases [101].

4.6 Challenges of PAD Management in Resource-Limited Settings

4.6.1 Awareness of PAD

Increased awareness of PAD in clinical settings should facilitate earlier detection of PAD, resulting in more aggressive risk factor control and initiation of guideline-appropriate therapies. However, multiple population-based studies have demonstrated low levels of knowledge of PAD in the general population, as well as in affected populations worldwide [2, 102, 103]. The First National PAD Public Awareness Survey reported major gaps in public knowledge of PAD, specifically regarding PAD terminology, associated risk factors, and leg symptoms including risk of amputation [2]. The general public was unaware that PAD is associated with high short-term risk of myocardial infarction, stroke, and death. In addition, only 14% of respondents associated PAD with a risk of amputation, and only 6% associated PAD with a risk of limb disability or walking impairment [2]. Knowledge gaps were the greatest in the populations at highest risk for PAD-associated morbidity and mortality, specifically in elderly and non-White participants. In addition, awareness of certain preventative treatment options such as smoking cessation was strikingly low [102]. Lower levels of education and lower SES were associated with more significant knowledge gaps around PAD, specifically regarding risk factors, symptoms, and outcomes [103].

4.6.2 Access to Medical Treatment

Essential vascular care functions are necessary to adequately address the growing burden of PAD in LMICs, where resources should be increasingly directed at preventing, detecting, and treating PAD. These include providing counseling for healthy diet and exercise routines, screening for and providing tobacco cessation counseling for smokers, screening patients at high risk for PAD, and treatment of major risk factors such as diabetes, hypertension, and dyslipidemia [104]. Multidrug therapy, including antiplatelet therapy, statin, and angiotensin-converting enzyme (ACE) inhibitor/angiotensin-receptor blocker (ARB) is cost-effective and essential in improving cardiovascular outcomes in patients at high risk for PAD [105]. The WHO offers model lists of essential medications, including those for the management of cardiovascular risk factors such as hypertension, diabetes, and dyslipidemia [106]. Despite this, very low rates of use of aspirin, statin, and blood pressure lowering agents have been observed in LMICs [107]. For example, the Prospective Urban Rural Epidemiology (PURE) study reported that in patients with known CHD in low-income countries, only 8.8% were taking an antiplatelet agent and 3.3% were taking a statin. Moreover, 69.3% of patients in lower middle-income countries, and 80.2% of patients in low-income countries received no drug therapy at all [107].

Clinical cohorts in LMICs have also demonstrated a low uptake of guideline-directed medical therapy in patients with PAD. A study by Okello et al. sampled 229 patients with diabetes aged >50 and reported a PAD prevalence of 24% using the ABI [108]. Only 11% of the patients with PAD were taking an aspirin and only one patient was taking a statin. Another study at a teaching hospital in Uganda reported a PAD prevalence of 39% in a cohort of patients with diabetes aged >35 years enrolled in the outpatient diabetes clinic. Approximately 41% of participants with PAD were asymptomatic. Only 22% were treated with antiplatelet agent and only 12% were taking a statin [109].

A subsequent analysis of the PURE study data examining availability and affordability of cardiovascular medicines revealed that combination therapy with a four-drug regimen (aspirin, beta-blocker, ACE-inhibitor, statin) for the secondary prevention of cardiovascular disease was not affordable for 33% of households in middle-income countries and 60% of households in low-income countries [110]. A meta-analysis of surveys from 36 countries analyzing access to five cardiovascular medicines of different classes reported that those were available in only 26% of public and 57% of private facilities [111]. Treatment for CVD in general was not affordable in most countries, particularly in low-income countries [111].

The international Reduction of Atherothrombosis for Continued Health Registry enrolled 68,236 patients over the age of 45 from 44 countries including 8322 patients with PAD [112]. PAD patients were less frequently in full-time employment (12.1% vs. 17.3%) and had a lower level of formal education (12.9% vs. 18.9%) compared to patients without PAD. PAD patients also had poorer risk factor control compared to patients with CHD or CVD but without PAD. A significant geographic variation was noted in the patterns of risk factor control, with 10.8% of patients with PAD in North America achieving good risk factor control, compared with only 5.6% in Japan, 4.9% in Latin America, 4.4% in Northern Europe, 4.2% in Australia, 3.3% in Eastern Europe, 3.1% in Asia, and 1.8% in the Middle East. PAD only patients and PAD patients with polyvascular disease with good risk factor control had fewer major CVD event rates after 1 year of follow-up [112].

4.6.3 Access to Vascular Surgical Care

An analysis of the World Bank and WHO data shows a marked scarcity of vascular surgeons in LMICs, including in the regions of Southeast Asia, Eastern Mediterranean, and Western Pacific, each of which have fewer than 3 vascular surgeons per ten million people [113]. There are approximately 101 vascular surgeons per ten million people in the United States and 72.7 per ten million in the United Kingdom, while in South Africa there are only 10.8 per ten million [114] and in Ethiopia there are 0.25 per ten million, 400 times fewer vascular surgeons per ten million people than in the United States [115]. In South Africa, it has been noted that a high percentage of patients present with CLI, in part due to a shortage of vascular surgical expertise in the country [114]. In Ghana, vascular disease resulted in a fourfold increase in DALYs per 100,000 people from 1990 to 2010. In addition, the death rate from vascular disease in this country doubled over the same time period [116]. Despite this, a nationwide assessment of vascular care capacity found that vascular surgical resources were severely lacking [116]. Specifically, skills to perform vascular procedures at the regional level were rare, vascular graft material were unavailable at all levels of care, and prosthetics for amputees were rarely available at the tertiary level of care. In addition, diagnostic/therapeutic angiography and computed tomography scans with lower extremity runoff protocols were unavailable at all hospitals. The main reasons for non-availability of vascular care included lack of equipment and supplies, technology breakage, lack of diagnostic capability, and lack of experienced surgeons to perform major vascular surgery procedures

[116]. Indeed, the absence of a vascular surgeon workforce in LMICs significantly limits access to vascular services. Notably, vascular surgery training programs in LMICs are limited, in part due to lack of funding, lack of access to proper equipment for training, and lack of infrastructure and supplies necessary for the education of vascular surgeons [117].

Other studies report that a major barrier in accessing vascular surgery services in LMICs is the lack of a suitable infrastructure, such as lack of operating rooms and inadequate surgical supplies and equipment [118]. Even in centers with access to operating rooms, a lack of access to angiography, imaging, and endovascular devices [119] are additional barriers to providing adequate vascular care. In addition, significant financial considerations exist in LMICs. For example, even if vascular surgery services are available, patients may be unable use them due to lack of affordability [118]. Additional limitations to seeking out surgical care include loss of income, lack of transportation, and needing to travel long distances to access surgical centers [120].

4.7 Prevention of PAD

Increased awareness of PAD and its risk factors at a population level is essential in the prevention of PAD and its complications, particularly in low-resource settings. This includes education of the general public on the effects of tobacco on arterial health, with programs aimed at screening for and providing tobacco cessation counseling. In addition, educational programs highlighting the effects of a sedentary lifestyle as well as implementation of dietary counseling and healthy exercise routines could help in the prevention of obesity, which would in turn reduce the risk of developing major PAD risk factors such as diabetes, hypertension, and dyslipidemia. Community-based exercise programs would also allow for additional screening for PAD risk factors, such as blood pressure measurement, glucose monitoring, and screening lipid level for all participants. Awareness among healthcare providers is also crucial. That will create a foundation for early and optimal treatment of hypertension, diabetes, and dyslipidemia, which would in turn help prevent PAD and its subsequent cardiovascular and limb outcomes.

4.8 Summary

PAD is a distinct atherosclerotic syndrome which is associated with a significantly increased risk of cardiovascular morbidity and mortality, as well as considerable disability and poor quality of life due to functional impairment and major adverse limb events. While PAD shares common risk factors with both coronary and cerebrovascular diseases [3], data has shown that individuals with PAD are at a greater risk for major adverse cardiovascular events compared to patients with CHD or stroke [6].

PAD has emerged as a global problem that is increasing in prevalence worldwide in both HICs and LMICs, likely due to an epidemiologic transition towards an older age distribution, and a resulting increase in risk factors such as smoking, diabetes, obesity, and hypertension, which are particularly striking in LMICs [17, 21]. Indeed, the burden of PAD has been increasing faster in LMICs and is expected to continue rising in the near future as the population ages and environmental changes, such as urbanization and industrialization, continue to accelerate [15, 16].

Despite its increasing prevalence, PAD continues to be underdiagnosed and undertreated due to a general lack of awareness by the general public and healthcare providers on a global level [2, 102, 103]. To address this, the ABI is a simple test that is considered a good indicator of PAD [78] and should be utilized more widely for the purposes of early detection and treatment of PAD, allowing for the implementation of targeted interventions aimed at managing risk factors and improving limb outcomes. Treatment of PAD at later stages of the disease is associated with increasing healthcare costs, placing a significant economic burden on health systems [11], and resulting in a substantial physical and psychosocial burden due to poor functional status, loss of mobility, and reduced quality of life [8, 9]. This is of particular concern in LMICs where PAD represents a major public health challenge and resources are limited. In those settings, government agencies and health care organizations should prioritize early detection of PAD in order to implement appropriate preventive and therapeutic interventions aimed at control of vascular risk factors, with the ultimate goal of improving cardiovascular and limb outcomes in this increasingly high-risk population.

Glossary

ABI The ratio of ankle systolic blood pressure to brachial systolic blood pressure.

Doppler waveforms Waveforms of the ankle arteries are collected using a Doppler probe.

Duplex ultrasound Imaging modality to evaluate blood flow and vascular structure using high-frequency sound waves.

Post-exercise ABI Ratio of ankle and brachial systolic blood pressures after exercise (usually treadmill but can be heel raise).

PVR Waveforms measured by cuffs inflated with a certain volume of air (usually ~60 mmHg).

TBI The ratio of great toe systolic blood pressure to brachial systolic blood pressure.

References

1. Hirsch AT, Criqui MH, Treat-Jacobson D, Regensteiner JG, Creager MA, Olin JW, Krook SH, Hunninghake DB, Comerota AJ, Walsh ME, McDermott MM, Hiatt WR. Peripheral arterial disease detection, awareness, and treatment in primary care. JAMA. 2001;286:1317–24.

2. Hirsch AT, Murphy TP, Lovell MB, Twillman G, Treat-Jacobson D, Harwood EM, Mohler ER III, Creager MA, Hobson RW II, Robertson RM, Howard WJ, Schroeder P, Criqui MH. Gaps in public knowledge of peripheral arterial disease: the first national PAD public awareness survey. Circulation. 2007;116:2086–94.
3. Bhatt DL, Steg PG, Ohman EM, Hirsch AT, Ikeda Y, Mas JL, Goto S, Liau CS, Richard AJ, Rother J, Wilson PW, REACH Registry Investigators. International prevalence, recognition, and treatment of cardiovascular risk factors in outpatients with atherothrombosis. JAMA. 2006;295:180–9.
4. Criqui MH, Langer RD, Fronek A, Feigelson HS, Klauber MR, McCann TJ, Browner D. Mortality over a period of 10 years in patients with peripheral arterial disease. N Engl J Med. 1992;326:381–6.
5. Abbott RD, Rodriguez BL, Petrovitch H, Yano K, Schatz IJ, Popper JS, Masaki KH, Ross GW, Curb JD. Ankle-brachial blood pressure in elderly men and the risk of stroke: the Honolulu Heart Program. J Clin Epidemiol. 2001;54:973–8.
6. Bonaca MP, Nault P, Giugliano RP, Keech AC, Pineda AL, Kanevsky E, Kuder J, Murphy SA, Jukema JW, Lewis BS, Tokgozoglu L, Somaratne R, Sever PS, Pedersen TR, Sabatine MS. Low-density lipoprotein cholesterol lowering with evolocumab and outcomes in patients with peripheral artery Disease. Circulation. 2018;137:338–50.
7. Matsushita K, Gao Y, Sang Y, Ballew SH, Salameh M, Allison M, Selvin E, Coresh J. Comparative mortality according to peripheral artery disease and coronary heart disease/stroke in the United States. Atherosclerosis. 2022;354:57–62.
8. Selvin E, Hirsch AT. Contemporary risk factor control and walking dysfunction in individuals with peripheral arterial disease: NHANES 1999–2004. Atherosclerosis. 2008;201:425–33.
9. McDermott MM, Greenland P, Guralnik JM, Liu K, Criqui MH, Pearce WH, Chan C, Schneider J, Sharma L, Taylor LM, Arseven A, Quann M, Celic L. Depressive symptoms and lower extremity functioning in men and women with peripheral arterial disease. J Gen Intern Med. 2003;18:461–7.
10. Regensteiner JG, Hiatt WR, Coll JR, Criqui MH, Treat-Jacobson D, McDermott MM, Hirsch AT. The impact of peripheral arterial disease on health-related quality of life in the Peripheral Arterial Disease Awareness, Risk, and Treatment: New Resources for Survival (PARTNERS) Program. Vasc Med. 2008;13:15–24.
11. Hirsch AT, Hartman L, Town RJ, Virnig BA. National health care costs of peripheral arterial disease in the Medicare population. Vasc Med. 2008;13:209–15.
12. Criqui MH, Denenberg JO, Langer RD, Fronek A. The epidemiology of peripheral arterial disease: importance of identifying the population at risk. Vasc Med. 1997;2:221–6.
13. Fowkes FG, Aboyans V, Fowkes FJ, McDermott MM, Sampson UK, Criqui MH. Peripheral artery disease: epidemiology and global perspectives. Nat Rev Cardiol. 2017;14:156–70.
14. World Health Organization. The world health report: 1999: making a difference. World Health Organization; 1999.
15. Yusuf S, Reddy S, Ounpuu S, Anand S. Global burden of cardiovascular diseases: Part I: General considerations, the epidemiologic transition, risk factors, and impact of urbanization. Circulation. 2001;104:2746–53.
16. Chockalingam A, Balaguer-Vintro I, Achutti A, de Luna AB, Chalmers J, Farinaro E, Lauzon R, Martin I, Papp JG, Postiglione A, Reddy KS, Tse TF. The World Heart Federation's white book: impending global pandemic of cardiovascular diseases: challenges and opportunities for the prevention and control of cardiovascular diseases in developing countries and economies in transition. Can J Cardiol. 2000;16:227–9.
17. Fowkes FGR, Rudan D, Rudan I, Aboyans V, Denenberg JO, McDermott MM, Norman PE, Sampson UKA, Williams LJ, Mensah GA, Criqui MH. Comparison of global estimates of prevalence and risk factors for peripheral artery disease in 2000 and 2010: a systematic review and analysis. Lancet. 2013;382:1329–40.
18. Matsushita K, Ballew SH, Sang Y, Kalbaugh C, Loehr LR, Hirsch AT, Tanaka H, Heiss G, Windham BG, Selvin E, Coresh J. Ankle-brachial index and physical function in older individuals: the Atherosclerosis Risk in Communities (ARIC) study. Atherosclerosis. 2017;257:208–15.

19. McDermott MM, Applegate WB, Bonds DE, Buford TW, Church T, Espeland MA, Gill TM, Guralnik JM, Haskell W, Lovato LC, Pahor M, Pepine CJ, Reid KF, Newman A. Ankle brachial index values, leg symptoms, and functional performance among community-dwelling older men and women in the lifestyle interventions and independence for elders study. J Am Heart Assoc. 2013;2:e000257.
20. McDermott MM, Fried L, Simonsick E, Ling S, Guralnik JM. Asymptomatic peripheral arterial disease is independently associated with impaired lower extremity functioning: the women's health and aging study. Circulation. 2000;101:1007–12.
21. Song P, Rudan D, Zhu Y, Fowkes FJI, Rahimi K, Fowkes FGR, Rudan I. Global, regional, and national prevalence and risk factors for peripheral artery disease in 2015: an updated systematic review and analysis. Lancet Glob Health. 2019;7:e1020–30.
22. He Y, Jiang Y, Wang J, Fan L, Li X, Hu FB. Prevalence of peripheral arterial disease and its association with smoking in a population-based study in Beijing, China. J Vasc Surg. 2006;44:333–8.
23. Woo J, Lynn H, Wong SY, Hong A, Tang YN, Lau WY, Lau E, Orwoll E, Kwok TC. Correlates for a low ankle-brachial index in elderly Chinese. Atherosclerosis. 2006;186:360–6.
24. Chuang SY, Chen CH, Cheng CM, Chou P. Combined use of brachial-ankle pulse wave velocity and ankle-brachial index for fast assessment of arteriosclerosis and atherosclerosis in a community. Int J Cardiol. 2005;98:99–105.
25. An W, Xian L, Zhao L, Detrano R, Criqui MH, Wu Y. Distribution of the ankle-brachial index and peripheral arterial disease in middle-aged and elderly Chinese: a population-based study of 18,000 men and women. Circulation. 2010;122:e43.
26. Desormais I, Aboyans V, Guerchet M, Ndamba-Bandzouzi B, Mbelesso P, Dantoine T, Mohty D, Marin B, Preux PM, Lacroix P, EPIDEMCA investigators. Prevalence of peripheral artery disease in the elderly population in urban and rural areas of Central Africa: the EPIDEMCA study. Eur J Prev Cardiol. 2015;22:1462–72.
27. Aboderin I, Ferreira M. Linking ageing to development agendas in sub-Saharan Africa: challenges and approaches. J Popul Ageing. 2008;1:51–73.
28. BeLue R, Okoror TA, Iwelunmor J, Taylor KD, Degboe AN, Agyemang C, Ogedegbe G. An overview of cardiovascular risk factor burden in sub-Saharan African countries: a socio-cultural perspective. Glob Health. 2009;5:10.
29. Dominguez LJ, Galioto A, Ferlisi A, Pineo A, Putignano E, Belvedere M, Costanza G, Barbagallo M. Ageing, lifestyle modifications, and cardiovascular disease in developing countries. J Nutr Health Aging. 2006;10:143–9.
30. Kalache A, Keller I. The greying world: a challenge for the twenty-first century. Sci Prog. 2000;83(Pt 1):33–54.
31. Matsushita K, Sang Y, Ning H, Ballew SH, Chow EK, Grams ME, Selvin E, Allison M, Criqui M, Coresh J, Lloyd-Jones DM, Wilkins JT. Lifetime risk of lower-extremity peripheral artery disease defined by ankle-brachial index in the United States. J Am Heart Assoc. 2019;8:e012177.
32. Zheng ZJ, Sharrett AR, Chambless LE, Rosamond WD, Nieto FJ, Sheps DS, Dobs A, Evans GW, Heiss G. Associations of ankle-brachial index with clinical coronary heart disease, stroke and preclinical carotid and popliteal atherosclerosis: the Atherosclerosis Risk in Communities (ARIC) Study. Atherosclerosis. 1997;131:115–25.
33. Low Wang CC, Blomster JI, Heizer G, Berger JS, Baumgartner I, Fowkes FGR, Held P, Katona BG, Norgren L, Jones WS, Lopes RD, Olin JW, Rockhold FW, Mahaffey KW, Patel MR, Hiatt WR, Committee ETE and Investigators. Cardiovascular and limb outcomes in patients with diabetes and peripheral artery Disease: the EUCLID Trial. J Am Coll Cardiol. 2018;72:3274–84.
34. Arya S, Binney Z, Khakharia A, Brewster LP, Goodney P, Patzer R, Hockenberry J, Wilson PWF. Race and socioeconomic status independently affect risk of major amputation in peripheral artery disease. J Am Heart Assoc. 2018;7:e007425.
35. Selvin E, Erlinger TP. Prevalence of and risk factors for peripheral arterial disease in the United States: results from the National Health and Nutrition Examination Survey, 1999–2000. Circulation. 2004;110:738–43.

36. McDermott MM, Liu K, Criqui MH, Ruth K, Goff D, Saad MF, Wu C, Homma S, Sharrett AR. Ankle-brachial index and subclinical cardiac and carotid disease: the multi-ethnic study of atherosclerosis. Am J Epidemiol. 2005;162:33–41.
37. Allison MA, Gonzalez F II, Raij L, Kaplan R, Ostfeld RJ, Pattany MS, Heiss G, Criqui MH. Cuban Americans have the highest rates of peripheral arterial disease in diverse Hispanic/Latino communities. J Vasc Surg. 2015;62:665–72.
38. Morrissey NJ, Giacovelli J, Egorova N, Gelijns A, Moskowitz A, McKinsey J, Kent KC, Greco G. Disparities in the treatment and outcomes of vascular disease in Hispanic patients. J Vasc Surg. 2007;46:971–8.
39. Krishnan MN, Geevar Z, Mohanan PP, Venugopal K, Devika S. Prevalence of peripheral artery disease and risk factors in the elderly: a community based cross-sectional study from northern Kerala, India. Indian Heart J. 2018;70:808–15.
40. Pande RL, Creager MA. Socioeconomic inequality and peripheral artery disease prevalence in US adults. Circ Cardiovasc Qual Outcomes. 2014;7:532–9.
41. Messiha D, Petrikhovich O, Lortz J, Mahabadi AA, Hering R, Schulz M, Rassaf T, Rammos C. Gender differences in outpatient peripheral artery disease management in Germany: a population based study 2009–2018. Eur J Vasc Endovasc Surg. 2022;63:714–20.
42. Vart P, Coresh J, Kwak L, Ballew SH, Heiss G, Matsushita K. Socioeconomic status and incidence of hospitalization with lower-extremity peripheral artery disease: atherosclerosis risk in communities study. J Am Heart Assoc. 2017;6:e004995.
43. Hirsch AT, Haskal ZJ, Hertzer NR, Bakal CW, Creager MA, Halperin JL, Hiratzka LF, Murphy WR, Olin JW, Puschett JB, Rosenfield KA, Sacks D, Stanley JC, Taylor LM Jr, White CJ, White J, White RA, Antman EM, Smith SC Jr, Adams CD, Anderson JL, Faxon DP, Fuster V, Gibbons RJ, Hunt SA, Jacobs AK, Nishimura R, Ornato JP, Page RL, Riegel B, American Association for Vascular Surgery, Society for Vascular Surgery, Society for Cardiovascular Angiography and Interventions; Society for Vascular Medicine and Biology; Society of Interventional Radiology; ACC/AHA Task Force on Practice Guidelines Writing Committee to Develop Guidelines for the Management of Patients With Peripheral Arterial Disease; American Association of Cardiovascular and Pulmonary Rehabilitation; National Heart, Lung, and Blood Institute; Society for Vascular Nursing; TransAtlantic Inter-Society Consensus; Vascular Disease Foundation. ACC/AHA 2005 Practice Guidelines for the management of patients with peripheral arterial disease (lower extremity, renal, mesenteric, and abdominal aortic): a collaborative report from the American Association for Vascular Surgery/ Society for Vascular Surgery, Society for Cardiovascular Angiography and Interventions, Society for Vascular Medicine and Biology, Society of Interventional Radiology, and the ACC/AHA Task Force on Practice Guidelines (Writing Committee to Develop Guidelines for the Management of Patients With Peripheral Arterial Disease): endorsed by the American Association of Cardiovascular and Pulmonary Rehabilitation; National Heart, Lung, and Blood Institute; Society for Vascular Nursing; TransAtlantic Inter-Society Consensus; and Vascular Disease Foundation. Circulation. 2006;113:e463–654.
44. Price JF, Mowbray PI, Lee AJ, Rumley A, Lowe GD, Fowkes FG. Relationship between smoking and cardiovascular risk factors in the development of peripheral arterial disease and coronary artery disease: Edinburgh Artery Study. Eur Heart J. 1999;20:344–53.
45. Ding N, Sang Y, Chen J, Ballew SH, Kalbaugh CA, Salameh MJ, Blaha MJ, Allison M, Heiss G, Selvin E, Coresh J, Matsushita K. Cigarette smoking, smoking cessation, and long-term risk of 3 major atherosclerotic diseases. J Am Coll Cardiol. 2019;74:498–507.
46. Olin JW, Sealove BA. Peripheral artery disease: current insight into the disease and its diagnosis and management. Mayo Clin Proc. 2010;85:678–92.
47. Jonason T, Bergstrom R. Cessation of smoking in patients with intermittent claudication. Effects on the risk of peripheral vascular complications, myocardial infarction and mortality. Acta Med Scand. 1987;221:253–60.
48. Mendez D, Alshanqeety O, Warner KE. The potential impact of smoking control policies on future global smoking trends. Tob Control. 2013;22:46–51.
49. Jha P, Ranson MK, Nguyen SN, Yach D. Estimates of global and regional smoking prevalence in 1995, by age and sex. Am J Public Health. 2002;92:1002–6.

50. Giovino GA, Mirza SA, Samet JM, Gupta PC, Jarvis MJ, Bhala N, Peto R, Zatonski W, Hsia J, Morton J, Palipudi KM, Asma S, GATS Collaborative Group. Tobacco use in 3 billion individuals from 16 countries: an analysis of nationally representative cross-sectional household surveys. Lancet. 2012;380:668–79.
51. Yang G, Fan L, Tan J, Qi G, Zhang Y, Samet JM, Taylor CE, Becker K, Xu J. Smoking in China: findings of the 1996 National Prevalence Survey. JAMA. 1999;282:1247–53.
52. Kumar A, Mash B, Rupesinghe G. Peripheral arterial disease—high prevalence in rural black South Africans. S Afr Med J. 2007;97:285–8.
53. Selvin E, Marinopoulos S, Berkenblit G, Rami T, Brancati FL, Powe NR, Golden SH. Meta-analysis: glycosylated hemoglobin and cardiovascular disease in diabetes mellitus. Ann Intern Med. 2004;141:421–31.
54. American Diabetes Association. Peripheral arterial disease in people with diabetes. Diabetes Care. 2003;26:3333–41.
55. Nordanstig J, Behrendt CA, Bradbury AW, de Borst GJ, Fowkes F, Golledge J, Gottsater A, Hinchliffe RJ, Nikol S, Norgren L. Peripheral arterial disease (PAD)—a challenging manifestation of atherosclerosis. Prev Med. 2023;171:107489.
56. Reddy KS. Cardiovascular diseases in the developing countries: dimensions, determinants, dynamics and directions for public health action. Public Health Nutr. 2002;5:231–7.
57. Boutayeb A, Boutayeb S. The burden of non communicable diseases in developing countries. Int J Equity Health. 2005;4:2.
58. Boutayeb A, Twizell EH, Achouayb K, Chetouani A. A mathematical model for the burden of diabetes and its complications. Biomed Eng Online. 2004;3:20.
59. Drewnowski A, Popkin BM. The nutrition transition: new trends in the global diet. Nutr Rev. 1997;55:31–43.
60. Popkin BM. The nutrition transition in low-income countries: an emerging crisis. Nutr Rev. 1994;52:285–98.
61. Grol ME, Halabi YT, Gerstenbluth I, Alberts JF, O'Niel J. Lifestyle in Curacao. Smoking, alcohol consumption, eating habits and exercise. West Indian Med J. 1997;46:8–14.
62. Danaei G, Singh GM, Paciorek CJ, Lin JK, Cowan MJ, Finucane MM, Farzadfar F, Stevens GA, Riley LM, Lu Y, Rao M, Ezzati M, Global Burden of Metabolic Risk Factors of Chronic Diseases Collaborating Group. The global cardiovascular risk transition: associations of four metabolic risk factors with national income, urbanization, and Western diet in 1980 and 2008. Circulation. 2013;127:1493–502, 1502e1–8.
63. Joosten MM, Pai JK, Bertoia ML, Rimm EB, Spiegelman D, Mittleman MA, Mukamal KJ. Associations between conventional cardiovascular risk factors and risk of peripheral artery disease in men. JAMA. 2012;308:1660–7.
64. Lloyd-Sherlock P, Beard J, Minicuci N, Ebrahim S, Chatterji S. Hypertension among older adults in low- and middle-income countries: prevalence, awareness and control. Int J Epidemiol. 2014;43:116–28.
65. Kearney PM, Whelton M, Reynolds K, Muntner P, Whelton PK, He J. Global burden of hypertension: analysis of worldwide data. Lancet. 2005;365:217–23.
66. Bosu WK. Epidemic of hypertension in Ghana: a systematic review. BMC Public Health. 2010;10:418.
67. Guerchet M, Aboyans V, Mbelesso P, Mouanga AM, Salazar J, Bandzouzi B, Tabo A, Clement JP, Preux PM, Lacroix P. Epidemiology of peripheral artery disease in elder general population of two cities of Central Africa: Bangui and Brazzaville. Eur J Vasc Endovasc Surg. 2012;44:164–9.
68. Hiatt WR, Hoag S, Hamman RF. Effect of diagnostic criteria on the prevalence of peripheral arterial disease. The San Luis Valley Diabetes Study. Circulation. 1995;91:1472–9.
69. Kou M, Ding N, Ballew SH, Salameh MJ, Martin SS, Selvin E, Heiss G, Ballantyne CM, Matsushita K, Hoogeveen RC. Conventional and novel lipid measures and risk of peripheral artery Disease. Arterioscler Thromb Vasc Biol. 2021;41:1229–38.
70. Ridker PM, Stampfer MJ, Rifai N. Novel risk factors for systemic atherosclerosis: a comparison of C-reactive protein, fibrinogen, homocysteine, lipoprotein(a), and standard cholesterol screening as predictors of peripheral arterial disease. JAMA. 2001;285:2481–5.

71. Chen Z, Peto R, Collins R, MacMahon S, Lu J, Li W. Serum cholesterol concentration and coronary heart disease in population with low cholesterol concentrations. BMJ. 1991;303:276–82.
72. Obsa MS, Ataro G, Awoke N, Jemal B, Tilahun T, Ayalew N, Woldegeorgis BZ, Azeze GA, Haji Y. Determinants of dyslipidemia in Africa: a systematic review and meta-analysis. Front Cardiovasc Med. 2021;8:778891.
73. Brook RD. Is air pollution a cause of cardiovascular disease? Updated review and controversies. Rev Environ Health. 2007;22:115–37.
74. Hoffmann B, Moebus S, Kröger K, Stang A, Möhlenkamp S, Dragano N, Schmermund A, Memmesheimer M, Erbel R, Jöckel KH. Residential exposure to urban air pollution, ankle-brachial index, and peripheral arterial disease. Epidemiology. 2009;20:280–8.
75. Tellez-Plaza M, Guallar E, Fabsitz RR, Howard BV, Umans JG, Francesconi KA, Goessler W, Devereux RB, Navas-Acien A. Cadmium exposure and incident peripheral arterial disease. Circ Cardiovasc Qual Outcomes. 2013;6:626–33.
76. Navas-Acien A, Selvin E, Sharrett AR, Calderon-Aranda E, Silbergeld E, Guallar E. Lead, cadmium, smoking, and increased risk of peripheral arterial disease. Circulation. 2004;109:3196–201.
77. Criqui MH, Aboyans V. Epidemiology of peripheral artery disease. Circ Res. 2015;116:1509–26.
78. Aboyans V, Criqui MH, Abraham P, Allison MA, Creager MA, Diehm C, Fowkes FG, Hiatt WR, Jönsson B, Lacroix P, Marin B, McDermott MM, Norgren L, Pande RL, Preux PM, Stoffers HE, Treat-Jacobson D. Measurement and interpretation of the ankle-brachial index: a scientific statement from the American Heart Association. Circulation. 2012;126:2890–909.
79. Wikström J, Hansen T, Johansson L, Lind L, Ahlström H. Ankle brachial index <0.9 underestimates the prevalence of peripheral artery occlusive disease assessed with whole-body magnetic resonance angiography in the elderly. Acta Radiol. 2008;49:143–9.
80. Flanigan DP, Ballard JL, Robinson D, Galliano M, Blecker G, Harward TR. Duplex ultrasound of the superficial femoral artery is a better screening tool than ankle-brachial index to identify at risk patients with lower extremity atherosclerosis. J Vasc Surg. 2008;47:789–92; discussion 792–3.
81. Tsuyuki K, Kohno K, Ebine K, Obara T, Aoki T, Muto A, Ninomiya K, Kumagai K, Yokouchi I, Yazaki Y, Watanabe S. Exercise-ankle brachial pressure index with one-minute treadmill walking in patients on maintenance hemodialysis. Ann Vasc Dis. 2013;6:52–6.
82. Hishida M, Imaizumi T, Menez S, Okazaki M, Akiyama S, Kasuga H, Ishigami J, Maruyama S, Matsushita K. Additional prognostic value of toe-brachial index beyond ankle-brachial index in hemodialysis patients. BMC Nephrol. 2020;21:353.
83. Gerhard-Herman MD, Gornik HL, Barrett C, Barshes NR, Corriere MA, Drachman DE, Fleisher LA, Fowkes FG, Hamburg NM, Kinlay S, Lookstein R, Misra S, Mureebe L, Olin JW, Patel RA, Regensteiner JG, Schanzer A, Shishehbor MH, Stewart KJ, Treat-Jacobson D, Walsh ME. 2016 AHA/ACC guideline on the management of patients with lower extremity peripheral artery disease: a report of the American College of Cardiology/American Heart Association task force on clinical practice guidelines. Circulation. 2017;135:e726–79.
84. Akhtar B, Siddique S, Khan RA, Zulfiqar S. Detection of atherosclerosis by ankle brachial index: evaluation of palpatory method versus ultrasound Doppler technique. J Ayub Med Coll Abbottabad. 2009;21:11–6.
85. Wang FM, Yang C, Ballew SH, Kalbaugh CA, Meyer ML, Tanaka H, Heiss G, Allison M, Salameh M, Coresh J, Matsushita K. Ankle-brachial index and subsequent risk of incident and recurrent cardiovascular events in older adults: the Atherosclerosis Risk in Communities (ARIC) study. Atherosclerosis. 2021;336:39–47.
86. Gupta DK, Skali H, Claggett B, Kasabov R, Cheng S, Shah AM, Loehr LR, Heiss G, Nambi V, Aguilar D, Wruck LM, Matsushita K, Folsom AR, Rosamond WD, Solomon SD. Heart failure risk across the spectrum of ankle-brachial index: the ARIC study (Atherosclerosis Risk In Communities). JACC Heart Fail. 2014;2:447–54.
87. Hicks CW, Al-Qunaibet A, Ding N, Kwak L, Folsom AR, Tanaka H, Mosley T, Wagenknecht LE, Tang W, Heiss G, Matsushita K. Symptomatic and asymptomatic peripheral artery dis-

ease and the risk of abdominal aortic aneurysm: the Atherosclerosis Risk in Communities (ARIC) study. Atherosclerosis. 2021;333:32–8.
88. Bonaca MP, Gutierrez JA, Creager MA, Scirica BM, Olin J, Murphy SA, Braunwald E, Morrow DA. Acute limb ischemia and outcomes with vorapaxar in patients with peripheral artery disease: results from the trial to assess the effects of vorapaxar in preventing heart attack and stroke in patients with atherosclerosis-thrombolysis in myocardial infarction 50 (TRA2 degrees P-TIMI 50). Circulation. 2016;133:997–1005.
89. Paskiewicz A, Wang FM, Yang C, Ballew SH, Kalbaugh CA, Selvin E, Salameh M, Heiss G, Coresh J, Matsushita K. Ankle-brachial index and subsequent risk of severe ischemic leg outcomes: the ARIC Study. J Am Heart Assoc. 2021;10:e021801.
90. Samba H, Guerchet M, Ndamba-Bandzouzi B, Kehoua G, Mbelesso P, Desormais I, Aboyans V, Preux PM, Lacroix P. Ankle brachial index (ABI) predicts 2-year mortality risk among older adults in the Republic of Congo: the EPIDEMCA-FU study. Atherosclerosis. 2019;286:121–7.
91. Luo Y, Li X, Li J, Wang X, Xu Y, Qiao Y, Hu D, Ma Y. Peripheral arterial disease, chronic kidney disease, and mortality: the Chinese ankle brachial index cohort study. Vasc Med. 2010;15:107–12.
92. Abboud H, Monteiro Tavares L, Labreuche J, Arauz A, Bryer A, Lavados PM, Massaro A, Munoz Collazos M, Steg PG, Yamout BI, Vicaut E, Amarenco P. Impact of low ankle-brachial index on the risk of recurrent vascular events. Stroke. 2019;50:853–8.
93. Guerchet M, Mbelesso P, Mouanga AM, Tabo A, Bandzouzi B, Clément JP, Lacroix P, Preux PM, Aboyans V. Association between a low ankle-brachial index and dementia in a general elderly population in Central Africa (Epidemiology of Dementia in Central Africa Study). J Am Geriatr Soc. 2013;61:1135–40.
94. Kim GY, Anderson MS, Brown CS, Powell C, Corriere MA. Gender disparities in major depression among patients with peripheral artery disease and associations with mortality. J Vasc Surg. 2021;74:e207–8.
95. McDermott MM, Greenland P, Liu K, Guralnik JM, Criqui MH, Dolan NC, Chan C, Celic L, Pearce WH, Schneider JR, Sharma L, Clark E, Gibson D, Martin GJ. Leg symptoms in peripheral arterial disease: associated clinical characteristics and functional impairment. JAMA. 2001;286:1599–606.
96. Grenon SM, Hiramoto J, Smolderen KG, Vittinghoff E, Whooley MA, Cohen BE. Association between depression and peripheral artery disease: insights from the heart and soul study. J Am Heart Assoc. 2012;1:e002667.
97. McDermott MM, Guralnik JM, Tian L, Kibbe MR, Ferrucci L, Zhao L, Liu K, Liao Y, Gao Y, Criqui MH. Incidence and prognostic significance of depressive symptoms in peripheral artery disease. J Am Heart Assoc. 2016;5:e002959.
98. Ruo B, Liu K, Tian L, Tan J, Ferrucci L, Guralnik JM, McDermott MM. Persistent depressive symptoms and functional decline among patients with peripheral arterial disease. Psychosom Med. 2007;69:415–24.
99. Arya S, Lee S, Zahner GJ, Cohen BE, Hiramoto J, Wolkowitz OM, Khakharia A, Binney ZO, Grenon SM. The association of comorbid depression with mortality and amputation in veterans with peripheral artery disease. J Vasc Surg. 2018;68:536–45.e2.
100. Onega T, Baron JA, Johnsen SP, Pedersen L, Farkas DK, Sørensen HT. Cancer risk and subsequent survival after hospitalization for intermittent claudication. Cancer Epidemiol Biomarkers Prev. 2015;24:744–8.
101. Mok Y, Ishigami J, Lutsey PL, Tanaka H, Meyer ML, Heiss G, Matsushita K. Peripheral artery disease and subsequent risk of infectious disease in older individuals: the ARIC Study. Mayo Clin Proc. 2022;97:2065–75.

102. Willigendael EM, Teijink JA, Bartelink ML, Boiten J, Moll FL, Buller HR, Prins MH. Peripheral arterial disease: public and patient awareness in The Netherlands. Eur J Vasc Endovasc Surg. 2004;27:622–8.
103. Lovell M, Harris K, Forbes T, Twillman G, Abramson B, Criqui MH, Schroeder P, Mohler ER III, Hirsch AT, Peripheral Arterial Disease Coalition. Peripheral arterial disease: lack of awareness in Canada. Can J Cardiol. 2009;25:39–45.
104. Stewart BT, Gyedu A, Giannou C, Mishra B, Rich N, Wren SM, Mock C, Kushner AL, Essential Vascular Care Guidelines Study Group. Consensus recommendations for essential vascular care in low- and middle-income countries. J Vasc Surg. 2016;64:1770–9.e1.
105. Gaziano TA, Opie LH, Weinstein MC. Cardiovascular disease prevention with a multidrug regimen in the developing world: a cost-effectiveness analysis. Lancet. 2006;368:679–86.
106. World Health Organization. The selection and use of essential medicines: report of the WHO Expert Committee, 2015 (including the 19th WHO Model List of Essential Medicines and the 5th WHO Model List of Essential Medicines for Children). World Health Organization; 2015.
107. Yusuf S, Islam S, Chow CK, Rangarajan S, Dagenais G, Diaz R, Gupta R, Kelishadi R, Iqbal R, Avezum A, Kruger A, Kutty R, Lanas F, Lisheng L, Wei L, Lopez-Jaramillo P, Oguz A, Rahman O, Swidan H, Yusoff K, Zatonski W, Rosengren A, Teo KK, Prospective Urban Rural Epidemiology Study Investigators. Use of secondary prevention drugs for cardiovascular disease in the community in high-income, middle-income, and low-income countries (the PURE Study): a prospective epidemiological survey. Lancet. 2011;378:1231–43.
108. Okello S, Millard A, Owori R, Asiimwe SB, Siedner MJ, Rwebembera J, Wilson LA, Moore CC, Annex BH. Prevalence of lower extremity peripheral artery disease among adult diabetes patients in southwestern Uganda. BMC Cardiovasc Disord. 2014;14:1–6.
109. Mwebaze RM, Kibirige D. Peripheral arterial disease among adult diabetic patients attending a large outpatient diabetic clinic at a national referral hospital in Uganda: a descriptive cross sectional study. PLoS One. 2014;9:e105211.
110. Khatib R, McKee M, Shannon H, Chow C, Rangarajan S, Teo K, Wei L, Mony P, Mohan V, Gupta R, Kumar R, Vijayakumar K, Lear SA, Diaz R, Avezum A, Lopez-Jaramillo P, Lanas F, Yusoff K, Ismail N, Kazmi K, Rahman O, Rosengren A, Monsef N, Kelishadi R, Kruger A, Puoane T, Szuba A, Chifamba J, Temizhan A, Dagenais G, Gafni A, Yusuf S, PURE Study Investigators. Availability and affordability of cardiovascular disease medicines and their effect on use in high-income, middle-income, and low-income countries: an analysis of the PURE study data. Lancet. 2016;387:61–9.
111. van Mourik MS, Cameron A, Ewen M, Laing RO. Availability, price and affordability of cardiovascular medicines: a comparison across 36 countries using WHO/HAI data. BMC Cardiovasc Disord. 2010;10:25.
112. Cacoub PP, Abola MTB, Baumgartner I, Bhatt DL, Creager MA, Liau C-S, Goto S, Röther J, Steg PG, Hirsch AT. Cardiovascular risk factor control and outcomes in peripheral artery disease patients in the Reduction of Atherothrombosis for Continued Health (REACH) Registry. Atherosclerosis. 2009;204:e86–92.
113. Bencheikh N, Zarrintan S, Quatramoni JG, Al-Nouri O, Malas M, Gaffey AC. Vascular surgery in low-income and middle-income countries: a state-of-the-art review. Ann Vasc Surg. 2023;95:297–306.
114. Cassimjee I, le Roux D, Pillai J, Veller M. Vascular surgery in South Africa in 2021. Eur J Vasc Endovasc Surg. 2021;61:719–20.
115. Lundgren F, Hodza-Beganovic R, Johansson M, Seyoum N, Tadesse M, Andersson P. A vascular surgery exchange program between Ethiopia and Sweden: a plus for both. IJS Global Health. 2020;3:e43.

116. Gyedu A, Stewart BT, Nakua E, Quansah R, Donkor P, Mock C, Hardy M, Yangni-Angate KH. Assessment of risk of peripheral vascular disease and vascular care capacity in low- and middle-income countries. Br J Surg. 2016;103:51–9.
117. Moreira RC. Critical issues in vascular surgery: education in Brazil. J Vasc Surg. 2008;48:87S–9S.
118. Bedwell GJ, Dias P, Hahnle L, Anaeli A, Baker T, Beane A, Biccard BM, Bulamba F, Delgado-Ramirez MB, Dullewe NP, Echeverri-Mallarino V, Haniffa R, Hewitt-Smith A, Hoyos AS, Mboya EA, Nanimambi J, Pearse R, Pratheepan AP, Sunguya B, Tolppa T, Uruthirakumar P, Vengadasalam S, Vindrola-Padros C, Stephens TJ. Barriers to quality perioperative care delivery in low- and middle-income countries: a qualitative rapid appraisal study. Anesth Analg. 2022;135:1217–32.
119. Rajaguru PP, Jusabani MA, Massawe H, Temu R, Sheth NP. Understanding surgical care delivery in Sub-Saharan Africa: a cross-sectional analysis of surgical volume, operations, and financing at a tertiary referral hospital in rural Tanzania. Glob Health Res Policy. 2019;4:1–9.
120. Chu K, Maine R, Duvenage R. We Asked the Experts: The Role of Rural Hospitals in Achieving Equitable Surgical Access in Low-Resourced Settings. World J Surg. 2021;45(10):3016–18. https://doi.org/10.1007/s00268-021-06271-5. PMID: 34338826; PMCID: PMC8327595.

Chapter 5
Global Experience of Self-Care in Cardiovascular Prevention

Barbara Riegel, Heleen Westland, Onome H. Osokpo, and Tiny Jaarsma

Cardiovascular disease (CVD) is the leading cause of death globally and continues to rise in economically underdeveloped countries [1]. The World Health Organization (WHO) estimates that 32% of all deaths globally were due to CVD in 2019 (17.9 million people), 85% of which were due to heart attack and stroke. Most CVD can be prevented by addressing individual-level behavioral risk factors (i.e., tobacco use, unhealthy diet, body weight management, physical inactivity, and excess alcohol intake) through self-care. In under-resourced countries, however, healthcare and system barriers can make self-care challenging. In this chapter, we define and describe self-care, focusing on how self-care is practiced in low- and low-middle-income countries, classified as such by the World Bank based on the national per capita health expenditure. Identifying these countries, we focused on the behavioral

B. Riegel (✉)
University of Pennsylvania School of Nursing, Philadelphia, PA, USA

Center for Home Care Policy and Research at VNS Health, New York, NY, USA
e-mail: briegel@nursing.upenn.edu

H. Westland
Julius Center for Health Sciences and Primary Care, University Medical Center Utrecht, Utrecht, The Netherlands
e-mail: H.Westland@umcutrecht.nl

O. H. Osokpo
University of Illinois Chicago, Chicago, IL, USA
e-mail: oosokpo@uic.edu

T. Jaarsma
Department of Health, Medicine and Caring Sciences, Linkoping University, Linkoping, Sweden
e-mail: tiny.jaarsma@liu.se

T. Romero et al. (eds.), *Global Challenges in Cardiovascular Prevention in Populations with Low Socioeconomic Status*,
https://doi.org/10.1007/978-3-031-79051-5_5

risk factors, gender differences, cultural practices, and beliefs about self-care. Healthcare focused and system focused factors enabling and supporting self-care are addressed. Finally, we explored the self-care interventions studied in low- and middle-income countries. We end the chapter with suggestions for policy changes that would support self-care across the world.

We have defined self-care in relation to chronic illnesses such as CVD as a process of maintaining health through health promoting practices and managing illness [2]. That is, self-care is required both when we are healthy and when we are ill. In reference to CVD, the known behavioral risk factors (e.g., physical inactivity) reflect insufficient self-care. Such behavior is common in young populations that perceive a robust time horizon [3]. It is often not until illness occurs that people begin to feel situationally pressed for time. At that point, behavior changes and self-care are adopted.

The WHO takes a broader view of self-care, defining it as "the ability of individuals, families and communities to promote their own health, prevent disease, maintain health, and to cope with illness and disability with or without the support of a health worker" [4]. They recognize individuals as active agents in managing their own health care, not to replace the health care system, but to provide choices and options for healthcare. Although the WHO talks about health promotion, disease prevention and control, self-medication, caregiving, rehabilitation, and palliative care, a careful review of their website illustrates the focus on sexual and reproductive care (e.g., antenatal care and postnatal care) and immunizations. Sections dealing with access to care come closest to a discussion of CVD prevention, but these two topics—CVD and access to care—are not clearly linked to the WHO website.

In many low- and middle-income countries such as most of those on the African continent, people who have little income rely on under-funded public health facilities. Only a small minority of the population has access to well-funded, quality private health care, so self-care is promoted as a form of "individual agency" said to support resilience in West and Central Africa [5]. Despite the prevalent lack of access to public health facilities, the WHO celebrated the increase by 10 years in healthy life expectancy between 2000 and 2019 in Africa at its 75th anniversary event in April 2023. However, these changes are due primarily to gains in reproductive, maternal, newborn, and child health, as well as progress in the fight against infectious diseases—not prevention of CVD.

As CVD remains the leading cause of death worldwide, and poor self-care behaviors are major contributors to CVD, self-care is particularly important in areas of the world where access to essential health services is lacking. Self-care is seen as an alternative to expanding access to universal health care in some low-income countries [6]. Over three quarters of CVD deaths take place in low- and middle-income countries, but relatively little is known about the multitude of barriers to the performance of self-care in most of these countries.

5.1 Facilitators and Barriers to Implementing Self-Care Strategies

The facilitators and barriers to self-care in low- and middle-income countries can be categorized as system-, provider-, and patient-level factors (Fig. 5.1). The main system-level factors that support self-care are health and fiscal policies put in place to facilitate local access to healthcare. In addition, the built environment plays an important role in supporting self-care.

At the healthcare provider-level, time and training are the main factors influencing the ability of providers to support self-care. An adequate number of knowledgeable and trained providers is needed to provide preventive care and early access when needed. Limited access to healthcare resources negatively impacts self-care for individuals with CVD in these countries [8]. Many physicians and nurses in low- and middle-income countries are overstretched, prioritizing acute illness conditions over the provision of self-care education to patients and their family caregivers [8, 9]. Another challenge faced by providers in fostering self-care is the lack of adequate training on effective strategies, such as motivational interviewing, to nudge patients living with CVD to engage in adequate self-care [9]. Scarce providers in rural areas, driven by migration to high-income countries for a better quality of life, exacerbate the problem. Another issue is poorly integrated services that hinder collaboration between acute care providers, primary care, and pharmacies [8]. In local governmental and non-governmental health centers, high out-of-pocket costs and long waiting times for healthcare impede the adoption of self-care practices, particularly for those living below the poverty line [8, 9].

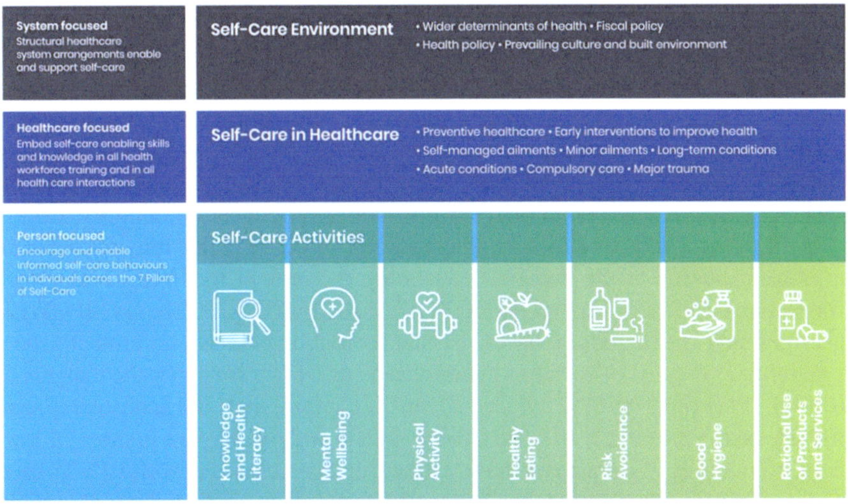

Fig. 5.1 Australian self-care alliance. The self-care matrix: a unifying framework for self-care. Adapted from El-Osta et al. [7]. Reprinted with permission

At the individual patient-level, many people lack resources for the purchase of recommended foods and prescribed medicines due to poverty [8]. Low income is a common reason for poor self-care. Furthermore, a limited understanding of the severity of asymptomatic conditions such as hypertension contributes to low self-care uptake [8, 9]. Another barrier is migration to urban areas, which has led to adoption of lifestyles that include unhealthy dietary habits and low levels of physical activity, as discussed further below [8]. Those who live in rural areas are challenged with having to develop their own self-help capacities (i.e., self-cultivation), issues of transportation, and access to health foods because of local agricultural resources. Individuals living in rural settings are less likely to self-medicate for minor illnesses compared to those in urban areas, perhaps because of poor health literacy, low levels of education, and/or family income disparities [10].

5.2 Behavioral Risk Factors for Cardiovascular Disease

As stated above, CVD can be effectively addressed through self-care practices. By addressing the behavioral risk factors of tobacco use, unhealthy diet, body weight management, physical inactivity, and excess alcohol intake, CVD could be prevented in a huge segment of the world's population. System-level policies in some countries support self-care behaviors, as described below.

5.2.1 Tobacco Use

Tobacco use refers to any habitual use of the tobacco plant leaf and its products—smoking, vaping, water pipe use, chewing, and sniffing. Smoking is most common and, as shown in Fig. 5.2, as of 2019, smoking was the most important behavioral contributor to death rates—primarily through CVD—worldwide [11]. It is estimated that 23% of the population worldwide smokes tobacco but the proportion of adults who smoke is falling in most countries. Unfortunately, about 80% of the world's 1.3 billion tobacco users live in low- and middle-income countries [12].

In 2007, the WHO introduced a practical, cost-effective policy initiative to scale up implementation of the demand reduction provisions of the WHO Framework Convention on Tobacco Control (WHO FCTC) called MPOWER. The six MPOWER measures are (1) to monitor tobacco use and prevention policies, (2) protect people from tobacco use, (3) offer help to quit tobacco use, (4) warn about the dangers of tobacco, (5) enforce bans on tobacco advertising, promotion, and sponsorship, and (6) raise taxes on tobacco. In Africa, the continent with the highest number of low-income countries, 44 countries have ratified or agreed to the WHO FCTC and tobacco use is lower in Africa than many other nations. A WHO press release highlights that, as of July 2023, 71% of the world's population is protected with at least

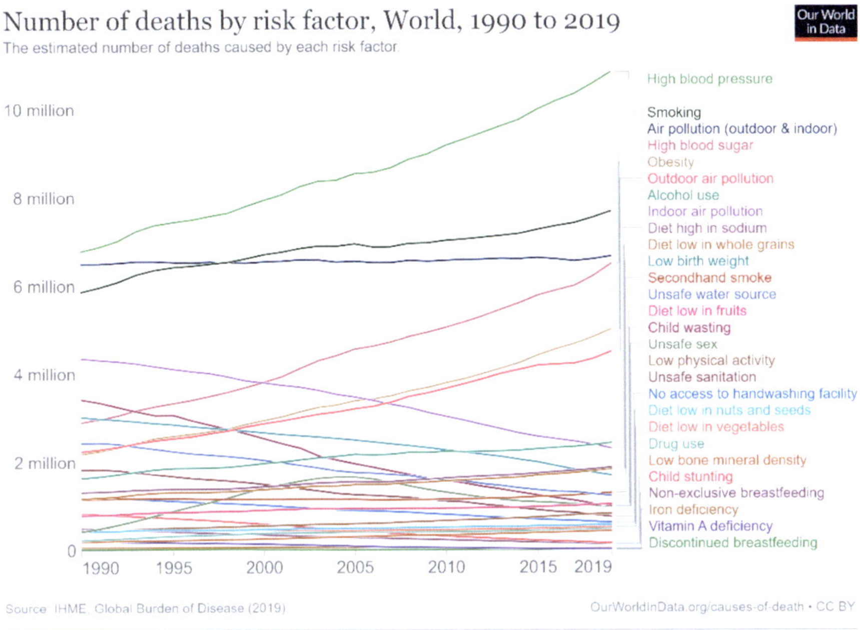

Fig. 5.2 Graphic illustration of the number of deaths by risk factor, worldwide, between 1990 and 2019. Source: The Institute for Health Metrics and Evaluation, Seattle, WA. Reprinted with permission

one best practice policy included in the WHO FCTC to help save lives from tobacco use; five times more than when the policy was introduced in 2007 [13].

5.2.2 *Unhealthy Diet*

An unhealthy diet is one that is high in sodium, sugar-sweetened beverages, and processed meats and low in whole grains, fruits, and vegetables. A 2019 study of the health effects of diet in 195 countries found that high intake of sodium and low intake of whole grains and fruits were the leading dietary risk factors for death and disability-adjusted life-years (DALYs) in many countries worldwide [14]. The impact of an unhealthy diet was highest for CVD compared to other causes of death and disability. Uzbekistan, a low-middle income country, had the highest rate of diet-related deaths but globally, consumption of nearly all healthy foods and nutrients was suboptimal in 2017, the year of data collection and analysis. The largest gaps between current and optimal intake were observed for nuts and seeds, milk, and whole grains while sugar-sweetened beverages, processed meat, and sodium intake were far above the optimal levels. The intake of legumes was high in the low- and low-middle income countries of western sub-Saharan Africa, and eastern sub-Saharan Africa.

The highest age-standardized rates of all diet-related deaths and DALYs were observed in countries with a low-middle and high-middle socio-demographic index (SDI), a summary measure calculated based on income, education, and fertility rate [15]. The four leading dietary risks for low SDI countries were a lack of intake of whole grains, fruit, nuts and seeds, and vegetables. Food prices appear to be responsible for the transition from unhealthy to healthy food choices [15].

5.2.3 *Weight Management*

Obesity, defined as a body mass index ≥30 kg/m^2, is a major risk factor for CVD, contributing directly to dyslipidemia, type 2 diabetes, hypertension, and sleep disorders [16]. Obesity is an independent risk factor for CVD mortality and is now a worldwide problem referred to as an "epidemic" by the WHO [17]. Obesity was originally prevalent in high-income countries but now the greatest number of people with obesity live in low- and middle-income countries [17]. Estimates found in the World Obesity Atlas [18] suggest that by 2030, 17.5% of the global population of adults will be obese. Further, the top ten countries with the most rapid rise in adult obesity prevalence over the past decades are almost exclusively low- and middle-income countries [18].

In many low- and middle-income countries, the population is still grappling with undernutrition. That is, undernutrition and obesity commonly co-exist within the same country, the same community, and the same household. Children in low- and middle-income countries are more vulnerable to malnutrition; yet these same children are exposed to high-fat, high-sugar, high-salt, energy-dense, and micronutrient-poor foods because these foods are often lower in cost. When these dietary patterns occur in conjunction with lower levels of physical activity, childhood obesity increases in the face of undernutrition.

Factors contributing to obesity include diet, lack of exercise, social determinants of health (i.e., the conditions in which we live, learn, work, and play), and genetics. Social determinants introduce inequities and deprivations that influence both health and the ability to perform self-care. Self-care is relevant to the balance of dietary intake and energy expenditure through physical activity. In most situations, obesity can be prevented by limiting intake of fats and sugars, increasing consumption of fruits, vegetables, legumes, whole grains, and nuts, and engaging in regular physical activity. However, limiting caloric intake to that which can be burned through activity is challenging. Stress and poor sleep cause some people to eat more. Therefore, policies that influence the built environment to improve access to parks, sidewalks, and affordable gyms are advocated to address obesity. Another important contributor to weight gain is oversized food portions. Food advertising encourages people to buy unhealthy foods, such as high-fat snacks and sugary drinks, and food deserts limit access to affordable healthy foods, such as fresh fruits and vegetables. Food preferences are developed in childhood, so much of the effort to address this issue is appropriately focused on childhood obesity.

5.2.4 Physical Inactivity

Physical activity guidelines differ by age, but adults should perform at least 150–300 min of moderate-intensity aerobic physical activity each week. Being physically active contributes in important ways to preventing and managing CVD. A recent study estimated that the population-level prevalence-based attributable risk for physical inactivity was comparable to that of tobacco use [19]. Yet, globally, at least 25% of adults fail to meet the recommended levels of physical activity and more than 80% of the world's adolescent population is insufficiently physically active [20]. Unfortunately, as countries develop economically, levels of activity decrease due to changing transport patterns, increased use of technology for work and recreation, cultural values as discussed further below, and increasing sedentary behaviors such as use of social media.

5.2.5 Excess Alcohol Intake

Alcohol comes in many forms that have been used in various cultures for centuries. Alcohol is a psychoactive substance with dependence-producing properties and powerful effects on the brain, producing pleasurable feelings and blunting negative feelings. These feelings motivate some people to drink alcohol routinely, despite the possibility that excessive alcohol intake can lead to high blood pressure, coronary artery disease, atrial fibrillation, peripheral arterial disease, cardiomyopathy, and stroke [21, 22]. Overall, the use of alcohol is responsible for 5.1% of the global burden of disease [23].

Alcohol use is known to be a major contributor to socioeconomic inequalities in health and mortality, with mortality rising with declines in socioeconomic status [24]. With economic growth, the prevalence and level of alcohol use have increased in low-income and middle-income countries [25]. The prevalence of heavy episodic drinking (≥5 drinks on one occasion) is thought to be >60% in some low- and middle-income countries [26]. A recent study of alcohol use in low- and middle-income countries found that the highest population-weighted prevalence of both current drinking and heavy episodic drinking was found in males [24].

Most recommendations for curbing alcohol intake are system-level policy recommendations rather than individual self-care practices. The WHO encourages policy-makers to regulate the marketing of alcoholic beverages, restrict the availability of alcohol, enact appropriate drink-driving policies, reduce demand through taxation and pricing mechanisms, raise awareness of the health and social problems for individuals and society at large caused by the harmful use of alcohol, ensure support for effective alcohol policies, provide accessible and affordable treatment for people with alcohol-use disorders, and implement screening and brief intervention programs for hazardous and harmful drinking [26]. Self-care is advocated in recovery from alcohol addiction [27].

5.3 Gender, Socioeconomic Status, and Health

Women of low socioeconomic status experience health disparities that contribute to poor outcomes. These disparities may be related to labor force participation, different family roles, societal expectations, and differences in the value given to health [28]. In a short-term perspective, as men are typically the family breadwinners, their health may be perceived as vital for family welfare. However, in long term, women's health is fundamental for the health and development of the family and future generations.

Self-care behaviors that are related to CVD prevention are known to differ in men and women irrespective of socioeconomic status [29, 30]. Obesity is more prevalent in women than men, and half of all women living with obesity live in 11 countries: the United States (U.S.), China, India, Brazil, Mexico, Russia, Egypt, Indonesia, Iran, Turkey, and Pakistan [18]. These countries span the full range of low- to high-income countries.

In Europe, a large registry sponsored by the European Society of Cardiology (EuroAspire V) provides insight into a gender by country–income interaction found for smoking behavior ($p < 0.001$). The EuroAspire V survey included cardiac patients from 27 different European countries with a large diversity in socioeconomic status. Significant gender differences in smoking were found in middle-income countries but not in high-income countries [31]. The prevalence of obesity was also found to vary between countries, with a significant gender by country–income interaction found for obesity ($p = 0.001$). Especially in middle-income European countries, the odds of not being obese were lower in women compared with men.

There are specific barriers and challenges to self-care that are gender specific and need tailoring of education and support. System-level policies serving as barriers for women are influenced by cultural norms so gender differences need to be contextualized to cultural norms, as described below [32].

5.4 Cultural Beliefs and Practices

Culture can be defined as the shared values, norms, feelings, and ways of thinking that are learned and transmitted to others in a particular group of people. These values, norms, feelings, and thoughts shape the beliefs and practices of the group [33, 34]. A variety of factors influence cultural beliefs and practices including country of residence, time spent in a place, family background and language, race and ethnicity, religious, spiritual, and social affiliations [34, 35]. These factors influence how people think, the beliefs they hold, theirs norms and values, behavioral preferences such as diet, and patterns of behavior [36]. Culture also influences how a person defines an illness, attributes a cause, chooses a treatment, and anticipates a cure [37]. Although culture clearly influences self-care choices, culture is rarely addressed in CVD prevention efforts [38].

Cultural norms significantly influence the use of tobacco products. In some countries, smoking is expected, especially for men. Religion is an important cultural influence on smoking. Some religions speak out against tobacco use while others encourage tobacco for spiritual purposes [39]. In a study of South Asian immigrants to the U.S., culturally specific tobacco products were considered beneficial [40]. In Ethiopia, the use of khat chewing is common and highly associated with smoking. Using these tobacco items may be seen as preserving cultural traditions and expressing ethnic identity in the new culture.

Dietary preferences are strongly influenced by culture because taste preferences develop in childhood and portion sizes and social eating norms are learned early in life [41]. These preferences are influenced by access to different kinds of foods and financial resources. Culture also appears to influence alcohol consumption of immigrant populations. Alcohol addiction is a problem for many people due to less opportunities in life but a connection to the culture of origin, traditional values and customs have been shown to have protective influences for alcohol use [42].

Beliefs about obesity are also influenced by culture. People in different countries may respond differently to weight gain because the association between obesity and socioeconomic status differs in various countries. For example, in countries where being overweight is associated with wealth and privilege, obesity is perceived as desirable [18]. Sub-Saharan Africans may equate higher weight with prestige, beauty, and happiness and lower weight with poverty and illness [43–45].

Cultural influences on physical activity include: (1) collectivism and cultural identity; (2) religiosity; (3) cultural attitudes and gender norms in regard to physical activity; (4) cultural perspectives on health in regard to physical activity; (5) cultural expectations of familism and lack of time; (6) lack of role models and motivation; (7) lack of culturally appropriate exercise facilities; and (8) cultural expectations of body image and physical appearance [46]. African immigrants to the U.S. have been found to perceive recommendations about physical activity to be inconsistent with their cultural norms and practices [47]. For example, riding a bicycle is perceived as a sign of poverty in some African nations [48–50]. Others perceived physical activities as dangerous to illness [48]. Walking and dancing were perceived as more culturally appropriate African practices than going to a gym [51].

At the provider-level, it should also be noted that the cultural background of health care providers may influence how they care for patients. In one study, health care providers reported that their own cultural background shaped their experiences and their practices with patients [52].

5.5 Successful Methods of Providing Self-care Support

System-level government policy plays a crucial role in incorporating structured self-care programs in routine care for patients with CVD, especially since the transition in low-income countries is away from infectious diseases toward chronic diseases, such as CVD, that require lifelong therapy [53, 54]. Such self-care programs are primarily focused on self-care education based on the WHO self-care guidelines. These programs typically include condition-specific self-care, addressing medication adherence, physical activity, weight management, low-salt diet, non-smoking, moderate alcohol usage, and adherence to diet and glycemic control in diabetes mellitus.

Access to care for patients who live in urban and rural areas surrounding the countryside may include visits to regional hospitals or clinics in urban and rural areas. In these settings, healthcare providers play an important role in providing self-care education during regular follow-up consultations. In studies evaluating self-care education programs, successful approaches have consisted of face-to-face group or individual sessions with videos, photographs, leaflets as well as interactive exercises in which participants can share experiences and learn by observing others, and telephone calls or SMS messaging [55–59]. Face-to-face and telephone support with printed education materials also suit the large number of illiterate patients found in low-income countries.

In providing self-care support, healthcare providers should take known risk factors for poor self-care into account, e.g., living in a rural area, low level of education, poor social support, long disease duration, poor knowledge, comorbidity, older age, low monthly income, widowed marital status, living a long distance from a healthcare institution, and lacking regular medical follow-up [60–66]. Recognizing these risks for poor self-care can alert the healthcare provider of potential problems with self-care that should be addressed.

5.6 Addressing Barriers to Self-Care

To address the system-, provider-, and individual-level barriers to self-care, a comprehensive approach is needed that incorporates strategies to enhance accessibility, affordability, education of patients, caregivers, and community leaders, and support for healthcare professionals. Strategies for facilitating the uptake of self-care behaviors are outlined here.

Systemic challenges are complex and difficult to address although certain strategies are known to address issues around affordability and accessibility to healthcare. Such strategies include enacting governmental healthcare policies targeted at retaining local providers [8, 9, 67], building low-cost community healthcare centers, and local pharmaceutical industries [8]. Governmental agencies need to develop policies, including tax incentives, to convince pharmaceutical industries to lower medication costs.

At the provider level, efforts are needed to promote effective coordination and collaboration among health care providers and services [68]. Adequate training and staffing would go a long way in enabling the workforce to support the efforts of individuals to engage in self-care.

At the individual level, it is critical to empower patients and their families and community leaders with the knowledge and tools needed to minimize illness complications and maintain health [8, 9, 67, 68]. However, these programs must be culturally sensitive and tailored to the community. These programs should address the impact of fast foods and physical inactivity on health. Healthcare providers can be supported by extension providers, patient-led support groups, and community workers working with faith and traditional leaders to increase community awareness regarding chronic illnesses and promote self-care uptake in low-and middle-income countries [69].

We previously described self-care interventions as those that focus on changing behavior by equipping the person with the knowledge and skills they need to actively engage in self-care maintenance, self-care monitoring, and self-care management [70]. Self-care maintenance involves the behaviors used to maintain physical and emotional stability. Eating a healthy diet and staying physically active are self-care maintenance behaviors. Self-care monitoring refers to the process of observing oneself for changes in signs and symptoms or body listening. Even someone healthy, without a chronic illness, needs to pay attention to themselves, listen to their body so that changes can be detected early. Self-care management is defined as the response to bodily changes—signs and —when they occur. A self-care intervention that addresses only self-care monitoring without addressing what to do with the information obtained is not a true self-care intervention because it is not holistic. Holistic, broad interventions are needed to capture the variety of issues related to health and illness. A true self-care intervention should address multiple components: (1) improving behaviors (e.g., tobacco use, diet, physical activity, and stress management), (2) encouraging independent monitoring or body listening, and (3) enhancing problem-solving and decision-making skills. We believe that interventions that emphasize behavior change without incorporating problem-solving and decision-making skills are not true self-care interventions [70].

5.7 Self-Care Interventions Tested in Low- and Low-Middle Income Countries

Some self-care interventions have been tested in low- and low-middle income countries. These studies are summarized briefly below to illustrate the CVD conditions studied and the approaches being used in these countries.

5.7.1 Africa

Few investigators are studying self-care intervention for CVD in Africa, but Ethiopia seems to be one place where self-care is being actively studied [60–66]. These studies are targeted at patients with hypertension and evaluated the association between self-care and associated factors at one time-point using questionnaires. Generally, they found that the level of knowledge on hypertension and self-care activities was low compared to the WHO standard. Particularly, self-care activities such as a low-salt diet intake, physical activity, managing weight, and taking medication to control hypertension were low [60–66]. In these studies, most participants were non-smokers and abstained from alcohol for religious reasons. Patients who were unable to read and write, older than 65 years, with uncontrolled hypertension, poor social support, comorbid conditions, and living a rural area were most likely to have poor self-care. In one study, patients were also interviewed about their self-care activities [63]. This study revealed that physical activity was a major challenge due to limited or lack of exercise facilities and patients' awareness and attitudes toward physical activity. Participants reported that the pressure during social events, preparing separate meals for one person in a family, and inadequate information on hypertension led to negligence of their hypertension. Dealing with temptations presented challenges for hypertension self-care practice. Together these studies illustrate how challenging individual-level approaches are when cultural and system-level factors like the built environment are not aligned with patient motivation.

Educational interventions are promising in locations where knowledge about how to prevent and manage illness is underdeveloped. So, it was not surprising that a self-care educational intervention based on social cognitive theory tested in Ethiopia with adults with chronic heart failure (HF) was effective in improving self-care [55]. These investigators conducted a clustered randomized control trial (RCT) of 186 patients. Intervention group participants received illustrated educational leaflets and an intensive 4-day training session with a 1-day follow-up session offered every 4 months. Self-care, measured using an instrument addressing primarily self-care maintenance behaviors, increased more in the intervention group compared to the control group ($p < 0.05$).

5.7.2 South Asia

Most of South Asia is classified as low-middle income (e.g., Pakistan, and India) except for Afghanistan, which is classified as a low-income country with a health system "on the brink of collapse" according to the WHO. A recent scoping review revealed that non-communicable diseases such as CVD are escalating in Afghanistan [71]. Little intervention research is being conducted in Afghanistan although one study of life skills training is based on self-care, improved mental health, and quality of life [72].

In India, several RCT of self-care interventions for diabetes have been conducted. One group of investigators studied the impact of a brief self-management intervention with education, relaxation skills, goal setting, and problem-solving [73]. They demonstrated improvements in HbA1c, quality of life, diet, exercise, medication adherence, glucose testing, perceived barriers, illness perceptions, personal control, beliefs in the effectiveness of treatment, understanding of the illness, depression, and anxiety. Another group conducted a pragmatic RCT in patients with depression and diabetes in India and significantly improved a composite measure of depressive symptoms and cardiometabolic disease at 24 months [56]. Another group studied the effect of text messaging with newly diagnosed adults with diabetes and found only a significant lowering of low density cholesterol levels in the intervention group [57]. Hypertension is also studied in India. A scalable group-based education and monitoring program tested in a cluster RCT significantly improved blood pressure control in the intervention group compared to the control group [74].

5.7.3 *Middle East*

Self-care is studied robustly in Iran, a low-middle income country in the middle east. One RCT conducted with 90 people with HF focused on improving symptom awareness and recognition, problem-solving, diet, exercise, and stress management [58]. Eight weeks after the intervention ended that they found significant improvement in the health status of patients in the intervention group.

Two other studies were performed with patients with diabetes. In one RCT, a structured educational program for improving lifestyle was conducted in 80 adults with type 2 diabetes [59]. Three months after the intervention, nutrition and physical activity improved more in the intervention group than the control group. HgA1c improved in both groups but achieving an HgA1c <7% was 10% more common in the intervention group compared to only 5% in the control group. In another RCT test, a telehealth approach providing care for adults with diabetes demonstrated significant decrease in fasting blood sugar and HgA1c in the intervention group after 3 months [75]. The authors explained their results as using telehealth allowed more time for self-care training.

Self-care interventions are also being used to address hypertension in Iran. Half of a sample of 56 older adults with hypertension were randomized to receive self-care education with written materials and four telephone follow-up visits [76]. After 3 months, normal blood pressure was achieved significantly more commonly in the intervention group compared to the control group. Finally, a 2-month home-based self-care education program was tested in an RCT conducted with 110 middle-aged adults with hypertension [77]. After 2 months, medication adherence, physical activity, adherence to a low-salt diet, and blood pressure control were better in the intervention group than the control group.

5.8 Conclusion

In this chapter, we have described self-care, an individual-level behavior that is strongly influenced by provider-level and system-level factors. The countries that have made the most strides are those that have implemented policy initiatives to address health needs and the built environment. Policy changes that would support self-care across the world are those that address healthcare access, the cost of care, and the built environment. Cultural- and gender-related factors have influenced self-care behaviors in various positive and negative ways. Throughout this chapter, we highlighted the efforts to improve self-care and address common risk factors for CVD in low- and low-middle countries. Notably, despite a lack of resources and the lack of focus on cardiovascular prevention by major organizations like the WHO, investigators in some countries are taking the initiative to address CVD locally. Clearly more effort is needed at both the policy level and by individuals if we are to stop and reverse the current rise in CVD worldwide [1].

Glossary

Culture The shared values, norms, feelings, and ways of thinking that are learned and transmitted to others in a particular group of people.

Healthcare provider-level factors that affect self-care Time, training, scarcity of providers, poorly integrated services, out-of-pocket costs, and long waiting times.

Individual patient-level factors that affect self-care Poverty, limited understanding of asymptomatic conditions, migration, rural residence, transportation, and access to healthy foods.

Individual-level behavioral risk factors Tobacco use, unhealthy diet, body weight management, physical inactivity, and excess alcohol intake.

Motivational interviewing A collaborative, goal-oriented style of communication with particular attention to the language of change. It is designed to strengthen personal motivation for and commitment to a specific goal by eliciting and exploring the person's own reasons for change within an atmosphere of acceptance and compassion.

Self-care The ability of individuals, families, and communities to promote their own health, prevent disease, maintain health, and to cope with illness and disability with or without the support of a health worker.

Self-care interventions Approaches that change behavior by equipping the person with the knowledge and skills they need to actively engage in self-care maintenance, self-care monitoring, and self-care management.

Social determinants of health The conditions in which we live, learn, work, and play.

System-level factors that affect self-care Health and fiscal policies and the built environment.

References

1. Roth GA, Mensah GA, Johnson CO, et al. Global burden of cardiovascular diseases and risk factors, 1990-2019: update from the GBD 2019 study. J Am Coll Cardiol. 2020;76(25):2982–3021.
2. Riegel B, Jaarsma T, Stromberg A. A middle-range theory of self-care of chronic illness. ANS Adv Nurs Sci. 2012;35(3):194–204.
3. Liao H-W, Carstensen LL. Future time perspective: time horizons and beyond. GeroPsych. 2018;31(3):163–7.
4. World Health Organization. Classification of self-care interventions for health: a shared language to describe the uses of self-care interventions. Geneva; 2021. Available from: https://apps.who.int/iris/handle/10665/350480
5. Worley H. How self-care can support resilience in west and central Africa: self-care approaches offer women more control over their lives. Washington, DC: Population Reference Bureau; 2022.
6. Nyatela A, Nqakala S, Singh L, Johnson T, Gumede S. Self-care can be an alternative to expand access to universal health care: what policy makers, governments and implementers can consider for South Africa. Front Reprod Health. 2022;4:1073246.
7. El-Osta A, Webber D, Gnani S, et al. The self-care matrix: a unifying framework for self-care. Self-Care Adv Study Underst Self-care. 2019;10(3):38–56.
8. Bekele H, Asefa A, Getachew B, Belete AM. Barriers and strategies to lifestyle and dietary pattern interventions for prevention and management of TYPE-2 diabetes in Africa, systematic review. J Diabetes Res. 2020;2020:7948712.
9. Suglo JN, Evans C. Factors influencing self-management in relation to type 2 diabetes in Africa: a qualitative systematic review. PLoS One. 2020;15(10):e0240938.
10. Gustafsson PE, San Sebastian M, Janlert U, Theorell T, Westerlund H, Hammarstrom A. Life-course accumulation of neighborhood disadvantage and allostatic load: empirical integration of three social determinants of health frameworks. Am J Public Health. 2014;104(5):904–10.
11. Reitsma MB, Kendrick PJ, Ababneh E, et al. Spatial, temporal, and demographic patterns in prevalence of smoking tobacco use and attributable disease burden in 204 countries and territories, 1990–2019: a systematic analysis from the Global Burden of Disease Study 2019. Lancet. 2021;397(10292):2337–60.
12. World Health Organization. WHO global report on trends in prevalence of tobacco use 2000–2025. Geneva; 2021.
13. Seven out of 10 people protected by at least one tobacco control measure [press release]. 2023 Jul 31.
14. Afshin A, Sur PJ, Fay KA, et al. Health effects of dietary risks in 195 countries, 1990–2017: a systematic analysis for the Global Burden of Disease Study 2017. Lancet. 2019;393(10184):1958–72.
15. Headey DD, Alderman HH. The relative caloric prices of healthy and unhealthy foods differ systematically across income levels and continents. J Nutr. 2019;149(11):2020–33.
16. Powell-Wiley TM, Poirier P, Burke LE, et al. Obesity and cardiovascular disease: a scientific statement from the American Heart Association. Circulation. 2021;143(21):e984–e1010.
17. World Health Organization. WHO acceleration plan to stop obesity. Geneva; 2023.
18. World Obesity Federation. World obesity atlas 2022. London; 2022.
19. Katzmarzyk PT, Friedenreich C, Shiroma EJ, Lee I-M. Physical inactivity and non-communicable disease burden in low-income, middle-income and high-income countries. Br J Sports Med. 2022;56(2):101–6.

20. Wold Health Organization. Global status report on physical activity. Geneva; 2022.
21. Larsson SC, Burgess S, Mason AM, Michaelsson K. Alcohol consumption and cardiovascular disease: a Mendelian randomization study. Circ Genom Precis Med. 2020;13(3):e002814.
22. Piano MR. Alcohol's effects on the cardiovascular system. Alcohol Res. 2017;38(2):219–41.
23. World Health Organization. Alcohol: key facts. Geneva; 2022.
24. Xu Y, Geldsetzer P, Manne-Goehler J, et al. The socioeconomic gradient of alcohol use: an analysis of nationally representative survey data from 55 low-income and middle-income countries. Lancet Glob Health. 2022;10(9):e1268–80.
25. Manthey J, Shield KD, Rylett M, Hasan OSM, Probst C, Rehm J. Global alcohol exposure between 1990 and 2017 and forecasts until 2030: a modelling study. Lancet. 2019;393(10190):2493–502.
26. World Health Organization. Global status report on alcohol and health. Geneva; 2018.
27. Melemis SM. Relapse prevention and the five rules of recovery. Yale J Biol Med. 2015;88(3):325–32.
28. Onarheim KH, Iversen JH, Bloom DE. Economic benefits of investing in women's health: a systematic review. PLoS One. 2016;11(3):e0150120.
29. Heo S, Moser DK, Lennie TA, Riegel B, Chung ML. Gender differences in and factors related to self-care behaviors: a cross-sectional, correlational study of patients with heart failure. Int J Nurs Stud. 2008;45(12):1807–15.
30. Graven LJ, Abbott L, Dickey SL, Schluck G. The influence of gender and race on heart failure self-care. Chronic Illn. 2021;17(2):69–80.
31. Vynckier P, Ferrannini G, Ryden L, et al. Gender gap in risk factor control of coronary patients far from closing: results from the European Society of Cardiology EUROASPIRE V registry. Eur J Prev Cardiol. 2022;29(2):344–51.
32. Dellafiore F, Arrigoni C, Pittella F, Conte G, Magon A, Caruso R. Paradox of self-care gender differences among Italian patients with chronic heart failure: findings from a real-world cross-sectional study. BMJ Open. 2018;8(9):e021966.
33. Airhihenbuwa CO. Health and culture: beyond the western paradigm. Sage; 1995.
34. Al-Bannay H, Jarus T, Jongbloed L, Yazigi M, Dean E. Culture as a variable in health research: perspectives and caveats. Health Promot Int. 2014;29(3):549–57.
35. Kagawa-Singer M, Dressler WW, George SM, Elwood WN. The cultural framework for health: an integrative approach for research and program design and evaluation. Bethesda, MD: National Institutes of Health: Office of Behavioral and Social Sciences Research; 2015.
36. Karimi M, Clark AM. How do patients' values influence heart failure self-care decision-making?: a mixed-methods systematic review. Int J Nurs Stud. 2016;59:89–104.
37. Arnault DS. Defining and theorizing about culture: the evolution of the cultural determinants of help-seeking, revised. Nurs Res. 2018;67(2):161–8.
38. Gallant MP, Spitze G, Grove JG. Chronic illness self-care and the family lives of older adults: a synthetic review across four ethnic groups. J Cross Cult Gerontol. 2010;25(1):21–43.
39. Culture and smoking: do cultural norms impact smoking rates? Tobacco Free Life; 2016. Available from: https://tobaccofreelife.org/resources/culture-smoking/
40. Mukherjea A, Morgan PA, Snowden LR, Ling PM, Ivey SL. Social and cultural influences on tobacco-related health disparities among South Asians in the USA. Tob Control. 2012;21(4):422–8.
41. Alloh F, Hemingway A, Turner-Wilson A. Exploring the experiences of west African immigrants living with type 2 diabetes in the UK. Int J Environ Res Public Health. 2019;16(19):3516.
42. Schwartz SJ, Unger JB, Des Rosiers SE, et al. Substance use and sexual behavior among recent Hispanic immigrant adolescents: effects of parent-adolescent differential acculturation and communication. Drug Alcohol Depend. 2012;125(Suppl 1):S26–34.
43. Agyemang C, Addo J, Bhopal R, Aikins Ade G, Stronks K. Cardiovascular disease, diabetes and established risk factors among populations of sub-Saharan African descent in Europe: a literature review. Glob Health. 2009;5:7.

44. Cooper Brathwaite A, Lemonde M. Health beliefs and practices of African immigrants in Canada. Clin Nurs Res. 2016;25(6):626–45.
45. Omenka OI, Watson DP, Hendrie HC. Understanding the healthcare experiences and needs of African immigrants in the United States: a scoping review. BMC Public Health. 2020;20(1):27.
46. Mathew Joseph N, Ramaswamy P, Wang J. Cultural factors associated with physical activity among U.S. adults: an integrative review. Appl Nurs Res. 2018;42:98–110.
47. Henry Osokpo O, James R, Riegel B. Maintaining cultural identity: a systematic mixed studies review of cultural influences on the self-care of African immigrants living with non-communicable disease. J Adv Nurs. 2021;77(9):3600–17.
48. Beune EJ, Haafkens JA, Agyemang C, Bindels PJ. Inhibitors and enablers of physical activity in multiethnic hypertensive patients: qualitative study. J Hum Hypertens. 2010;24(4):280–90.
49. Kindarara DM, McEwen MM, Crist JD, Loescher LJ. Health-illness transition experiences with type 2 diabetes self-management of sub-Saharan African immigrants in the United States. Diabetes Educ. 2017;43(5):506–18.
50. Nyaaba GN, Agyemang C, Masana L, et al. Illness representations and coping practices for self-managing hypertension among sub-Saharan Africans: a comparative study among Ghanaian migrants and non-migrant Ghanaians. Patient Educ Couns. 2019;102(9):1711–21.
51. Ilunga Tshiswaka D, Ibe-Lamberts KD, Whembolua GS, Fapohunda A, Tull ES. "Going to the gym is not Congolese's culture": examining attitudes toward physical activity and risk for type 2 diabetes among Congolese immigrants. Diabetes Educ. 2018;44(1):94–102.
52. Jönsson A, Cewers E, Ben Gal T, Weinstein JM, Strömberg A, Jaarsma T. Perspectives of health care providers on the role of culture in the self-care of patients with chronic heart failure: a qualitative interview study. Int J Environ Res Public Health. 2020;17(14):5051.
53. Geneau R, Stuckler D, Stachenko S, et al. Raising the priority of preventing chronic diseases: a political process. Lancet. 2010;376(9753):1689–98.
54. Beaglehole R, Yach D. Globalisation and the prevention and control of non-communicable disease: the neglected chronic diseases of adults. Lancet. 2003;362(9387):903–8.
55. Dessie G, Burrowes S, Mulugeta H, et al. Effect of a self-care educational intervention to improve self-care adherence among patients with chronic heart failure: a clustered randomized controlled trial in Northwest Ethiopia. BMC Cardiovasc Disord. 2021;21(1):374.
56. Ali MK, Chwastiak L, Poongothai S, et al. Effect of a collaborative care model on depressive symptoms and glycated hemoglobin, blood pressure, and serum cholesterol among patients with depression and diabetes in India: the INDEPENDENT randomized clinical trial. JAMA. 2020;324(7):651–62.
57. Vinitha R, Nanditha A, Snehalatha C, et al. Effectiveness of mobile phone text messaging in improving glycaemic control among persons with newly detected type 2 diabetes. Diabetes Res Clin Pract. 2019;158:107919.
58. Aghamohammadi T, Khaleghipour M, Shahboulaghi FM, Dalvandi A, Maddah SSB. Effect of self-management program on health status of elderly patients with heart failure: a single-blind, randomized clinical trial. J Acute Dis. 2019;8(5):179–84.
59. Sanaeinasab H, Saffari M, Yazdanparast D, et al. Effects of a health education program to promote healthy lifestyle and glycemic control in patients with type 2 diabetes: a randomized controlled trial. Prim Care Diabetes. 2021;15(2):275–82.
60. Tebelu DT, Tadesse TA, Getahun MS, Negussie YM, Gurara AM. Hypertension self-care practice and its associated factors in Bale Zone, Southeast Ethiopia: a multi-center cross-sectional study. J Pharm Policy Pract. 2023;16(1):20.
61. Worku Kassahun C, Asasahegn A, Hagos D, et al. Knowledge on hypertension and self-care practice among adult hypertensive patients at University of Gondar Comprehensive Specialized Hospital, Ethiopia, 2019. Int J Hypertens. 2020;2020:5649165.
62. Tadesse DB, Gerensea H. Self-care practice among hypertensive patients in Ethiopia: systematic review and meta-analysis. Open Heart. 2021;8(1):e001421.

63. Assefa B, Zeleke H, Sergo T, Misganaw M, Mekonnen N. Self-care practice and associated factors among hypertensive follow-up patients at East Gojam zone public hospitals, North West Ethiopia, 2021. J Hum Hypertens. 2023;37:854–61.
64. Gelaw S, Yenit MK, Nigatu SG. Self-care practice and associated factors among hypertensive patients in Debre Tabor Referral Hospital, Northwest Ethiopia, 2020. Int J Hypertens. 2021;2021:3570050.
65. Hussen FM, Adem HA, Roba HS, Mengistie B, Assefa N. Self-care practice and associated factors among hypertensive patients in public health facilities in Harar Town, Eastern Ethiopia: a cross-sectional study. SAGE Open Med. 2020;8:2050312120974145.
66. Wondmieneh A, Gedefaw G, Getie A, Demis A. Self-care practice and associated factors among hypertensive patients in Ethiopia: a systematic review and meta-analysis. Int J Hypertens. 2021;2021:5582547.
67. Stephani V, Opoku D, Beran D. Self-management of diabetes in Sub-Saharan Africa: a systematic review. BMC Public Health. 2018;18(1):1148.
68. Otieno P, Agyemang C, Wao H, et al. Effectiveness of integrated chronic care models for cardiometabolic multimorbidity in sub-Saharan Africa: a systematic review and meta-analysis. BMJ Open. 2023;13(6):e073652.
69. Sanya RE, Johnston ES, Kibe P, et al. Effectiveness of self-financing patient-led support groups in the management of hypertension and diabetes in low- and middle-income countries: systematic review. Trop Med Int Health. 2023;28(2):80–9.
70. Riegel B, Westland H, Freedland KE, et al. Operational definition of self-care interventions for adults with chronic illness. Int J Nurs Stud. 2022;129:104231.
71. Neyazi N, Mosadeghrad AM, Afshari M, Isfahani P, Safi N. Strategies to tackle non-communicable diseases in Afghanistan: a scoping review. Front Public Health. 2023;11:982416.
72. Shovaz FA, Zareei Mahmoodabadi H, Salehzadeh M. Effectiveness of life skills training based on self-care on mental health and quality of life of married Afghan women in Iran. BMC Womens Health. 2022;22(1):296.
73. Abraham AM, Sudhir PM, Philip M, Bantwal G. Efficacy of a brief self-management intervention in type 2 diabetes mellitus: a randomized controlled trial from India. Indian J Psychol Med. 2020;42(6):540–8.
74. Gamage DG, Riddell MA, Joshi R, et al. Effectiveness of a scalable group-based education and monitoring program, delivered by health workers, to improve control of hypertension in rural India: a cluster randomised controlled trial. PLoS Med. 2020;17(1):e1002997.
75. Ravari ASA, Mirzaei T, Raeisi M, Hassanshahi E, Kamiab Z. Effect of tele-nursing on blood glucose control among the elderly with diabetes: a randomized controlled trial. Evidence Based Care J. 2021;11:54.
76. Farahmand F, Khorasani P, Shahriari M. Effectiveness of a self-care education program on hypertension management in older adults discharged from cardiac-internal wards. ARYA Atheroscler. 2019;15(2):44–52.
77. Hazrati Gonbad S, Zakerimoghadam M, Pashaeypoor S, Haghani S. The effects of home-based self-care education on blood pressure and self-care behaviors among middle-aged patients with primary hypertension in Iran: a randomized clinical controlled trial. Home Health Care Manag Pract. 2021;34(1):9–16.

Chapter 6
Environment, Cardiovascular Health, and Local and Global Inequities

Pablo Ruiz-Rudolph and Karla Yohannessen

When thinking about the environment, we usually recall images of deteriorated territories that greatly concern us. We remember images of factories releasing hazardous wastes and trucks emitting air pollutants, and more recently, images of wildfires occurring during heat waves, as a likely consequence of global warming. The environment, however, can be even more complex and is also found in our cities, in how they are built, in the presence of green-spaces, or lack of them, and more broadly, in all places where we live, play, learn, and work. In these environments, each component can affect our health in different and complex ways; consider motor vehicles, they release air pollutants that can affect your health directly, when you inhale them, but also indirectly through greenhouse gases and their effects on global warming. The environment can also include the biosphere, which affects us and can be affected by our actions, and ultimately, the whole earth, in what is understood as planetary health [1]. From this point of view, we can meditate in how our societies and economies are structured, how they can be drivers of the way that cities are built and ultimately determine the environments we live, affecting us both locally, for instance, by the presence of infrastructure to do exercise, and globally, for instance, as sources of persistent chemicals or greenhouse gases.

Cardiovascular diseases (CVD), on the other hand, are one the main contributors to global mortality and disability and are quite unevenly distributed around the globe [2]. Cardiovascular diseases encompass many different major diseases such as ischemic heart disease and stroke and affect different organs, but they can all be related in their origin, as they are produced when affecting some general

P. Ruiz-Rudolph (✉)
Epidemiology Program, Institute of Population Health, Faculty of Medicine,
University of Chile, Santiago, Chile
e-mail: pabloruizr@uchile.cl

K. Yohannessen
Environmental Health Program, Institute of Population Health, Faculty of Medicine,
University of Chile, Santiago, Chile

T. Romero et al. (eds.), *Global Challenges in Cardiovascular Prevention in Populations with Low Socioeconomic Status*,
https://doi.org/10.1007/978-3-031-79051-5_6

physio-pathological routes such as endothelial dysfunction or oxidative stress [3–5]. In this way, when one route is stressed, many diseases could result as an outcome. We are all at risk of suffering cardiovascular diseases as they are produced by very common and widely spread individual risk-factors, such as obesity and cigarette smoking, that stress these routes. The question guiding this chapter is whether the environment could be a cause of CVD. The environment might be affecting similar mechanisms as the "traditional" CVD risk-factors, thus compounding their effects. Another question guiding this article is whether the environment can affect to a greater extent a particular group of individuals, raising an equity problem. We will consider this question from the traditional person-time-place perspective: Who–when–where are the most affected? Women, the poor; now, in the future; in some parts of a city, countries in the southern hemisphere? Would some already burdened individuals suffer even a larger burden due to the environment? A final question we will attempt to address is what can be done about all this. In facing this question, we will see that there are "synergistic loops" between cardiovascular health, the environment and social inequities that seem to operate in an interrelated way compounding the health impacts; and behind many of these causes, we can recognize societal drivers that ultimately push the stress in our environment and our health.

The chapter is organized in four main sections. The first deals with our understanding of the environment and present three main stressors affecting CVD: air pollution, climate change, and the urban environment. We show how these stressors are interrelated both by their drivers and effects. The second section reviews the current understanding of how these stressors affect CVD, describing the main mechanisms postulated and how these mechanisms usually overlap, compounding the risks. The third starts reviewing concepts of equity and environmental justice and presents how some populations, seen from a local and global perspective, might be more affected by environmental stressors. We close with a section of recommendations of how to prevent these impacts. We review main recommendations that can be found in the literature, along with the challenges to improve health, now and in the future, presented by the presence of these "synergistic loops" and societal drivers presented throughout the chapter.

6.1 What Do We Understand by Environment and What Are the Relevant Environmental Stressors for Cardiovascular Health?

The concept of environment, and its relationship with health, has many rich sources [6, 7]. Some quite intuitive, dictionary definitions of environment point to all circumstances, objects, and conditions that surround us. Historically, the concept has mutated from an early twentieth century understanding of the environment as a natural, pristine, healthy place, such as a national park, to a mid-twentieth century one where the environment is more usually associated with chemical pollutants, produced in factories or by combustion sources, which are unintendedly present in our air, water, soil, or food [8]. Two well-known examples are the contamination by asbestos used as insulating material and lead used in gasoline as an anti-knock. More recent definitions also recognize the importance of urban environments as promoter of health and well-being and the impacts of global environmental degradation in future generations. Last, it is important to remark the contribution of the environmental justice movement that made a paradigmatic shift moving the concept of the environment from natural, pristine, distant places, to the actual places where we live, play, learn, and work. This shift puts at the center the surrounding where communities develop and where they can thrive or get sick [8, 9].

Many environmental stressors have been identified as risk-factors of CVD. Here we will focus in three major ones: air pollution, climate change, and the urban environment, as they have been recognized as major contributors of CVD mortality and burden of disease [2–5, 10–12], there have been calls for action from several scientific societies [13–17], and they have quite interrelated dynamics that make interesting cases when sources, projections, and likely solutions are considered. In any case, many other environmental stressors have been identified [18]; with many of them, i.e., microplastics and deforestation, being currently major matters of concern.

A critical point when thinking about how to prevent the effects of these environmental stressors is to think about the underlying causes of these manifestations. In public health, a useful conceptual framework is the social determinants of health, which points to ascertain the "causes of the causes" for a given health effect [19]. In this view, determining that smoking increases CVD risks is not enough, but aims to understand the social conditions that drive low-income teenage Chilean girls to start smoking [20]. This framework has been particularly applied to environmental problems, generating the DPSEEA model (Driving forces-Pressures-State-Exposure-Effects-Actions) by the World Health Organization (WHO) [7]. The model links environmental stressors with health effects but also with the underlying drivers, the underlying social determinants. This facilitates decision-making as driving forces become main target for intervention. We can exemplify it with traffic air pollution. Driving forces might be population growth, urban design (i.e., a sprawled, highway oriented city) and energy options. This would generate pressures to the environment in the form of emissions of air pollutants, which in turn modify the state, the actual concentrations in air. This deterioration in the state would threaten health only when people are actually exposed to pollutants, because they spend time in traffic or are downwind from major highways. Actions could be targeted to any of the levels: we could use masks to decrease exposures, we could move highways away from populated centers, we could put filters in the exhausts, but from a public health point of view the most effective action is to modify the drivers, for instance, changing a city orientation so to decrease traffic. Even more, in the next sections, we will see that many stressors share driving forces.

6.1.1 Air Pollution

Essentially, air pollutants are gases and particles suspended in air that can be inhaled and produce health effects [21, 22]. From all known air pollutants, three have been identified as of major concern by monitoring programs due to their ubiquity and demonstrated health impacts: particulate matter of size below 2.5 μm ($PM_{2.5}$), ozone (O_3), and nitrogen oxides (NO_X) [23]. Air pollutants can be directly emitted from sources and are known as primary pollutants. Examples are sulfur dioxide (SO_2) emitted from coal-fired power-plants, carbon monoxide (CO) from motor vehicles, and $PM_{2.5}$ from residential wood-combustion [24–26]. Pollutants can also be produced in the atmosphere through chemical reactions from gaseous precursors and are known as secondary pollutants. Major examples are O_3 formed from volatile organic compounds and NO_X, and $PM_{2.5}$ which can be formed from reactions of SO_2, NO_X, or volatile organic compounds (VOCs) [22, 27–30]. Consequently, in order to control secondary pollutants, O_3, or secondary $PM_{2.5}$, we should control their gaseous precursors. Main sources of air pollutants worldwide are vehicular and industrial emissions, particularly large combustion sources for energy production, such as coil- and oil-fired power plants [3, 31, 32]. More recently, and due to energy crisis, the use of biomass burning for heating and cooking has been greatly expanded [24, 25, 33–35].

To have effects, people need to be in contact—being exposed—and inhale these pollutants. People can be exposed because the pollutants accumulate in a city or because they are in the vicinity of emissions. For instance, high exposures to CO, $PM_{2.5}$, NO_X, and ultrafine particles (UFP) have been observed within meters of traffic emissions [36–38], and to $PM_{2.5}$ in neighborhoods with large presence of residential wood-burning for heating [39–41]. Worldwide, a case that provokes particularly large exposures to $PM_{2.5}$ and CO are household air pollution (HAP) produced by unvented indoor biomass burning. These emissions, happening mostly in very disadvantage populations, accumulate in close, kitchen microenvironments, leading to very high concentrations of pollutants that are later inhaled, mainly by women and their children [42–44]. Sources can also have impacts at a regional scale, for instance, power plants or smelters emissions can affect cities hundreds of kilometers away [27, 31, 32]; and even at a transcontinental or global scale [45], as the most notorious impacts of dust storms, which can increase the concentrations of particulate matter thousands of kilometers away from their origin [46].

Global exposures to air pollutants are high; for $PM_{2.5}$, the global annual mean concentration was 42.6 μg/m^3, much higher than the WHO annual guideline of 2005 of 10 μg/m^3 or the revised 5 μg/m^3 guidelines 2021 [22, 26]. Exposures are also highly unequal globally with lower concentrations in North America and Europe and higher concentrations in East, Central, and South Asia; North Africa and the Middle East; and Southern and Western sub-Saharan Africa and Central America, with inequalities being even increased when HAPs are considered [2]. Trajectories of air pollution exposures also vary widely worldwide depending on technological and economic development, being more notorious the rise in emission by China and

India with the concomitant reduction in North America and Europe [47]. Forecasting future exposures is highly dependent on available technologies, levels of production and most important, the links to reduction due to the climate change mitigation efforts [48, 49].

6.1.2 Climate Change

Climate change refers to long-term changes in temperatures and weather patterns [50]. These changes may be due to natural internal processes, such as changes in the activity of the sun or large volcanic eruptions; however, since the nineteenth century, human activities have been the main driver of climate change through persistent anthropogenic changes in the composition of the atmosphere and in land use [51]. Human activities that produce persistent changes in the composition of the atmosphere are those activities that produce greenhouse gases (GHG), the deforestation and destruction of marine ecosystems that absorb GHGs, and the increase in population that consumes more and more natural resources, which has led to overwhelming urbanization and the constant demand of products of animal origin [12, 52]. The main GHGs in the Earth's atmosphere are water vapor (H_2O), carbon dioxide (CO_2), nitrous oxide (N_2O), methane (CH_4), and ozone (O_3), which can all be emitted naturally; however, the constant and progressive anthropogenic emission of GHG due to the combustion of fossil fuels and large-scale production of products of animal origin, added to the deforestation and changes in land use for residential use or agricultural production, has produced an increase in these gases in the atmosphere [45, 52, 53]. In addition, in the atmosphere, there are a number of GHGs entirely produced by man, such as halocarbons and other substances containing chlorine and bromine, hydrofluorocarbons (HFCs), and perfluorocarbons (PFCs) [53].

As a result of all these anthropogenic emissions, heat is trapped in the atmosphere, and significant variations in the climate are occurring that would not occur naturally; the last decade (2011–2020) was the warmest ever recorded and, currently, the temperature of the Earth is 1.1 °C higher than at the end of the nineteenth century [10, 12, 53, 54]. Global warming alters the water cycle which has led to the emergence of droughts and desertification, ocean acidification, melting of the poles and rising sea levels, as well as an increase in the frequency and intensity of extreme weather events. All these phenomena are having devastating consequences in our planet with evident damage to ecosystems, loss of biodiversity, extinction of species, and general decrease in natural resources with their corresponding impact on the health, well-being, and living conditions of the population, while at the same time striking a difficult blow to the society and the local, regional, and global economy [12, 55].

Climate change alters atmospheric conditions and harms the processes of dilution, dispersion, and elimination of atmospheric pollutants from the ecosystem. In general, densely populated areas may be particularly and disproportionately affected by climate-mediated worsening air quality. For example, global warming is causing changes in precipitation patterns and other climate anomalies, which have resulted in drier conditions that may increase the frequency and intensity of wildfires and dust storms that simultaneously emit or produce toxic air pollutants. Furthermore, higher temperatures, decreased precipitation, and air stagnation are favorable conditions to promote the formation and accumulation of secondary pollutants; and inversely, some pollutants such as O_3 are greenhouse gases themselves and can even increase the temperatures during heatwaves [10]. For these reasons, the concept of "climate penalty" arises, which refers to the greater formation of secondary pollutants, such as O_3 at ground level (tropospheric), with the increase in temperatures and the alteration of meteorological conditions caused by the climate change [10, 55].

6.1.3 Urban Environment

According to the World Bank, in 2022, the global urban population will exceed 55% of the world's total population, and 7 out of 10 people are projected to live in cities by 2050. Once a city is built, the physical structure and land use patterns may be impossible to change over generations, leading to an unsustainable expansion [56]. Within a city, the built environment is understood as the totality of the places and the infrastructure created, such as buildings, streets, and parks, are the main settings where we live, work, study, and play. An important phenomenon that appeared in the twentieth century was urban sprawl, which refers to the uncontrolled expansion of urban areas, usually through low density developments in the suburbs, which dramatically changes the quality of the built environment, and involves the consumption of large amounts of land and natural resources, such as fossil fuels to fuel motor vehicles and power generation, water lost through runoff from extensive impervious surfaces, consumer goods to fill large houses, and increased time dedicated to travel [56, 57]. These two urban aspects can become environmental stressors as they can facilitate or impede physical activity, improve or degrade air quality, provide or impede access to healthy foods, and promote social interaction or aggravate social isolation, among many others [57].

The urban environment relates to physical activity through the incentive, or lack of it, for the population to commute using active transportation. The combination of land use, density, connectivity, and design play an important role in walkability and physical activity levels in communities [57, 58]. When different land uses (for example, residential, schools, workplaces, and retail) are located close to each other, travel distances are shortened, allowing people to move from one place to another by walking or cycling, and increasing physical activity as part of the daily routine. On the contrary, when distances are long, car use is encouraged along sedentary behavior. People who use public transportation typically walk to and from transit stops, systematically adding minutes of physical activity to their daily routine.

Urban sprawl, with their low-density developments, is associated with fewer people walking or cycling, as well as a lack of public transport, which favors the use of the car [57–59]. Other urban design features, such as connectivity, bike lines, shade, perceptions of safety, and natural amenities such as trees and landscapes, also affect decisions about outdoor activities, including walking and cycling for walking and commuting [57, 58].

Urban design can also affect us through other paths. Air pollution is affected through urbanization and transportation patterns. Emissions from the transportation sector include GHGs and toxic air pollutants. Exposures to emissions from cars and trucks are larger near busy roads [36, 37, 60], which are often located in low-income neighborhoods that also face other environmental and social health threats. Good urban and transportation planning can reduce miles traveled, GHG emissions, and air pollution concentration in a city or neighborhood [57–59]. Public parks and green spaces provide places where people can engage in physical activity, enjoy contact with nature and other people, and relax, contributing to the quality of life of a city's residents [57–59]. Additionally, green spaces improve air quality, reduce noise, and improve biodiversity while moderating temperatures during hot periods and providing cool, shaded areas [61, 62]. For these reasons, the World Health Organization recommends that all people reside within 300 m of green spaces. Healthy food environment in communities includes the location of food stores and the availability of healthy, affordable foods, where evidence has been consistent in reporting that readily available fresh foods improve health [61, 62].

6.1.4 Compound Impacts

We finish the section alerting in how these impacts may be compounded, which is highly likely as they share many drivers, increasing the risks not only for CVD but for many other health outcomes. We will illustrate the point through climatic extreme events. These events can occur compounded (compound events) or in cascade (several events happening consecutively), increasing the impacts in the environment, the population, and society. For instance, higher temperatures can increase the frequency of heat waves and also, alter global water cycles, which can lead to more frequent episodes of heavy rains and more intense hurricanes. In turn, more precipitations exacerbate the risk of flooding and landslides. Risk of flooding in coastal regions is amplified by sea-level rise, threatening costal infrastructure. As other case, increasing temperatures can also increase the frequency, severity, and duration of heat waves and droughts, which in turn increase the risk of wildfires. Droughts, heat waves, wildfires, and floods often occur as product of several interlinked physical processes, which in isolation might not be extreme, but combined can provoke very significant impacts [55].

6.2 How Environmental Stressors Affect Health?

6.2.1 Air Pollution Effects

Air pollution is the fourth cause of illness and death in the world [11]. The World Health Organization (WHO) estimated that 91% of the world's population lives in places where average annual air pollution levels exceed recommended levels for PM [3, 5]. According to the Global Burden of Disease (GBD) study, air pollution was responsible for 9 million deaths worldwide in 2019, of which 61.9% were due to cardiovascular diseases, including ischemic heart disease (32%) and stroke (28%) [5]. Air pollutants can cause cardiovascular toxic effects through complex and varied mechanisms. The main categories have been identified: initiating mechanisms, effector pathways, and development of risk factors. Once pollutants had entered the body, they can initiate mechanisms by triggering processes such as inflammation, activation of neural reflex arcs, and ligation of pattern recognition receptors. Effector mechanisms involve the subsequent activation of rapid neuronal pathways and the release of biologically active substances such as inflammatory cytokines, oxidized lipids, immune cells, microparticles, and microRNAs. Last, the development of risk factors, such as hypertension and type 2 diabetes, is a result of chronic oxidative stress and inflammation induced by the pollutants [5, 10].

Many studies have consistently shown that short-term exposure to daily levels of $PM_{2.5}$ (between hours and days) is associated with an increased risk of myocardial infarction, stroke, and death from cardiovascular disease, increasing the mortality risk by up to 1% per each increase of 10 μg/m^3 of $PM_{2.5}$ [3–5, 10]. Air pollution has also been associated with an increased risk of atrial fibrillation and ventricular arrhythmias. On the other hand, long-term exposure to $PM_{2.5}$ (1–5 years) has been associated with elevated mortality from ischemic heart disease and an increased risk of hospitalization or death from heart failure [3, 5]. These effects have been observed even at very low exposure levels, below the 10 μg/m^3 annual WHO air quality guideline for $PM_{2.5}$, unveiling that most air quality standards are not sufficient protect the cardiovascular health of the population [3, 5]. Biological factors such as advanced age, previous cardiovascular disease, cardiovascular risk factors, lung diseases, and immunosuppression can increase a person's susceptibility to air pollution [5]. A very important risk groups are those apparently healthy at-risk individuals, which includes a large population of people with asymptomatic peripheral vascular or coronary disease, who could be seriously affected by an episode of air pollution [3].

Air pollution has also been causally related to other risk factors for cardiovascular diseases, particularly hypertension and diabetes mellitus; in many cases, sharing their physio-pathological paths, thus compounding their effects [3–5]. Short-term increases in $PM_{2.5}$ levels have been associated with alterations in vascular tone, increases in blood pressure up to 10 mm of Hg, while long-term exposures have been associated with increased incidence of new-onset hypertension, and increases in carotid intima-media thickness, coronary artery calcification, abdominal aortic calcification, and susceptibility to atherosclerotic plaque formation [3]. Furthermore, evidence from experimental and epidemiological studies had linked $PM_{2.5}$ exposures with insulin resistance and type 2 diabetes. Even more, these associations have been observed at very low $PM_{2.5}$ exposures, below 5 $\mu g/m^3$ [4, 5]. Finally, we highlight that these mechanisms can induce not only CVD but many other health effects [63].

Other pollutants, which might originate from similar sources as air pollutants, have also been associated with the risk of cardiovascular disease. Lead exposure, which might originate from smelters, is a known risk factor for hypertension and is associated with mortality from cardiovascular causes. Exposure to methylmercury, which can originate from coal-combustion, has been associated with an increased risk of death from cardiovascular disease and nonfatal myocardial infarction. Consistent dose-response associations have also been found between arsenic exposure, which can originate from copper smelters, and coronary heart disease, peripheral artery disease, and type 2 diabetes [5]. Additionally, pollutants from manufactured chemicals such as halogenated hydrocarbons (polychlorinated biphenyls, dioxins, brominated flame retardants, and organochlorine pesticides), perfluoroalkyl substances, and plastic-associated chemicals (bisphenol A and phthalates) have been implicated in increased disease risk and cardiovascular risk factors due to its association with diabetes mellitus, dyslipidemia, insulin resistance, and obesity [5].

6.2.2 Climate Change Effects

Climate change has been considered the greatest challenge to global public health of the twenty-first century. Climate change may worsen cardiovascular health or lead to premature deaths from cardiovascular diseases through direct and indirect pathways. Direct pathways include exposure to extreme heat and poor air quality due to the formation of secondary pollutants, forest fires, and dust storms [10]. Indirect pathways involve multiple and complex mechanisms, including access to healthy food and clean water, transportation, housing, electricity, communication systems, healthcare infrastructure, and other social determinants of health, all of which are essential for maintaining good cardiovascular health [4, 10].

From the direct pathways, events of extreme heat or heat waves are the ones most easily associated with climate change. Extreme heat can have serious implications for cardiovascular health, especially in people with pre-existing conditions. Body responses, which include dehydration, increased metabolic demand, hypercoagulability, electrolyte imbalances, and systemic inflammatory response, can put significant pressure on the cardiovascular system, resulting in increased risks of ischemic heart disease, stroke, heart failure, and arrhythmia. Several studies have shown a 15% increase in mortality from cardiovascular diseases during heat waves. Furthermore, some at-risk patients using diuretics as treatment for some base cardiovascular disease can have exacerbated dehydration states and electrolyte imbalances [4, 64]. Higher temperatures can also contribute to the climate penalty through increased levels of O_3

formation, which in turn could increase local temperatures [4]. Additionally, the synergistic effect between air pollution and high temperatures on the cardiovascular system has been observed, with increased heat-related cardiovascular mortality when high concentrations of $PM_{2.5}$ or ozone are present [10].

Droughts are associated with extremely low rainfall, high evaporation, and high temperatures, increasing the risk of dust storms, water insecurity, wildfires, food shortages, and other health-related events [12]. The forest fire season and burning time in some areas have been extended due to drought and low rainfall. Direct health impacts of wildfires include burns, injuries, mental health effects, and premature deaths [12]. Exposure to wildfire smoke causes increased cardiovascular morbidity and mortality, particularly among older people [65]. Sand and dust storms have been associated with increased mortality and cardiovascular morbidity when comparing days with dust storms to days without this event, specifically, an increase in cardiovascular hospitalizations and emergency department visits for ischemic heart disease and stroke [4, 10].

Other phenomena that have increased with climate change are heavy rains, hurricanes, storms, and rising sea levels that can cause devastating floods. In addition to deaths and injuries, threats continue after floods as people lose their homes, sewer overflows can contaminate drinking water and agricultural soils, increasing the risk of infectious, water-, soil-, and vector-borne diseases. Studies have shown an increased risk of short- and long-term mortality and worsening of non-communicable diseases in populations affected by floods during the first year, as well as the occurrence of post-traumatic stress disorders, depression, anxiety, and stress, which have been described as cardiovascular risk factors [12]. As an indirect pathway, climate change is expected to negatively affect food production and security in all aspects of the food system (availability, access, utilization, and stability) and their interactions. This will have serious consequences for human health due to a lack of sufficient nutrients to sustain life or a greater susceptibility to infectious diseases. However, healthy eating, which is closely related to cardiovascular health, will also be affected by food insecurity [12]. Although the entire planet is being affected by climate change, the impact is uneven according to socioeconomic, demographic, and environmental factors, so that children, the elderly women, the poor, and those living in coastal regions are particularly susceptible to climate change [12].

Although the effects of air pollution and climate change on cardiovascular health may appear independent, they are closely interrelated ecologically. Climate change and air pollution exist in vicious feedback loops, where each exacerbates the other. To start, GHGs and air pollutants largely come from the same sources. GHG emissions, mainly from the burning of fossil fuels, contribute to climate change, and conversely, climate change leads to an increase in ground-level $PM_{2.5}$ and O_3. As part of climate change and global warming, extreme weather conditions will contribute to more substantial acute increases in air pollution [3]. For example, climate change generates extreme heat events, which intensify in large cities where urban heat islands are created by replacing trees and vegetation with buildings and pavements that absorb heat instead of reflecting it. These high temperatures also increase the demand for electricity for air conditioning, which in turn increases the burning of fossil fuels and pollution [5, 10].

6.2.3 *Effects of the Urban Environment*

With rapid urbanization, the urban environment is receiving increased attention as it can be a promoter or a threat to health. At the neighborhood level, the urban environment is characterized by similar social positions, demographics, and housing characteristics, and it is the most appropriate spatial unit to predict residents' exposures [57, 59]. Within a neighborhood, consistent evidence showing that the protective effects of green (trees, grass, forests, and parks) and blue spaces (lakes, rivers, and coastal waters) on multiple non-communicable disease outcomes, including respiratory diseases, diabetes, stroke, coronary heart disease, ischemic heart disease, and cardiovascular diseases have been found. Green and blue spaces additionally provide regulatory services and health-related benefits including urban heat regulation, noise reduction, improved air quality and moderation of climate extremes, pollination, pest regulation, seed dispersal, and global climate regulation, which are commonly considered protective factors for cardiovascular disease and other outcomes. Neighborhood with a higher walkability can effectively reduce the risk of diabetes. Green spaces and walk-friendly built environments also promote physical activity, social interactions, and psychological well-being, thereby benefiting the overall health of urban residents [59].

Conversely, proximity to major highways, industries and landfills can pose serious threats to human health. Proximity to major roads has deleterious effects on cardiovascular diseases, lung cancer, and type 2 diabetes. Leukemia and lung cancer can also be induced by prolonged exposure to industrial sites. Additionally, residential proximity to landfills is associated with cardiovascular disease, respiratory diseases, and some types of cancer. Pathways may be related to ambient air toxins emitted from industrial sites and major highways [59]. Climate change represents a threat to urban infrastructure and the built environment. Coastal and low-lying geographic areas, as well as densely populated cities with poor infrastructure services and a lack of green spaces, offer less protection against the potential health risks associated with extreme weather events, contributing to vulnerability to climate change [4].

6.3 Environmental Inequities as Determinants of Cardiovascular Health Inequities

It has been long recognized that social determinants and inequities can affect the health of populations [66, 67]. Social determinants usually associated with health outcomes are socioeconomical position, race or ethnicity, networks of social support, culture and language, access to care, and residential environment [68]. Extensive literature demonstrates the disparities in cardiovascular health for different groups [20, 68, 69]. A couple of topics that are mainstream in this area are: first, how upstream social determinants, such governance and policies, determine health disparities, and the second, how these social differences are embodied in people, how they "get under the skin." It can be argued that our surrounding, our neighborhoods, the air we breathe might be involved [67].

The concepts of environmental justice point directly to these environmental inequities and how they can affect our health [9]. Environmental justice put the light in the unequal spatial distribution, where we live, play, learn, and work, of the environmental risks and benefits of societal activities, and how these burdens disproportionately fall upon some social groups. This disproportion in understood at many levels: in the first macro level, as the lack of political voice so to influence politically in the distribution process, in the second communitarian level, as spatial segregation of people and the spatial accumulation of risks in their surroundings, and in the third individual level, as the individual vulnerability and lack of capacity to cope with the extra burden experienced [9]. Thus, some marginalized groups might not have the political voice to avoid the location of toxic waste in their surroundings; their neighborhood would deteriorate, increasing their exposures to pollutants, resulting in many already vulnerable individuals getting sick, which is aggravated by the lack of access to good health care to cope with it. This traditional view of environmental justice has been enriched to encompass a global perspective, contrasting the global north and the global south. It put the focus in the disproportion, at the global level, of where extraction, production, consumption, and disposal happen; in summary, who, get the benefits and who bears the burdens. Additionally, new perspectives on sustainability, climate justice, and interspecies and intergenerational justice have been moved to the front line [8, 70].

Air pollution is a good example of environmental inequity. Large number of studies have compared exposures to air pollution by social determinants, finding large disproportions by socioeconomical status, particularly in the US [71]. These disproportionate exposures occur not only for air pollutants but for many other chemical pollutants, affecting vulnerable populations near industrial sites, major roadways, and agricultural operations [72]. A well-known example in Chile is the Quintero-Puchuncaví industrial area, where 12 companies have gathered since the 1960s emitting all type of pollutants to the nearby populations [73–75]. Another particularly interesting example of air pollution and CVD inequities was reported by Bevan et al. Using US counties as unit of observation, they found higher exposures to $PM_{2.5}$ in counties with higher social deprivation, and at the same time, stronger associations between CVD and $PM_{2.5}$ in these counties [76]. In another study, Mujahid et al. found that black adults living in neighborhoods that have been historically "redlined," a form of historical discrimination sanctioned by governments, presented lower indexes of cardiovascular health [77].

At the global level, large differences in exposures have been seen between regions as mentioned in Sect. 6.1.1 [2, 47]. Additionally, evidence of disparities by social determinants in regions other than North America and Europe can be found but are scanter [71]. In Latin America, for example, evidence is not abundant and is limited to three countries (Chile, Brazil, and México); most important, authors highlight the lack of studies analyzing race or ethnicity considering the colonial and slavery historical past of the region [78]. In general, there is a paucity of studies of environmental risks and inequities from the global south [71, 78, 79].

Besides being the major threat facing our generation [80–82], climate change stands out for the high inequity that entails both its causes and impacts. There is a large disproportion in greenhouse emissions causing climate change, with some countries (EEUU, Europe, China, India) leading by far. This disproportion is increased and shifted to rich countries of the global north when emissions are considered in terms of consumption, i.e., not attributing the emission to where a product is manufactured but where they are consumed [83, 84]. The impacts, not only to health but to ecosystems, the economy, and other societal outcomes, are also greatly disproportionate between the global north and the global south but in the opposite direction as with the emissions [85].

Within the cities, many low-income residents could only afford to live in informal setting, exposed to high risks that may add to their already fragile health. Additionally, a disproportionate distribution of environmental stressors is expected as urban heat islands, urban green, environmental hazards and pollutants, and access to healthy waterways [86]. Vulnerable populations, including children, the elderly, people with disabilities, racial and ethnic minorities, and people of low socioeconomic status, are at particular risk for adverse health impacts due to poorly designed urban environment. These people may have less access to parks, green areas, and open spaces for physical activity and to healthy food stores. They may live near busy roads that make walking difficult and contribute to high noise levels and poor air quality. They may not have a car and public transportation may be poor, limiting their access to many of the goods and services available to other members of society [57, 62].

Urban population is expected to rise in the range of billion in the next decades, with most of the growth happening in cities of the global south [87]. At the same time much of the impacts of climate change will happen in these cities, which are chronically underfunded for the required adaptation efforts. Within-city inequities might even increase, as adaptation plans will likely differ between affluent parts of the city and their less affluent counterpart [87]. This can be illustrated by the luxury effect [86], where affluent neighborhoods, with greater discretionary income and capital, could afford greener and more biodiverse surrounding, which in turn, could protect them of heat waves, air pollution, and other environmental hazards.

Two final comments on inequities are regarding the concepts of degrowth and intergenerational justice. Regarding the first, Scheidel et al. denounce that many large economies have developed by fostering an unsustainable and unjust growth [88]. In what is called the "imperial way of life," rich economies have prospered through the unlimited appropriation of resources and work force. From this diagnostic emerge degrowth movements that point to a radical change in ways of production, away from industrial, capitalistic profiles. From the global south, on the other hand, the stress is put in justice. Many countries of the region have suffered scarcity and are not convened by degrowth, asking: degrowth of what? In part it could be understood that countries living an imperial way of life should reduce their consumption, but many regions in the global south will need to grow in infrastructure and other benefits of modernization to attain a decent quality of life [89]. For intergenerational justice or intergenerational responsibility, a driving idea is that our generation must pass our world intact to the next generation. In this view, we are custodians, not masters, of the biosphere, and warns us of the suffering and tragic choices that we will pass to our descendants [70] that could come from our inaction.

6.4 Recommendations to Face Environmental Challenges in Highly Unequal Contexts

Several recommendations have been emanated from medical and scientific societies and from major reviews, particularly to face the air pollution and climate change threats. Some of the statements stress the benefits of individual actions such as use of filtrations systems to protect individuals against air pollution, the use of air quality indexes and maps so people can avoid exposures, and heat warning systems to avoid the effects of heat waves [3, 16, 23]. Others point to a somehow more collective action of the health care personnel through the direct action in reducing the healthcare sector emissions and through research and education, to practitioners and patients, of the impacts of the environment on health so it can translate in public advocacy. Some of the major review, on the other hand, stress the point of collective action and highlight that individual measures are unlikely to solve the problems and argue for cross-level global actions that encompass actions to control air pollution, the effects of climate change, considering inequalities [4]. Some of the points raised are supporting the work of the air quality standards and comply with the Paris agreements, the need of an energy transition with the phase-out of fossil fuels, reorient city design to decrease car use, increase public transport and walkability, increase green space and in general create people oriented cities, besides arguing for a plant-based diet and creation of adaptation plans for climate change with a focus on vulnerable people [4, 5, 12]. Shi et al. are even more comprehensive when considering urban adaptation to climate change and propose that plans should include citizen participation, funding at a global scale, and apply multilevel and multi-scalar approaches, integrating justice criteria for infrastructure financing of rapid grow, low budget cities [87].

We conclude with a final reflection regarding a broader view of the problem and solutions. Throughout the chapter, we have seen how all issue regarding the environment, health, and equity are quite interlinked among them usually exacerbating their impacts (Fig. 6.1). It is not only CVD that are impacted by these environmental stressors but many other diseases. It is not only that we affect our nearby environment, but also of other species and ultimately the whole planet. It is not only us now, but the ones to come. And the ones already burdened will be even more. In this context we urge to consider broader measures to tackle the problem, modifying the driving forces to get out of the loops as presented previously.

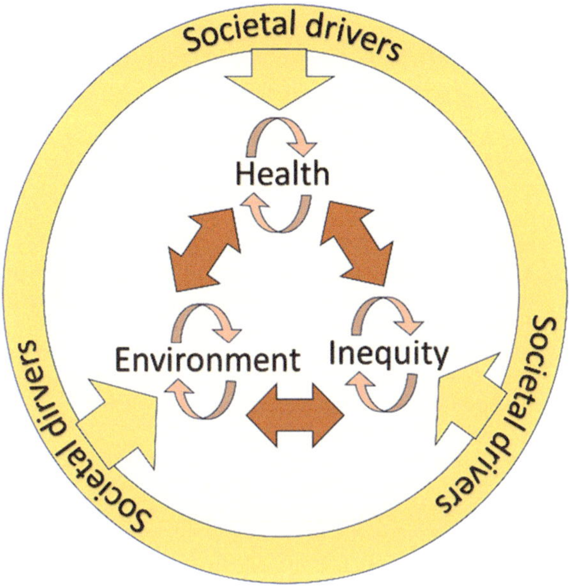

Fig. 6.1 Synergistic loops between environment, health, and equity

Glossary

Air pollution Gases and particles suspended in air that can be inhaled and produce health effects.

Built environment Totality of the places and the infrastructure created, such as buildings, streets, and parks, are the main settings where we live, work, study, and play.

Climate change Refers to long-term changes in temperatures and weather patterns.

Environment Circumstances, objects, or conditions by which one is surrounded.

Environmental justice The fair treatment and meaningful involvement of all people regardless of race, color, national origin, or income, with respect to the development, implementation, and enforcement of environmental laws, regulations, and policies.

Environmental stressors They are components of the natural or altered environment that could interact with organisms triggering a response that can lead to impaired health.

Green spaces An area of grass, trees, or other vegetation set apart for recreational or aesthetic purposes in an otherwise urban environment.

Greenhouse gases (GHGs) The gases in the atmosphere that raise the surface temperature of planets such as the Earth.

Urban environment An area with an increased density of human-created structures in comparison to the areas surrounding it.

References

1. Haines A, Frumkin H. Planetary health. Cambridge University Press; 2021. https://doi.org/10.1017/9781108698054.
2. Roth GA, Mensah GA, Johnson CO, Addolorato G, Ammirati E, Baddour LM, Barengo NC, Beaton AZ, Benjamin EJ, Benziger CP, Bonny A, Brauer M, Brodmann M, Cahill TJ, Carapetis J, Catapano AL, Chugh SS, Cooper LT, Coresh J, et al. Global burden of cardiovascular diseases and risk factors, 1990–2019. J Am Coll Cardiol. 2020;76(25):2982–3021. https://doi.org/10.1016/j.jacc.2020.11.010.
3. Al-Kindi SG, Brook RD, Biswal S, Rajagopalan S. Environmental determinants of cardiovascular disease: lessons learned from air pollution. Nat Rev Cardiol. 2020;17(10):656–72. https://doi.org/10.1038/s41569-020-0371-2.
4. Khraishah H, Alahmad B, Ostergard RL, AlAshqar A, Albaghdadi M, Vellanki N, Chowdhury MM, Al-Kindi SG, Zanobetti A, Gasparrini A, Rajagopalan S. Climate change and cardiovascular disease: implications for global health. Nat Rev Cardiol. 2022;19(12):798–812. https://doi.org/10.1038/s41569-022-00720-x.
5. Rajagopalan S, Landrigan PJ. Pollution and the heart. N Engl J Med. 2021;385(20):1881–92. https://doi.org/10.1056/nejmra2030281.
6. Frumkin H. Introduction. In: Environmental health: from global to local. 2nd ed. Jossey-Bass; 2010. p. XXIX–LVII.
7. Frumkin H. Introduction to environmental health. In: Environmental health: from global to local. 3rd ed. Jossey-Bass; 2016. p. 45–68.
8. Fragkou MC. Environmental justice. In: The Wiley Blackwell encyclopedia of urban and regional studies. Wiley; 2019. p. 1–6. https://doi.org/10.1002/9781118568446.eurs0091.
9. Kruize H, Droomers M, van Kamp I, Ruijsbroek A. What causes environmental inequalities and related health effects? An analysis of evolving concepts. Int J Environ Res Public Health. 2014;11(6):5807–27. https://doi.org/10.3390/ijerph110605807.
10. Alahmad B, Khraishah H, Althalji K, Borchert W, Al-Mulla F, Koutrakis P. Connections between air pollution, climate change, and cardiovascular health. Can J Cardiol. 2023;39(9):1182–90. https://doi.org/10.1016/j.cjca.2023.03.025.
11. Murray CJL, Aravkin AY, Zheng P, Abbafati C, Abbas KM, Abbasi-Kangevari M, Abd-Allah F, Abdelalim A, Abdollahi M, Abdollahpour I, Abegaz KH, Abolhassani H, Aboyans V, Abreu LG, Abrigo MRM, Abualhasan A, Abu-Raddad LJ, Abushouk AI, Adabi M, et al. Global burden of 87 risk factors in 204 countries and territories, 1990–2019: a systematic analysis for the Global Burden of Disease Study 2019. Lancet. 2020;396(10258):1223–49. https://doi.org/10.1016/S0140-6736(20)30752-2.
12. Zhao Q, Yu P, Mahendran R, Huang W, Gao Y, Yang Z, Ye T, Wen B, Wu Y, Li S, Guo Y. Global climate change and human health: pathways and possible solutions. Eco Environ Health. 2022;1(2):53–62. https://doi.org/10.1016/j.eehl.2022.04.004.
13. Brook RD, Franklin B, Cascio W, Hong Y, Howard G, Lipsett M, Luepker R, Mittleman M, Samet J, Smith SC, Tager I. Air pollution and cardiovascular disease. Circulation. 2004;109(21):2655–71. https://doi.org/10.1161/01.CIR.0000128587.30041.C8.
14. Brook RD, Rajagopalan S, Pope CA, Brook JR, Bhatnagar A, Diez-Roux AV, Holguin F, Hong Y, Luepker RV, Mittleman MA, Peters A, Siscovick D, Smith SC, Whitsel L, Kaufman JD. Particulate matter air pollution and cardiovascular disease. Circulation. 2010;121(21):2331–78. https://doi.org/10.1161/CIR.0b013e3181dbece1.
15. Gulati M. The role of the preventive cardiologist in addressing climate change. Am J Prev Cardiol. 2022;11:100375. https://doi.org/10.1016/j.ajpc.2022.100375.
16. Kaufman JD, Elkind MSV, Bhatnagar A, Koehler K, Balmes JR, Sidney S, Burroughs Peña MS, Dockery DW, Hou L, Brook RD, Laden F, Rajagopalan S, Bishop Kendrick K, Turner JR. Guidance to reduce the cardiovascular burden of ambient air pollutants: a policy statement from the American Heart Association. Circulation. 2020;142(23) https://doi.org/10.1161/CIR.0000000000000930.

17. Peters A, Schneider A. Cardiovascular risks of climate change. Nat Rev Cardiol. 2021;18(1) https://doi.org/10.1038/s41569-020-00473-5.
18. Münzel T, Hahad O, Daiber A, Landrigan PJ. Soil and water pollution and human health: what should cardiologists worry about? Cardiovasc Res. 2023;119(2):440–9. https://doi.org/10.1093/cvr/cvac082.
19. Rose G. Strategy of preventive medicine. Oxford University Press; 1993.
20. Powell-Wiley TM, Baumer Y, Baah FO, Baez AS, Farmer N, Mahlobo CT, Pita MA, Potharaju KA, Tamura K, Wallen GR. Social determinants of cardiovascular disease. Circ Res. 2022;130(5):782–99. https://doi.org/10.1161/CIRCRESAHA.121.319811.
21. Thurston GD, Kipen H, Annesi-Maesano I, Balmes J, Brook RD, Cromar K, De Matteis S, Forastiere F, Forsberg B, Frampton MW, Grigg J, Heederik D, Kelly FJ, Kuenzli N, Laumbach R, Peters A, Rajagopalan ST, Rich D, Ritz B, et al. A joint ERS/ATS policy statement: what constitutes an adverse health effect of air pollution? An analytical framework. Eur Respir J. 2017;49(1) https://doi.org/10.1183/13993003.00419-2016.
22. World Health Organization. Air quality guidelines: global update 2005. 2005.
23. Brauer M, Casadei B, Harrington RA, Kovacs R, Sliwa K, Brauer M, Davaakhuu N, Hadley M, Kass D, Miller M, Escamilla Nunez MC, Ta-Chen Su DP, Vaartijes ICH, Vedanthan R. Taking a stand against air pollution—the impact on cardiovascular disease. Circulation. 2021;143(14):E800–4. https://doi.org/10.1161/CIRCULATIONAHA.120.052666.
24. Blanco E, Rubilar F, Quinteros ME, Cayupi K, Ayala S, Lu S, Jimenez RB, Cárdenas JP, Blazquez CA, Delgado-Saborit JM, Harrison RM, Ruiz-Rudolph P. Spatial distribution of particulate matter on winter nights in Temuco, Chile: studying the impact of residential wood-burning using mobile monitoring. Atmos Environ. 2022;286:119255. https://doi.org/10.1016/j.atmosenv.2022.119255.
25. Quinteros ME, Blanco E, Sanabria J, Rosas-Diaz F, Blazquez CA, Ayala S, Cárdenas-R JP, Stone EA, Sybesma K, Delgado-Saborit JM, Harrison RM, Ruiz-Rudolph P. Spatio-temporal distribution of particulate matter and wood-smoke tracers in Temuco, Chile: a city heavily impacted by residential wood-burning. Atmos Environ. 2023;294:119529. https://doi.org/10.1016/j.atmosenv.2022.119529.
26. World Health Organization. Air quality guidelines 2021. 2021. https://apps.who.int/iris/handle/10665/345329.
27. Hewitt CN. The atmospheric chemistry of sulphur and nitrogen in power station plumes. Atmos Environ. 2001;35(7):1155–70. https://doi.org/10.1016/S1352-2310(00)00463-5.
28. Kanakidou M, Seinfeld JH, Pandis SN, Barnes I, Dentener FJ, Facchini MC, Van Dingenen R, Ervens B, Nenes A, Nielsen CJ, Swietlicki E, Putaud JP, Balkanski Y, Fuzzi S, Horth J, Moortgat GK, Winterhalter R, Myhre CEL, Tsigaridis K, et al. Organic aerosol and global climate modelling: a review. Atmos Chem Phys. 2005;5(4):1053–123. https://doi.org/10.5194/acp-5-1053-2005.
29. Ruiz PA, Gupta T, Kang CM, Lawrence JE, Ferguson ST, Wolfson JM, Rohr AC, Koutrakis P. Development of an exposure system for the toxicological evaluation of particles derived from coal-fired power plants. Inhal Toxicol. 2007;19(8):607–19. https://doi.org/10.1080/08958370701353148.
30. Ruiz PA, Lawrence JE, Wolfson JM, Ferguson ST, Gupta T, Kang CM, Koutrakis P. Development and evaluation of a photochemical chamber to examine the toxicity of coal-fired power plant emissions. Inhal Toxicol. 2007;19(8):597–606. https://doi.org/10.1080/08958370701353361.
31. Prieto-Parra L, Yohannessen K, Brea C, Vidal D, Ubilla CA, Ruiz-Rudolph P. Air pollution, PM 2.5 composition, source factors, and respiratory symptoms in asthmatic and nonasthmatic children in Santiago, Chile. Environ Int. 2017;101:190–200. https://doi.org/10.1016/j.envint.2017.01.021.
32. Ruiz-Rudolph P, Arias N, Pardo S, Meyer M, Mesías S, Galleguillos C, Schiattino I, Gutiérrez L. Impact of large industrial emission sources on mortality and morbidity in Chile: a small-areas study. Environ Int. 2016;92–93:130–8. https://doi.org/10.1016/j.envint.2016.03.036.
33. Karanasiou A, Alastuey A, Amato F, Renzi M, Stafoggia M, Tobias A, Reche C, Forastiere F, Gumy S, Mudu P, Querol X. Short-term health effects from outdoor exposure to bio-

mass burning emissions: a review. Sci Total Environ. 2021;781 https://doi.org/10.1016/j.scitotenv.2021.146739.
34. Naeher LP, Brauer M, Lipsett M, Zelikoff JT, Simpson CD, Koenig JQ, Smith KR. Woodsmoke health effects: a review. Inhal Toxicol. 2007;19(1):67–106. https://doi.org/10.1080/08958370600985875.
35. Sigsgaard T, Forsberg B, Annesi-Maesano I, Blomberg A, Bølling A, Boman C, Bønløkke J, Brauer M, Bruce N, Héroux ME, Hirvonen MR, Kelly F, Künzli N, Lundbäck B, Moshammer H, Noonan C, Pagels J, Sallsten G, Sculier JP, Brunekreef B. Health impacts of anthropogenic biomass burning in the developed world. Eur Respir J. 2015;46(6):1577–88. https://doi.org/10.1183/13993003.01865-2014.
36. Hoek G, Brunekreef B, Goldbohm S, Fischer P, van den Brandt PA. Association between mortality and indicators of traffic-related air pollution in the Netherlands: a cohort study. Lancet. 2002;360(9341):1203–9. https://doi.org/10.1016/S0140-6736(02)11280-3.
37. Suárez L, Mesías S, Iglesias V, Silva C, Cáceres DD, Ruiz-Rudolph P. Personal exposure to particulate matter in commuters using different transport modes (bus, bicycle, car and subway) in an assigned route in downtown Santiago, Chile. Environ Sci Process Impacts. 2014;16(6):1309–17. https://doi.org/10.1039/c3em00648d.
38. Zhu Y, Hinds WC, Kim S, Shen S, Sioutas C. Study of ultrafine particles near a major highway with heavy-duty diesel traffic. Atmos Environ. 2002;36(27):4323–35. https://doi.org/10.1016/S1352-2310(02)00354-0.
39. Larson T, Su J, Baribeau AM, Buzzelli M, Setton E, Brauer M. A spatial model of urban winter woodsmoke concentrations. Environ Sci Technol. 2007;41(7):2429–36. https://doi.org/10.1021/es0614060.
40. Quinteros ME, Blazquez C, Ayala S, Kilby D, Cárdenas-R JP, Ossa X, Rosas-Diaz F, Stone EA, Blanco E, Delgado-Saborit J-M, Harrison RM, Ruiz-Rudolph P. Development of spatio-temporal land use regression models for fine particulate matter and wood-burning tracers in Temuco, Chile. Environ Sci Technol. 2023; https://doi.org/10.1021/acs.est.3c00720.
41. Su JG, Allen G, Miller PJ, Brauer M. Spatial modeling of residential woodsmoke across a non-urban upstate New York region. Air Qual Atmos Health. 2013;6(1):85–94. https://doi.org/10.1007/s11869-011-0148-1.
42. McCracken JP, Wellenius GA, Bloomfield GS, Brook RD, Tolunay HE, Dockery DW, Rabadan-Diehl C, Checkley W, Rajagopalan S. Household air pollution from solid fuel use: evidence for links to CVD. Glob Heart. 2012;7(3):223. https://doi.org/10.1016/j.gheart.2012.06.010.
43. Yucra S, Tapia V, Steenland K, Naeher LP, Gonzales GF. Association between biofuel exposure and adverse birth outcomes at high altitudes in Peru: a matched case-control study. Int J Occup Environ Health. 2011;17(4):307–13. https://doi.org/10.1179/107735211799041869.
44. Yucra S, Tapia V, Steenland K, Naeher LP, Gonzales GF. Maternal exposure to biomass smoke and carbon monoxide in relation to adverse pregnancy outcome in two high altitude cities of Peru. Environ Res. 2014;130:29–33. https://doi.org/10.1016/j.envres.2014.01.008.
45. Burney J, Persad G, Proctor J, Bendavid E, Burke M, Heft-Neal S. Geographically resolved social cost of anthropogenic emissions accounting for both direct and climate-mediated effects. Sci Adv. 2022;8(38) https://doi.org/10.1126/sciadv.abn7307.
46. Zhang X, Zhao L, Tong D, Wu G, Dan M, Teng B. A systematic review of global desert dust and associated human health effects. Atmosphere. 2016;7(12):158. https://doi.org/10.3390/atmos7120158.
47. Cohen AJ, Brauer M, Burnett R, Anderson HR, Frostad J, Estep K, Balakrishnan K, Brunekreef B, Dandona L, Dandona R, Feigin V, Freedman G, Hubbell B, Jobling A, Kan H, Knibbs L, Liu Y, Martin R, Morawska L, et al. Estimates and 25-year trends of the global burden of disease attributable to ambient air pollution: an analysis of data from the Global Burden of Diseases Study 2015. Lancet. 2017;389(10082):1907–18. https://doi.org/10.1016/S0140-6736(17)30505-6.
48. Lelieveld J, Evans JS, Fnais M, Giannadaki D, Pozzer A. The contribution of outdoor air pollution sources to premature mortality on a global scale. Nature. 2015;525(7569):367–71. https://doi.org/10.1038/nature15371.

49. Park S, Allen RJ, Lim CH. A likely increase in fine particulate matter and premature mortality under future climate change. Air Qual Atmos Health. 2020;13(2):143–51. https://doi.org/10.1007/s11869-019-00785-7.
50. United Nations. What is climate change? 2023. https://www.un.org/en/climatechange/what-is-climate-change.
51. IPCC. Global warming of 1.5°C: annex I. Cambridge University Press; 2022. https://doi.org/10.1017/9781009157940.
52. Lelieveld J, Klingmüller K, Pozzer A, Burnett RT, Haines A, Ramanathan V. Effects of fossil fuel and total anthropogenic emission removal on public health and climate. Proc Natl Acad Sci. 2019;116(15):7192–7. https://doi.org/10.1073/pnas.1819989116.
53. IPCC. Summary for policymakers. In: Climate change 2022—impacts, adaptation and vulnerability. Cambridge University Press; 2023. p. 3–34. https://doi.org/10.1017/9781009325844.001.
54. NOAA. Annual 2022 global climate report. 2023. https://www.ncei.noaa.gov/access/monitoring/monthly-report/global/202213.
55. AghaKouchak A, Chiang F, Huning LS, Love CA, Mallakpour I, Mazdiyasni O, Moftakhari H, Papalexiou SM, Ragno E, Sadegh M. Climate extremes and compound hazards in a warming world. Annu Rev Earth Planet Sci. 2020;48(1):519–48. https://doi.org/10.1146/annurev-earth-071719-055228.
56. World Bank. Urban development. 2023. https://www.worldbank.org/en/topic/urbandevelopment/overview.
57. Dannenberg AL, Capon AG. Healthy communities. In: Frumkin H, editor. Environmental health: from global to local. 3rd ed. Jossey-Bass; 2016.
58. Hall CM, Ram Y. Walk score® and its potential contribution to the study of active transport and walkability: a critical and systematic review. Transp Res D Transp Environ. 2018;61:310–24. https://doi.org/10.1016/j.trd.2017.12.018.
59. Zhang Y, Liu N, Li Y, Long Y, Baumgartner J, Adamkiewicz G, Bhalla K, Rodriguez J, Gemmell E. Neighborhood infrastructure-related risk factors and non-communicable diseases: a systematic meta-review. Environ Health. 2023;22(1) https://doi.org/10.1186/s12940-022-00955-8.
60. Cepeda M, Schoufour J, Freak-Poli R, Koolhaas CM, Dhana K, Bramer WM, Franco OH. Levels of ambient air pollution according to mode of transport: a systematic review. Lancet Public Health. 2017;2(1):e23–34. https://doi.org/10.1016/S2468-2667(16)30021-4.
61. Kondo M, Fluehr J, McKeon T, Branas C. Urban green space and its impact on human health. Int J Environ Res Public Health. 2018;15(3):445. https://doi.org/10.3390/ijerph15030445.
62. World Health Organization. Urban green space and health: intervention impacts and effectiveness: report of a meeting. 2016.
63. Pope CA, Dockery DW. Health effects of fine particulate air pollution: lines that connect. J Air Waste Manage Assoc. 2006;56(6):709–42. https://doi.org/10.1080/10473289.2006.10464485.
64. Desai Y, Khraishah H, Alahmad B, Chan HTH. Heat and the heart. Yale J Biol Med. 2023;96:197.
65. Chen H, Samet JM, Bromberg PA, Tong H. Cardiovascular health impacts of wildfire smoke exposure. Particle Fibre Toxicol. 2021;18(1):2. https://doi.org/10.1186/s12989-020-00394-8.
66. Krieger N. Epidemiology and the people's health. Oxford University Press; 2011. https://doi.org/10.1093/acprof:oso/9780195383874.001.0001.
67. Palmer RC, Ismond D, Rodriquez EJ, Kaufman JS. Social determinants of health: future directions for health disparities research. Am J Public Health. 2019;109:S70–1. https://doi.org/10.2105/AJPH.2019.304964.
68. Havranek EP, Mujahid MS, Barr DA, Blair IV, Cohen MS, Cruz-Flores S, Davey-Smith G, Dennison-Himmelfarb CR, Lauer MS, Lockwood DW, Rosal M, Yancy CW. Social determinants of risk and outcomes for cardiovascular disease: a scientific statement from the American Heart Association. Circulation. 2015;132(9):873–98. https://doi.org/10.1161/CIR.0000000000000228.
69. Teshale AB, Htun HL, Owen A, Gasevic D, Phyo AZZ, Fancourt D, Ryan J, Steptoe A, Freak-Poli R. The role of social determinants of health in cardiovascular diseases: an umbrella review. J Am Heart Assoc. 2023;12(13) https://doi.org/10.1161/JAHA.123.029765.

70. Foster A, Cole J, Petrikova I, Farlow A, Frumkin H. Planetary health ethics. In: Myers S, Frumkin H, editors. Planetary health: protecting nature to protect ourselves. Island Press; 2020. p. 453–74. https://doi.org/10.5822/978-1-61091-966-1.
71. Hajat A, Hsia C, O'Neill MS. Socioeconomic disparities and air pollution exposure: a global review. Curr Environ Health Rep. 2015;2(4):440–50. https://doi.org/10.1007/s40572-015-0069-5.
72. Solomon GM, Morello-Frosch R, Zeise L, Faust JB. Cumulative environmental impacts: science and policy to protect communities. Annu Rev Public Health. 2016;37(1):83–96. https://doi.org/10.1146/annurev-publhealth-032315-021807.
73. Gayo EM, Muñoz AA, Maldonado A, Lavergne C, Francois JP, Rodríguez D, Klock-Barría K, Sheppard PR, Aguilera-Betti I, Alonso-Hernández C, Mena-Carrasco M, Urquiza A, Gallardo L. A cross-cutting approach for relating anthropocene, environmental injustice and sacrifice zones. Earths Future. 2022;10(4) https://doi.org/10.1029/2021EF002217.
74. Martínez Órdenes M. Cerrar Ventanas para abrir puertas: propuesta ética para la investigación en salud pública en zonas de alta vulnerabilidad climática. Salud Ciencia Tecnol. 2023;3:417. https://doi.org/10.56294/saludcyt2023417.
75. Ruiz Rudolph P. Escrito sobre relación de causalidad en el caso de daño ambiental por emisiones del Complejo Industrial Ventanas. Cuadernos Médico Sociales. 2023;63(2):93–109. https://doi.org/10.56116/cms.v63.n2.2023.1429.
76. Bevan GH, Freedman DA, Lee EK, Rajagopalan S, Al-Kindi SG. Association between ambient air pollution and county-level cardiovascular mortality in the United States by social deprivation index. Am Heart J. 2021;235:125–31. https://doi.org/10.1016/j.ahj.2021.02.005.
77. Mujahid MS, Gao X, Tabb LP, Morris C, Lewis TT. Historical redlining and cardiovascular health: the multi-ethnic study of atherosclerosis. Proc Natl Acad Sci. 2021;118(51) https://doi.org/10.1073/pnas.2110986118.
78. Gouveia N, Slovic AD, Kanai CM, Soriano L. Air pollution and environmental justice in Latin America: where are we and how can we move forward? Curr Environ Health Rep. 2022;9(2):152–64. https://doi.org/10.1007/s40572-022-00341-z.
79. AghaKouchak A, Huning LS, Chiang F, Sadegh M, Vahedifard F, Mazdiyasni O, Moftakhari H, Mallakpour I. How do natural hazards cascade to cause disasters? Nature. 2018;561(7724):458–60. https://doi.org/10.1038/d41586-018-06783-6.
80. Perera ATD, Nik VM, Chen D, Scartezzini J-L, Hong T. Quantifying the impacts of climate change and extreme climate events on energy systems. Nat Energy. 2020;5(2):150–9. https://doi.org/10.1038/s41560-020-0558-0.
81. Romanello M, McGushin A, Di Napoli C, Drummond P, Hughes N, Jamart L, Kennard H, Lampard P, Solano Rodriguez B, Arnell N, Ayeb-Karlsson S, Belesova K, Cai W, Campbell-Lendrum D, Capstick S, Chambers J, Chu L, Ciampi L, Dalin C, et al. The 2021 report of the lancet countdown on health and climate change: code red for a healthy future. Lancet. 2021;398(10311):1619–62. https://doi.org/10.1016/S0140-6736(21)01787-6.
82. Vicedo-Cabrera AM, Scovronick N, Sera F, Royé D, Schneider R, Tobias A, Astrom C, Guo Y, Honda Y, Hondula DM, Abrutzky R, Tong S, de Sousa Zanotti Stagliorio Coelho M, Saldiva PHN, Lavigne E, Correa PM, Ortega NV, Kan H, Osorio S, et al. The burden of heat-related mortality attributable to recent human-induced climate change. Nat Clim Chang. 2021;11(6):492–500. https://doi.org/10.1038/s41558-021-01058-x.
83. Haines A, Frumkin H. Sustaining urban health in the anthropocene epoch. In: Planetary health: safeguarding human health and the environment in the anthropocene. Cambridge University Press; 2021. p. 291–309. https://doi.org/10.1017/9781108698054.
84. Pichler P-P, Zwickel T, Chavez A, Kretschmer T, Seddon J, Weisz H. Reducing urban greenhouse gas footprints. Sci Rep. 2017;7(1):14659. https://doi.org/10.1038/s41598-017-15303-x.
85. Timmons Roberts J. The international dimension of climate justice and the need for international adaptation funding. Environ Just. 2009;2(4):185–90. https://doi.org/10.1089/env.2009.0029.
86. Schell CJ, Dyson K, Fuentes TL, Des Roches S, Harris NC, Miller DS, Woelfle-Erskine CA, Lambert MR. The ecological and evolutionary consequences of systemic racism in urban environments. Science. 2020;369(6509) https://doi.org/10.1126/SCIENCE.AAY4497.

87. Shi L, Chu E, Anguelovski I, Aylett A, Debats J, Goh K, Schenk T, Seto KC, Dodman D, Roberts D, Roberts JT, Van Deveer SD. Roadmap towards justice in urban climate adaptation research. Nat Clim Chang. 2016;6(2):131–7. https://doi.org/10.1038/nclimate2841.
88. Scheidel A, Schaffartzik A. A socio-metabolic perspective on environmental justice and degrowth movements. Ecol Econ. 2019;161:330–3. https://doi.org/10.1016/j.ecolecon.2019.02.023.
89. Rodríguez-Labajos B, Yánez I, Bond P, Greyl L, Munguti S, Ojo GU, Overbeek W. Not so natural an alliance? Degrowth and environmental justice movements in the global south. Ecol Econ. 2019;157:175–84. https://doi.org/10.1016/j.ecolecon.2018.11.007.

Chapter 7
COVID-19 Pandemia, Socio-economic Status, Limitations, and Outcomes Observed in the Access to Health Care

Luis Fidel Avendaño, Mauricio Canals, Carolina Nazzal Nazal, and Faustino Alonso

Subtitles

1. Virological Aspects

1.1. History of epidemics impact in the human communities. Pandemics have ever existed and currently viruses are the principal responsible agents.

1.2. Factors participating in the emergence of outbreaks and pandemics. Although factors depending on agent, environment, and host always participate, those referred to the agent are of principal importance.

1.3. Viral participation in the generation of pandemics. Historically viruses have caused the majority of pandemics because its biologic characteristic enables their genetic variations. The RNA viruses are the main candidates for future pandemics.

1.4. The COVID-19 pandemic. The SARS-CoV-2 jumped in 2019 from an animal reservoir to the men and it acquired the capacity of easy transmission through the air. And it has continued mutating and so evading the control measures that science is recommending.

2. COVID-19 pandemic: The case of Chile. This is a long and narrow country with 19,500,000 inhabitants living in the southwest of South America. Their social status is characterized by a life expectancy at birth of around 80 years, infant mortality of 6.5/1000 alive newborns, general mortality of 6.5/1000 inhabitants: in relation to the latter, deaths from cerebrovascular disease (48.3/100,000) and myocardial ischemic disease (45.7/100,000) account for the two more frequent specific causes.

L. F. Avendaño (✉)
Faculty of Medicine, University of Chile, Santiago, Chile
e-mail: lavendan@uchile.cl

M. Canals · C. N. Nazzal · F. Alonso
Faculty of Medicine, School of Public Health, University of Chile, Santiago, Chile
e-mail: mcanals@uchile.cl; cnazzal@uchile.cl; falonso@uchile.cl

T. Romero et al. (eds.), *Global Challenges in Cardiovascular Prevention in Populations with Low Socioeconomic Status*,
https://doi.org/10.1007/978-3-031-79051-5_7

Low-income poverty affects 15% of the inhabitants and the average schooling reached 11.7 years in 2020.

2.1 Measures adopted in Chile to mitigate the effects of COVID-19. The prompt and permanent access to different vaccines allowed high immunization coverage, which hopefully reduced the lethality of severe cases. Also, the treatment for severe hospitalized cases improved with a larger supply of new personnel and equipment support.

2.2. Impact of COVID-19 in health outcomes. Most of the health resources were destined to severe COVID cases and many out-patient health actions were delayed.

2.2.1. Hospitalizations. There was a great demand for intensive care units for COVID, but it was resolved with a 243% increase in the number of beds and with most O_2 supplementation in many wards.

2.2.2. Cardiovascular impact. Despite the decline of the primary healthcare consecutive to the priority to COVID management, the universal coverage for acute myocardial infarction implemented in Chile in the 90s was effective enough in preventing an increase in AMI lethality during the pandemic.

2.2.3. Health expenditures. A brief comment on expenses increment for pandemic management is done.

3. **Lessons and Challenges for Future Pandemics**

In Chile, the Public Health System traditionally responds promptly. Under the risk of the emerging COVID 19 pandemic, in March 2020 after the first case was reported, efforts for controlling its diffusion were initiated. The permanent information and counseling of WHO and PAHO helped the government authorities to assign personnel and resources to combat the pandemic. Chile was one of the first countries in producing worthy statistics related to the local impact and in adopting pandemic control measures, acquiring as soon as possible the vaccines commercially available as described in point 2. Health and Science Ministries and Universities collaborated in testing and evaluating many possible vaccines. Significant vaccination efforts were undertaken to achieve a herd immunity in the country; however, this goal was hindered by the permanent appearance of virus variants of concern causing the increase of new cases. National Health Service was permanently incrementing the personnel and equipment, mostly mounting new intensive care units (ICU) and coordinating the public and private health systems to satisfy the rising health demands.

The lesson for the future is that rapid diagnostic tests are necessary for measuring the factual magnitude of the problem, while science identifies the agent and starts the vaccine development race. In the meanwhile, it is necessary to implement non-pharmaceutical interventions to reduce COVID-19 mortality and healthcare demand.

We think that the humankind has learnt a lot with the COVID-19 experience and is better prepared to contest a future pandemic emergence.

7.1 Virological Aspects

7.1.1 History of Epidemics Impact in the Human Communities

The epidemic and pandemic emergences have historically had a great influence on the human community according to accreditable information. They have been caused by bacteria, parasites, and viruses, the latter the more frequent agents. The control of those events has represented a great advance because the decreasing death rates has contributed to a significant increase in the population [1].

Smallpox, produced by a Poxvirus, has probably infected the human beings since10,000 years BC, being responsible for around 50% of lethality among the infected people and causing more than 300 million of deaths. The impact of the smallpox transmission during the Americas discovery in the fifteenth century has been extensively reported. The WHO concluded that the smallpox eradication by using a live smallpox vaccine had already occurred in 1980.

It has been historically estimated that *measles* virus has caused more than 200 million deaths through local and worldwide outbreaks and pandemics. However, its actual control also using a live virus vaccine represents other example of effective public health intervention. Its massive application has eliminated the infection in many countries and regions, but so far it has not been eradicated.

During the Middle Age, the *bubonic plague* or "black death," caused by the *Yersinia pestis* bacteria and transmitted by rats and fleas as vectors, produced 75 million of deaths, equivalent to 30–60% of the European population, taking advantage of the low socio-economic status in those times.

The *Spanish influenza* caused by influenza A virus (H1N1) in 1918, killed about 50 million people, far more than lost their lives in the whole First World War. Although vaccines and antiviral drugs have been developed so far, influenza viruses continue causing human and animal outbreaks and pandemics of variable magnitude. Their frequent mutation ability, supported by their particular molecular biology, represents a permanent threat of pandemic emergence as the epidemic history has clearly shown.

The *human immunodeficiency virus (HIV)*, starting from 1981, is today the principal pandemic responsible agent in the world, accounting for more than 25 million of deaths. Furthermore, in the twenty-first century another *influenza A* pandemic emerged (Hsw1N1-2009), despite the high scientific and technological advances (vaccines, antiviral, communications, transport, health systems, and others) and caused around 200,000 deaths, emphasizing that despite their relative simplicity and small size, the microbial agents are very difficult to control and combat. In the meanwhile, other outbreaks and pandemics have emerged, like dengue, Yellow fever, Zika virus, West Nile virus, Chikungunya virus, coronavirus, monkeypox, without provoking great international concern [2].

The present COVID-19 pandemia will be further analyzed to learn from the experience acquired through 3 years of public and private efforts trying to neutralize and avoid its effects.

7.1.2 Agents, Host, and Environmental Factors in the Emergence of Outbreaks and Pandemics

Factors depending on the agent, the host, and the environment participate in the etiology and pathogenesis of epidemics in different moments and proportions. During the Middle Ages and the Antiquity, probably the low socio-economic status facilitated the emergence of infectious diseases and the unawareness about their etiology, the ways of combating them and the persistence of inappropriate attitudes and habits contributed to prolong their diffusion.

The successive advances in science, technology, education, and other aspects permitted to progress in the socio-economic conditions for improving the public health care and decreasing their impact.

However, the modern way of life often includes human individual or group travelers to new territories, interacting with animals and plants and certainly new microbial agents for which there is not immunity, and a threat of emergence of new diseases.

Thus, in 2019 a new variant of SARS coronavirus made a host species jump from a bat through another animal (pangolin, *Manis javanica*) to a human being. However, some studies have suggested that many other vertebrates could have been the intermediate host in this species jump like palm civets, bamboo rats, raccoon dogs (*Nyctereutes procyonoides*), being probably the latter who transmitted the virus to the human specie. This kind of animal is commercially available in Wuhan as pet or food. And the virus got the necessary new mutations permitting its efficient transmission among humans evading the control measures to stop its diffusion and upsetting the entire humanity [3].

Therefore, we ought to analyze the microbial agents—mostly the viruses—considered today as the principal factor responsible for the emergence of outbreaks and pandemics.

7.1.3 Viral Participation in the Generation of Pandemics

Viruses are traditionally classified from a syndromic point of view, which is easy to understand by health professionals: respiratory viruses, enteric viruses, viruses that affect nervous system or cardiovascular system, viruses of sexual or vertical transmission, and so on. But the current classification is done according to the viral structure. Thus, the first main consideration is the type of viral genome (DNA or RNA). Then, the presence of a lipoproteic membrane: nude or enveloped virus. Furthermore, some genome characteristics (one or two strands; linear, circular, segmented, positive or negative sense strand) and other properties are considered.

This classification needs more complete information about viruses because their pathogenesis depends on those characteristics. The virulence and transmissibility of the infectious agents do not necessarily have direct relationship with the site demarcated as "target organ," but with other stepladders on the course of the infection. For example, patients can die from severe measles because of encephalitis or pneumonia rather than skin manifestation, or the severity of herpes simplex infection resides in the possibility of getting an encephalitis.

The structural classification allows to emphasize two very important facts in the pathogenesis of viral infections. First, viruses just need to keep themselves in nature as species, independently if this fact implies benefit or damage to other living organisms. Viruses are strict intracellular parasites because their replication depends on the host metabolic machinery: animal or vegetable cell, bacteria (phagos), amoeba or other virus (hepatitis D virus). Secondly, the way of replication depends on their type of genome and the need for a polymerase enzyme activity for copying the original genomic sequence (Baltimore classification scheme) [4].

The DNA viruses use a DNA-dependent DNA polymerase to replicate its genome, a function normally performed by animal cells during their replication. However, the RNA viruses need the action of RNA-dependent RNA polymerase (transcriptase), which does not normally exist. Therefore, they have just two possibilities to achieve its genome multiplication: (I) to carry the RNA polymerase as a structural protein or (II) to have the polymerase sequence codified in its RNA genome for being transcripted and translated by the host machinery during the replication process.

Mutations during viral replication due to insertion or removal of nucleotides are not uncommon. They are more frequent in RNA than in DNA viruses because of the low fidelity of the RNA transcriptase and the absence of a proof-reading/correction ability as compared to the DNA replication process. Consequently, in RNA viruses may exist countless genetics variant mixtures, with different genetic and antigenic composition (quasi species), which under environmental pressure for viral evolution can survive as new different viruses. Since among viruses affecting human beings, seven DNA virus families are mentioned versus 14 RNA virus families, the mutation phenomenon could represent a natural survivability mechanism for the RNA virus species. Most of the emerging viral epidemics correspond to RNA viruses [4].

Another factor favoring the emergence of viral variants is the presence of non-human host reservoir, like animals, where their control is normally not possible. This biological advantage has difficulty preventing outbreaks and pandemics, and the influenza viruses have been the best historical example. They have RNA genome consisting in eight fragments and it can undergo gene swapping or reassortment when a cell is infected simultaneously by two different viruses and the progeny virions may contain mixtures of each parent's genes (antigenic shift) resulting in new viruses to whom the population have no immunity. Thus, after the influenza A H1N1 (Spain, EEUU 1918), new mutations continued causing pandemics like influenza A H2N2 (China, 1957) H3N2 (Hong Kong, 1968), Hsw1N1 (EEUU), and outbreaks related to pigs, horses, or avian reservoirs which have not been able to produce human epidemics. These animal influenza viruses need more mutations to be efficiently transmissible to humans, eluding the specie barrier [5] (Table 7.1).

Table 7.1 Epidemics and pandemics for influenza viruses occurred from 1918

Year	Virus designation	Place	Source
1918	H1N1	Spain (USA)	Avian
1957	H2N2	Asia (China)	Avian/swine
1968	H3N2	Hong Kong (China)	Avian/swine
1976	Hsw1N1	Fort Dix—USA	Swine
1977	H1N1a	Russia (China)	Human/avian
1995	H7N7	England	Avian
1997	H5N1	Hong Kong (China)	Avian
1999	H9N2	Hong Kong (China)	Avian
2002	H7N2	Virginia, USA	Avian
2003	H7N7	The Netherlands	Avian
2003	H9N2	Hong Kong	Avian
2003	H5N1c	China, Sud East	Avian
2003	H1N2	Europe, Asia, America	Human
2003	H5N1c	Asia, Africa	Avian
2003	H7N2	New York, USA	Avian
2004	H7N3	Canada	Avian
2004	H5N1c	Thailand, Vietnam	Avian
2004	H10N7	Egypt	Avian
2009	Hsw1N1	Mexico/USA	Swine

Source: Avendaño LF, Ferrés M, Luchsinger V, Spencer E. Virología Clínica. 2ª Ed. Mediterráneo, Santiago, 2018

The viral transmission depends also upon the environmental stability because climatic factors (humidity, temperature, wind, rains), overcrowding, urban/rural settings, and other conditions may affect the contagion effectiveness. The enveloped viruses are usually unstable out of the cell because their lipoproteic membrane is sensible to environmental conditions; therefore, to survive they must be transmitted rapidly to a new host. Thus, enveloped viruses like many respiratory viruses, HIV, measles, and others must find prompt new hosts to infect, while nude viruses like enteroviruses, adenoviruses, rotavirus, and hepatitis A viruses can survive weeks or months in the environment.

7.1.4 The COVID-19 Pandemic

Emergence of a new virus, pandemic emergence, worldwide efforts for containment; effects of diseases and control measures over population; socio-economic impact in health budgets, vaccine development.

The emergence in December 2019 of a new coronavirus specie responsible for the COVID-19 pandemic has caused unprecedented disruption of human society and represented a great scientific and social challenge for the pandemic control [6].

The *Coronaviridae* family includes many enveloped RNA viruses. They are classified into alpha through delta *Coronaviridae* subfamilies. The former discovered coronaviruses were mostly associated with mild human respiratory infections like common cold diseases (hCoV 229E, hCoV NL 63, hCoV OC 43, and hCoV HKU1). However, coronaviruses can also infect mammals (canines, felines, pigs, cattle, bats) and birds. The last emerging coronaviruses have been associated with severe respiratory disease outbreaks, like the earlier SARS (Severe Acute Respiratory Syndrome, 2002–2003) and MERS (Middle East Respiratory Syndrome, 2012) viruses.

Coronaviruses are pleomorphic, ranging from 120 to 140 nm in diameter. Their envelope has large heavily glycosylated spikes (S) giving to the virion the appearance of a crown. The genome is a positive-sense single helical strand of RNA, 30 kb in size and is 5′ capped and 3′ polyadenylated. The RNA is translated directly into two large proteins, to be lately cleaved to form an RNA polymerase. This enzyme transcribes a large negative RNA strand, which will be transcribed both to a full-length virion-positive strand (genome) and to a set of subgenomic mRNA, to be translated to surface (S), membrane (M), envelope (E), and nucleoprotein (N) proteins. Also, functional proteins (ORF) are synthesized (Fig. 7.1).

The replication of SARS-CoV-2 and the pathogenesis of the disease can show points considered potential targets for intervention through vaccines, antivirals, and other containment measures. Since just a few antiviral drugs have shown clinical usefulness, most efforts have been directed to the vaccine development which has constituted the main tool for epidemic control.

The viral source of infection is usually an infected person, and pre-symptomatic or subclinical cases are supposed to be responsible for at least 50% of infections. The virus transmission occurs mostly by respiratory secretions transported in small (aerosol) and large droplets, and seldom by fomites. It gets to the epithelial cells of the upper respiratory tract, attaches its S glycoprotein to the ACE-2 cell receptor, and starts viral replication. Inflammation, edema, and exudation occur in the first week, and little fever, cough, sore throat, rhinitis, and general compromise are the main symptoms. Since there are ACE-2 receptors in the intestine, diarrhea can also arise. Around 80% of cases are asymptomatic or mild, with little fever, coughs, sore throat, and rhinitis. Around 5% of patients present with high fever, cough, myalgia, and breathlessness and X-ray study may show pneumonia, suggesting the patient may require admission to an intensive care unit (ICU) because of his severity. The lethality is around 1% considering the cases confirmed by laboratory tests. Since there are ACE-2 receptors in cardiovascular, renal, vascular endothelium, and other body territories, the patient aggravation can take place through an immune generalized hyper reaction, being very severe or fatal.

Their viral structure as an RNA virus with high mutation frequency plus the presence of an animal reservoir (bats, pangolin, and others) represents two effective strategies for surviving in nature almost impossible to control. Although their RNA polymerase has some proof-reading/correction capability, it is not efficient enough to avoid the mutation emergence and the detection of many new strains has been a paradigmatic problem to combat in the COVID-19 pandemia [7] (Table 7.2).

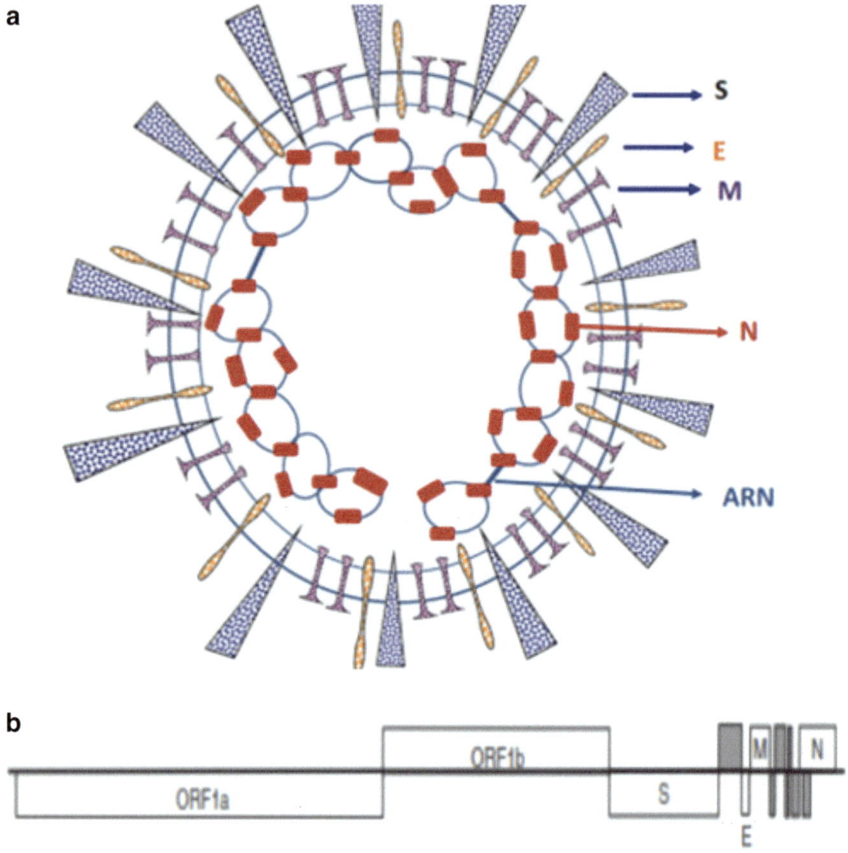

Fig. 7.1 Structure of SARS-CoV-2. (**a**) The virus has one RNA helical genome strain surrounded by the nucleocapside protein N. The viral membrane glycoproteins (M) and envelope (E) are embedded in the host membrane-derived lipidic bilayer, where emerges the spike glycoprotein (S) which mediates interaction with cell receptor ACE-2. (**b**) RNA (+) genome where open reading frames (ORF) for functional proteins (ORF 1a-1b, 3a, 3b, 6, and others) and structural proteins S, E, M, N are displayed

After the initial human contagion in China from an animal reservoir—equivalent to intermediate host—it was promptly transmitted directly from human to human generating an outbreak and by this way persisting as a new specie in nature. This mutagenic change had consisted in a variation of the viral envelop glycoprotein S, facilitating the viral attachment to the cell receptor ACE-2, mostly in the respiratory mucosa. The infection induces an immune response allowing to eliminate or ameliorate the infection and to prevent a new infection for some time. The development of vaccines could also generate immunity to the virus and is one of the principal tools to combat the outbreak. Both, the natural infection and the vaccine-induced immunity in the community contribute to develop a herd immunity to prevent new infections. However, the viral mutation could change the efficiency of the immune

Table 7.2 SARS-COV-2 circulating variants of concern

Lineage	Synonyms	Emergence
Alpha	B.1.1.7, 201/501.Y.V1,VOC 202012/01	UK, Sep 2020
Beta	B.1.351, 20H/501Y.V2	South Africa, Aug 2020
Gamma	P.1, B.1.1.28.1, 20J/501Y.V3	Brazil, Jul 2020
Epsilon	B.1, 427 California (CA) B.1.429, CAL 20C	USA, Sep 2020
Zeta	P.2, B.1.1.28.2	Brazil, Oct 2020
Lota	B.1.526,21F	USA, Nov 2020
Delta	B.1.617.2, 21J	India, Dec 2020
Eta	B 1.525, 20A/S:484K	Worldwide, Dec 2020
Lambda	C 37, B.1.1.1.C37	Peru, Dec 2020
Theta	P.3,B.1.1.28.3,21E	Philippines, Jan 2021
Kappa	B.1.617.1, 20A/S:154K	India, Oct 2021
Omicron BA 1	BA 1 (previously B.1.1.529), 21K	South Africa, Dec 2021
Omicron BA 2	BA.2, 21L	South Africa, Dec 2021
Omicron BA. 2.12.1	BA.2.12.1, 22C	North-America, Dec 2021
Omicron BA.2.75	BA.4, 22A	South Africa, Jan 2022
Omicron BA.4	BA.4, 22A	South Africa, Jan 2022
Omicron BA.5	BA.5, 22B	South Africa, Jan 2022
Omocron BQ. 1.1	BQ. 1.1, 22E	Nigeria, Jul 2022
Omicron XBB. 1.5	XBB. 1.5, 23A	USA, Nov 2022

Source: https://viralzone.expasy.org/9556

response and some viral characteristics of the infection, like transmissibility, strain virulence, sensitivity to health interventions so the health authorities are performing diagnostic methods, vaccine efficacy, and antiviral sensitivity measurements for containment [8].

The new virus was detected and identified during the first moments of their emergence—Chinese scientists published its full sequence on Jan. 11, 2020—and the World Health Organization declared on January 30th a Public Health Emergency of International Concern (PHEIC), the highest alert level and 1 month later announces the status of pandemic (11-3-2020). Nevertheless, these actions and recommendations did not impede the worldwide pandemic diffusion.

The emergence of a new virus pandemic can be explained because the biologic characteristics of the SARS-CoV-2 makes very difficult to control its progression. It is hard to accept that despite the great advances in science and socio-economic development the humanity is not able to beat a simple virus.

The success in smallpox, polio, measles, and rubella control has been possible because these viruses have only human reservoirs. Furthermore, attenuated live vaccines were developed and applied, which prevent the viral diffusion, not only the infection severity and lethality. The infection by Ebola virus is much more severe but less contagious because the transmission through direct contact starts when the patient has clinical symptoms and does not occur by respiratory secretions as in coronavirus infection. Furthermore, the contagion in SARS-CoV-2 arises 2 days before having symptoms and more than 50% of transmission is due to contact with asymptomatic cases.

To demonstrate the difficulties in controlling the advance of the pandemia, we cite the Imperial College London's long list of public health measures aimed at reducing contact rates in the population and thereby reducing transmission of the virus to limit the COVID-19 impact through non-pharmaceutical interventions (NPIs).

The global impact of COVID-19 has been profound, and the public health threat represents the most serious episode seen in a respiratory virus since the 1918 H1N1 influenza pandemic. In the absence of a COVID-19 vaccine, we should trust in the potential role of several public health measures—the so-called non-pharmaceutical interventions (NPIs)—aimed at reducing contact rates in the population and thereby reducing transmission of the virus. But by observing the evolution of the pandemic it should be concluded that the effectiveness of these interventions is likely too limited, requiring multiple interventions to be combined to have a substantial impact on transmission.

Two fundamental possible strategies have been proposed: (a) mitigation, which focuses on slowing but not necessarily stopping epidemic spread—reducing peak healthcare demand while protecting those most at risk of severe disease from infection, and (b) suppression, which aims to reverse epidemic growth, reducing case numbers to low levels and maintaining that situation indefinitely. Each policy has major challenges. Probably optimal mitigation policies (combining home isolation of suspect cases, home quarantine of those living in the same household as suspect cases, and social distancing of the elderly and others at most risk of severe disease) might reduce peak healthcare demand by two-third and deaths by half. However, the resulting mitigated epidemic would still likely result in hundreds of thousands of deaths and health systems (most notably intensive care units) being overwhelmed many times over. For countries able to achieve it, this leaves suppression as the preferred policy option [9].

In the UK and US context, suppression will minimally require a combination of social distancing of the entire population, home isolation of cases, and household quarantine of their family members. This may need to be supplemented by school and university closures though it should be recognized that such closures may have negative impacts on health systems due to increased absenteeism. The major challenge of suppression is that this type of intensive intervention package—or something equivalently effective at reducing transmission—will need to be maintained until a vaccine becomes available (potentially 18 months or more)—it is predictable that transmission will quickly rebound if interventions are relaxed. While experience in China and in South Korea showed that suppression is possible in the short term, it remains to demonstrate whether it is possible long term, and whether the social and economic costs of the interventions adopted thus far can be reduced. Furthermore, the policy of zero COVID case in China has failed and recently they had a big population contagion, probably because they did not complement it with a massive enough vaccination program.

From the viral point of view, the efficacy of NPIs seems to be limited. The vaccine development has four steps for evaluating immune dose schemes, efficacy, and safety comparing the vaccinated people with a control group and finally the effectiveness after their use in the community [10]. The NPIs measures do not have those evaluation steps to qualify their effectiveness. Is it possible to evaluate the correct use of facemasks, the impact of closing nurseries, schools, universities, the social distancing, closing the borders, and other measures? Also, the contact tracing is done usually late because the contagion starts before having symptoms or from an asymptomatic case.

The most effective prevention measure is vaccination. However, a great number of vaccines developed against COVID-19 are mostly efficient in decreasing the disease severity and lethality, but no more than 50% achieve prevention of the infection contagion (Table 7.3).

It is necessary to consider that the mutant generation process in SARS-CoV-2 can generate strains with different transmissibility, virulence, vaccine, and antiviral sensitivity.

The forenamed considerations do not explain the amazing observation that this pandemic has coincided with a disappearance of the habitual cold season respiratory virus circulation. It is almost incredible for us to observe that RSV and influenza epidemics disappeared for 2 years (Fig. 7.2).

We think that the temporal application of some NPIs (e.g., facemask, people circulation restriction, social distancing, closure of nurseries and schools) was responsible for that effect. The pandemic is teaching this strategy for future consideration when it was necessary to isolate some people with immune suppression, pre-term children, and other conditions because of high risk of contagion.

Table 7.3 Vaccines granted emergency use listing (EUL) by WHO

Inactivated	
Bharat Biotech	Covaxin
Sinopharm	Covilo
Sinovac	Coronavac
Protein subunit	
Serum Institute of India:	COVOVAX (Novavax formulation)
Novavax	Nuvaxovid
RNA	
Moderna	Spikeva
Pfizer BionTech	Comirnaty
Non-replicating viral vector	
CanSino	Convidecia
Janssen (Johnson & Johnson)	Jcovden
Oxford/AstraZeneca	Vaczevria
Serum Institute of India	Covishield (Oxford/AstraZeneca formulation)

Source: © 2023 VIPER Group COVID19 Vaccine Tracker Team https://covid19.trackvaccines.org/agency/who/

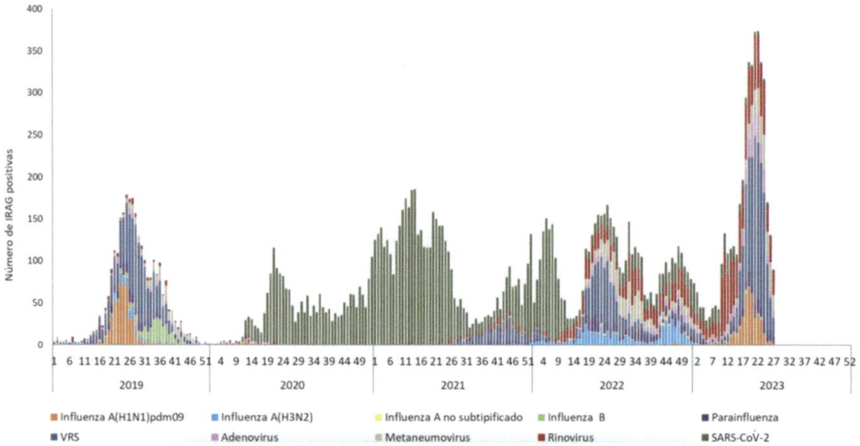

Fig. 7.2 Viral surveillance in acute respiratory severe hospitalized cases in Chile. 2019 to 22 week 2023. (Source: Depto. Epidemiología. MINSAL. Chile)

Since the start of the pandemic 3 years ago, WHO has recorded close to seven million deaths from COVID-19 though the real death toll from the pandemic may be three times higher. A few thousand deaths are still being reported to the agency every week, and some models estimate that excess mortality is still at about 10,000 deaths a day worldwide.

The WHO declared on May 15, 2023, the end to the emergency phase of the COVID-19 pandemic and it likely will usher the world into a new phase of disease monitoring with a scaling back of surveillance and available resources to fight COVID-19 [11].

7.2 COVID-19 Pandemic: The Case of Chile

Chile is located at the southwestern end of South America and its long and narrow territory of 756,700 m^2 is divided into 16 regions. Santiago, localized in the metropolitan region, is the capital of the country. According to National Statistics Institute (INE) protections, the total population in 2023 was estimated in 19,493,184, being 41.9% of people concentrated in the metropolitan region.

The birth rate for 2022 has been estimated in 10.03 live births/1000 inhabitants, and the total fertility rate in 1.3 children per woman of childbearing age. The population density is 22.8 inhabitants/km^2, reaching 451 inhabitants/km^2 in the metropolitan region; the urban population reaches 87% at all. The masculinity index is 95.9 men for every 100 women [12]. In relation to the distribution according to age groups, 18.6% of the population is under 15 years of age, 71.6% is between 15 and 64 years, and 12.7% are over 64, which generates an old age index of 68.3 over 64 years for every 100 children under 15 [12].

The review of some social determinants of health indicates that 7% of the population declares belonging to some ethnic group. Total poverty affects 15% of the inhabitants, with a percentage of indigence that reaches 4%. The average autonomous income of households is US $1500 (approx.), with a relationship of 15.7 between the income of the fifth and the first quintile (20/20 index) and a Gini coefficient of 0.47 [12]. The Average schooling reaches 11.7 years in 2020 (CASEN).

In relation to the health situation, the life expectancy at birth was reported as 82.1 years for women and 77.3 years for men during the period from 2015 to 2020. General mortality has exhibited a consistent downward trend over the past several years, reaching 6.5 deaths per 1000 inhabitants in 2020 [12]. Additionally, infant mortality has significantly decreased in recent decades, culminating in an overall figure of 6.5 deaths per 1000 live births for children under 1 year of age. In relation to general mortality, deaths from cerebrovascular disease (48.3/100,000) and myocardial ischemic disease (45.7/100,000) account for the two more frequent specific causes [13]. Despite the importance of this group of causes of death and the growing aging of the population, in recent years the lethality due to circulatory diseases in the country has decreased and, in comparison to the rest of the world, the Chilean rate can still be considered low, not reaching the levels observed in more developed countries.

7.2.1 Measures Adopted to Mitigate the Effects of COVID-19

These measures proposed by the government to control the pandemics and their effects can be described in several aspects:

1. Pandemic containment. The mostly considered measures were the mobility restrictions, the use of facemasks, and the closure and control of borders, among others.
2. Measures to avoid the interruption of supply chains. The objective was to avoid the hoarding of essential goods and inputs, the increase in the availability of basic supplies, and the prohibition of the suspension of the electrical supply and state subsidies.
3. Health. To increase the access and affordability of COVID-19 diagnosis, adaptation and strengthening of the national health system, complementation of public and private system for preventive and curative medicine, vaccine implementation according to the evolution of the pandemic and the availability of new vaccines.
4. Employment benefits. Increase of personnel and equipment for covering the COVID-19 ambulatory and hospital setting requirements.
5. Social benefits such as the COVID-19 Emergency Bonus, Emergency Family Income, and Middle-Class Bonus.
6. Educational policies settings, such as closure of educational centers, continuing by alternative means of teaching processes and food support at schools.

7. Economic reactivation measures such as employment subsidies.

Among the most important epidemiologic interventions, we remark quarantines, diagnostic tests, implementation of a trace-treat-isolate strategy, vaccines, and adaptation/strengthening of the health system [14, 15]. The implementation of quarantines has many problems because it has important effects on the population, such as access to work and to financial resources, and also the confinement can have severe effects on mental health. In Chile, while vaccines were not available, quarantine was the most important mitigation measure. Dynamic quarantines only at the beginning of the pandemic incorporated a large population number, but in the metropolitan region were mostly applied in small units (communes), which made difficult their effectiveness [16].

The quarantines were incorporated into the so-called step-by-step plan that considered five successive stages: (A) quarantine, (B) transition, (C) preparation, (D) initial opening, and (E) advanced opening, whose restrictive mechanisms were: the quarantine of communes, restriction of mobility, restriction of recreational and social activities, restriction of classes and curfew [17].

Diagnostic tests: PCR systems were the first pandemic diagnostic/control measure implemented against the COVID-19 pandemic since it was the most effective tool to detect and then isolate and treat people who suffered from the disease in an opportune way. Testing makes it possible to protect the health, to reduce the rate of contagion in the community and to protect the health systems, being part of the trace-treat-isolate strategy (TTI). To guarantee universal access to diagnosis, the first policy implemented was to categorize the reverse polymerase chain reaction test (RT-PCR) in the Health Benefits Tariff. This allowed both the National Health Fund (FONASA) and the Social Security Health Institutions (ISAPRE) to offer the corresponding coverage to all their beneficiaries. In Chile, more than 65,000 tests were performed in a single day in 2021. The traceability problem in Chile was the delay time between diagnosis and isolation implementation. Furthermore, since most of contagions occurred from asymptomatic or pre-symptomatic cases, the tracing contact moment remains always late for applying efficiently the isolation strategy, seriously affecting their effectiveness. Also, the proportion of patients who were traced in the system within the first 3 days remained below 60% during 2020 and 2021, the hardest years of the pandemic [18].

Vaccine development: It was an essential strategy in the fight against COVID-19, and Chile participated in its development through the implementation of Phase 3 clinical trials, which aim to evaluate the efficacy of vaccines in the disease prevention. The first clinical trial conducted in Chile began in August 2020 and was led by the Catholic University and the Sinovac laboratory. For the implementation, there was a contribution of public resources of $2600 million [19]. The study aimed to evaluate the efficacy, safety, and immunogenicity of two vaccination schedules with CoronaVac, an inactivated vaccine against SARS-CoV-2 infection, in adults developed in China. Other Phase 3 clinical trials of vaccines against COVID-19 that were being implemented in Chile corresponded to collaborations between the University of Chile and Janssen/Johnson & Johnson; the University of Chile and the Las Condes Clinic with AstraZeneca; and the Universidad de la Frontera with the CanSino Laboratory [19].

In September 2020, the Government of Chile announced an agreement with COVAX, a global initiative led by the WHO and the European Union, which would allow access to eight million doses of a vaccine that had WHO validation. That same month, another agreement was also confirmed with the Pfizer BioNTech laboratory to access ten million doses of its vaccine from 2021 [19].

The "National Vaccine Plan against COVID-19" began in December 2020, having as its main objective the inoculation of 15 million people as the initial target population. The initial strategy consisted of immediately vaccinating the health personnel and people at risk, and then the target population [18]. The behavior of the population was excellent, rapidly reaching high coverage. Studies of the effectiveness of vaccines (pharmacological intervention) in Chile did not focus on transmission, but on the probability that individuals vaccinated with different doses were hospitalized, entered the ICU, or die. These studies clearly determined that during 2021 there was a differential admission to hospitalization or ICU and a differential mortality between those vaccinated versus unvaccinated. Thus, for example, an effectiveness of the CoronaVac vaccine was reported in Chile among people with complete vaccination of 65.9% for acquiring COVID-19, 87.5% for hospitalization, 90.3% for admission to the ICU and 86.3% for deaths associated with COVID-19 [26]. Also, the complete vaccine schedule and the third and fourth doses with different schedules, mainly AstraZeneca and Pfizer, showed even better effectiveness, over 90% for deaths [20]. By March 2022, a total of 54,745,764 COVID vaccine doses had already been administrated to the Chilean target population (E. Paris, Health Secretary. Personnel communication, May 2022). The vaccination program has gone ahead until now.

Health Service: Finally, another very important aspect was the plasticity of the National Health system to adapt to the pandemic requirements. The COVID-19 pandemic caused a sharp increase in the demand for health care, such as diagnostics, hospitalizations, and intensive care units. To avoid the collapse of the healthcare network in Chile, an effort was made to fortify the operational capacity of the health system, reinforcing human resources in health and the space and supplies available for medical care. Thus, the Health Services were able to hire new personnel and the entire healthcare network, both public and private healthcare providers, were coordinated. Thus, by means of a special resolution of the Ministry of Health, private providers were incorporated into the public network of the Health Services according to their geographic location and assigned territory. Therefore, the complete organization of this national network, known as the COVID-19 Integrated Network, was conducted by the directors of each Health Services [19]. Then, to increase the supply, the Ministry of Health used resources for the implementation of additional beds. To accomplish this task, the presence of a national centralized bed management (CMB) system, created in 2009, which integrates public and private hospitals was essential to optimize the use of beds when the system was overstressed. CBM was implemented to overcome access and opportunity restrictions to hospital admission in the context of the Chilean mixed health system, with public and private components (insurance and healthcare providers).

Specifically, in relation to accessibility to Intensive Care Unit (ICU) beds, the opening and complexity of the ICU allowed to increase their number by 243%

through the conversion of beds [17]. In fact, according to the Ministry of Health, the number of ICU beds from the pandemic beginning in January 2020 to June 2021 increased by 339%, while the increment from 2010 to 2019 had been only 64% (E. Paris. Health Secretary. Personal communication, May 2022).

7.2.2 *Impact of COVID-19 in Health Outcomes*

Chile experienced for 2 years an epidemic with a high impact on the population with high lethality and mortality and a great impact on the health system. In the COVID-19 epidemic curve (cases/day) since its beginning, four epidemic periods can be recognized: (1) the first epidemic concentrated mainly on the metropolitan region (5/13–8/15/2020); (2) a 20/21 epidemic with the participation of all regions (12/13/2020–7/16/2021), (3) a short-term outbreak associated with the δ variant (11/4–5/12–2021), and (4) a large epidemic outbreak associated with the Omicron variant (1/5/2022 to date) [18, 20] (Fig. 7.3).

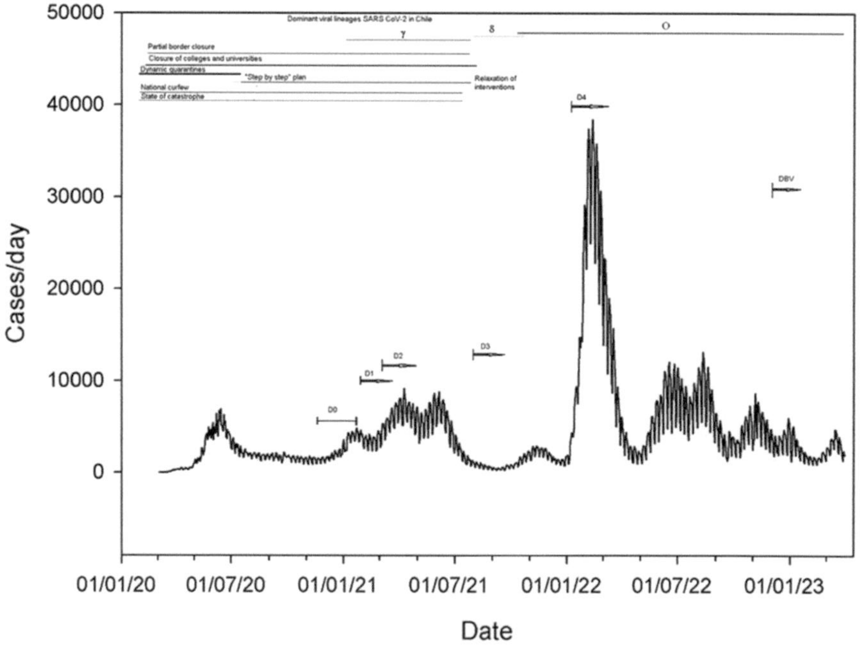

Fig. 7.3 Evolution of the incidence (reported cases/day) of COVID-19 in Chile, from 3/3/2020 to 3/31/2023. The letters γ, δ, and O, with the respective lines show the periods in which the Gama, Delta, and Omicron variants were dominant. The lines associated with the interventions show the duration of each of them. D0 indicates the vaccination period for health personnel and patients at risk. D1, D2, D3, D4, and D5, with their respective arrows, indicate the start of the mass vaccination period with the first, second, third, fourth, and fifth (bivalent) doses

Viral variants of SARS CoV-2 have played an important role in viral transmission, with variant of concerns (VOCs) dominating in major outbreaks; the original variant (WIV04/2019), and the α variant (UK; B.1.1.7) in the 2020 epidemic, the γ variants (P.1) and the Andean variant (λ; C.37) in the epidemic 20/21 and the δ and O variants in the last two outbreaks, these last variants being the ones with the highest reproductive numbers reported (Fig. 7.3).

The transmission dynamics have been influenced by the usual social movements of Chile, especially by vacation periods (January–February), festivities, crowds, and overcrowding in transportation media and work locations, which are typical of the start of activities, schools, and universities in March. The impact on the health system has been direct in hospitalizations, especially on ICU occupancy and a great collateral effect on medical consultations, well-child care, surgery waiting lists, and care for patients with chronic diseases such as cardiovascular diseases (CVD) and cancer [21–23] (Fig. 7.4).

The rapid removal of restrictions in 2021 assumed that population immunity acquired through vaccination would allow an incidence that would not saturate health systems. Non-pharmacological interventions only had a clear effect when five million people were quarantined in the metropolitan region in 2020 [24], while dynamic quarantines did not demonstrate adequate efficacy, being insufficient to control increases in incidence [16]. Due to the entry and re-entry of infections from neighboring communes and, on the other hand, because the most vulnerable population did not have the conditions to carry out adequate quarantines, being the most affected and the one that decreased their mobility the least during the quarantines

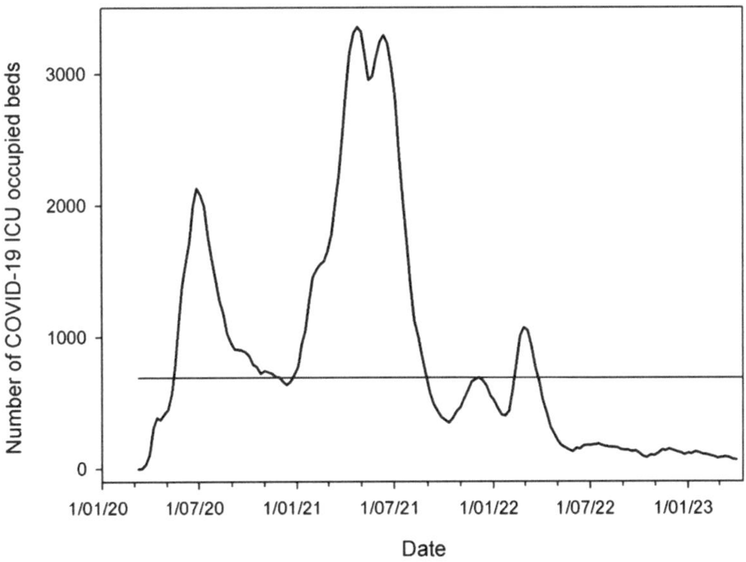

Fig. 7.4 Number of ICU beds occupied by patients diagnosed with COVID-19. The straight line represents the initial number of ICU beds available in the public service

[25]. Li et al. [16] show that in Chile small quarantines in interconnected areas have little effect on reducing transmission although have a good effect in isolated localities and when considering large areas and a large population.

Vaccination had a rapid and high coverage. However, the moderate effectiveness of vaccines and the appearance of new variants disallowed achieving herd immunity (Fig. 7.5).

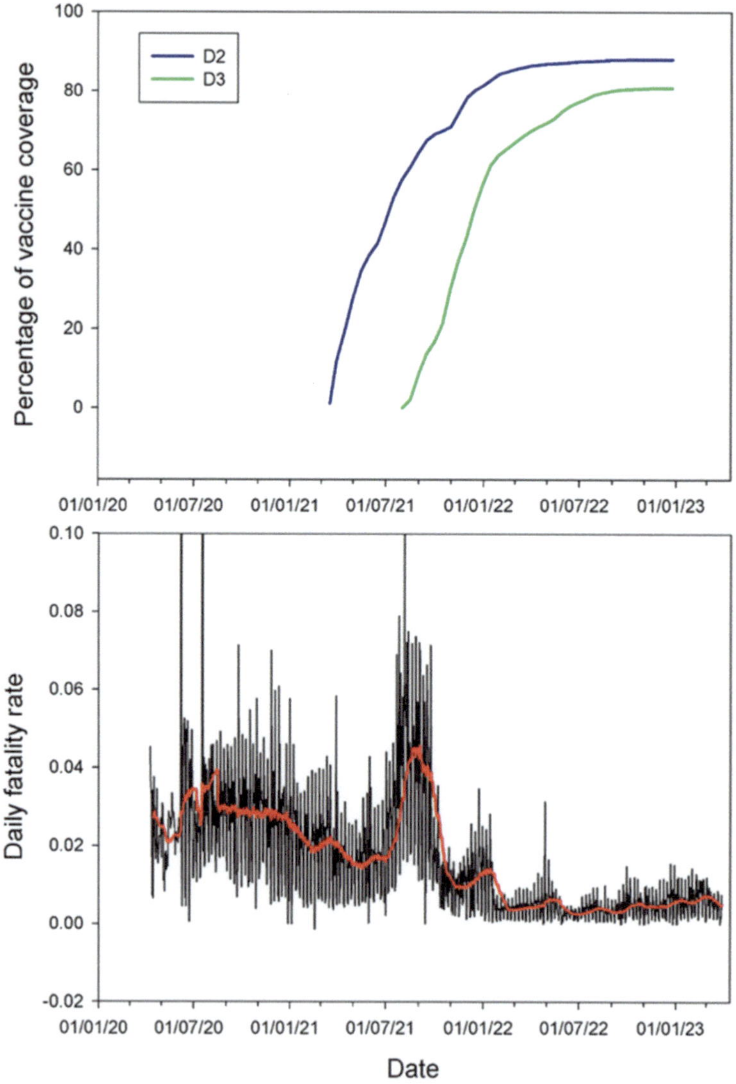

Fig. 7.5 Evolution of vaccination coverage with full dose (two doses; D2) and booster dose (D3) for SARS CoV-2 and daily lethality of COVID-19 in Chile from 4/1/2020 to 31/3/2023. The red line corresponds to the moving average of order 30 of the lethality (30 days)

The total case fatality and daily case fatality have been decreasing over time, following higher vaccine coverage and improved patient management. While the entry of the δ variant produced an increase in daily lethality in Chile, the O variant produced a clear drop in daily lethality in Chile and in the world, estimated at values close to those of influenza [26–28].

Hospitalizations

During this pandemic, in the world, associated with the increase in health care due to COVID-19, hospitalizations for different diseases such as acute coronary syndrome [29, 30], acute myocardial infarction [31], and cerebrovascular accidents have decreased [32–36]. An increase in out-of-hospital cardiorespiratory arrest events (OHCA) has also been reported [37, 38], which could be explained by reduced access to health care during the pandemic.

Cardiovascular Impact

In the case of acute myocardial infarction (AMI), Chile presented a distinct situation as compared to other countries worldwide. In the first year of the COVID-19 pandemic (2020), both admissions and mortality rates related to AMI experienced a slight decline. However, the contribution of AMI-related deaths to overall mortality remained constant when deaths attributed to COVID-19 were excluded, as illustrated in Table 7.4. Given that Chile has universal health coverage for AMI patients, which was maintained during the pandemic, it was effective in providing opportune health care for AMI, in contrast to other health problems that experienced major interruptions in access to hospital care.

Table 7.4 Distribution of hospital discharges and deaths due to acute myocardial infarction (AMI), Chile 2019–2020

	Total	AMI					
Year	*N*	*N*	Relative importance (%)	Age (mean)	Age (SD)	Men (%)	Rate[a]
Hospital discharges							
2019	1,667,180	13,275	0.80	64.1	13.2	69.7	69.5[b]
2020	1,330,447	12,598	0.98[c]	63.9	12.7	70.9	64.7
Mortality							
2019	109,658	6062	5.53	72.7	14.2	62.7	31.7
2020	126,169	6161	5.60[c]	73.2	14.6	61.0	31.7

[a] Hospitalization and mortality rate expressed per 100,000 inhabitants
[b] $p = 0.017$ (comparison of hospitalization rate 2019 vs. 2020)
[c] The relative importance was estimated excluding hospitalizations and deaths from COVID-19, respectively (hospitalizations = 47,996 and deaths = 16,189, according to DEIS databases) to correct the effect of COVID. p value = 0.45

The analysis of the pandemic's impact on emergency room visits in the public sector in Chile revealed a decrease in the overall number of visits for various causes. However, notably, the number of visits by patients with AMI and their access to medical care remained unaffected. This factor contributed to the significant observation that the mortality rate from this cause did not increase significantly and highlights the effectiveness of the emergency network as a critical component of the Chilean healthcare system [39, 40].

It is noteworthy that public hospitals efficiently managed the demand generated by AMI, optimizing the length of stay by reducing it by 1 day. This achievement was, in part, a consequence of the extensive use of the Centralized Bed Management System, which effectively distributed excess healthcare demand for COVID-19 primarily to private providers. This strategy allowed the entire healthcare system to continue caring for other prioritized conditions throughout 2020 (Fig. 7.6).

When comparing the years 2019 and 2020 in Chile, it is evident that deaths due to AMI remained relatively constant (6062 vs. 6121). Excluding deaths from COVID-19, the relative importance of AMI among the total death toll also remained constant (5.53% vs. 5.60%), as shown in Table 7.3. What exhibited more variation was the location of these deaths, largely influenced by lockdowns and the fear of the population of leaving homes. There was a notable increase in deaths occurring at the decedent's home, rising from 45.3 to 52.0% ($p < 0.001$). In contrast, deaths in hospitals decreased from 35.8% to 33.4% ($p = 0.006$). Deaths in "other places of death," including primary care clinics, emergency facilities, nursing homes, and on the streets, also experienced a decrease from 18.9% to 14.6% ($p < 0.001$).

Considering the factors previously discussed, such as the existence of universal coverage for AMI care, the centralized bed system, and the functioning of the emergency network, it is noteworthy that the overall AMI case-fatality rate did not exhibit significant variation between the pre-pandemic year and the pandemic year in Chile. Specifically, the in-hospital case fatality increased from 6.0 to 6.6% ($p = 0.08$). However, a notable increase in case fatality was observed among patients admitted to private hospitals (Fig. 7.7).

The observed difference in case fatality can be attributed to the transfer of patients from public to private centers facilitated by the centralized bed system. Historically, patients treated in the public sector in Chile have been associated with a higher risk and worse prognosis, due to their baseline clinical and sociodemographic characteristics, including a higher prevalence of diabetes, hypertension, obesity, older age, and lower socio-economic status [41]. Additionally, private hospitals had to manage a significant burden of COVID-19 cases, which placed substantial stress on their healthcare resources [42].

The case of Chile demonstrates that prioritizing AMI patients within a universal health coverage system and integrating public and private healthcare providers were likely highly effective in reducing the impact of the COVID-19 pandemic on hospital admissions for AMI.

However, in primary care, the management of patients at risk for cardiovascular disease (CVD) was significantly disrupted, raising concerns about potential long-term effects. This poses a challenge for the management of future pandemics.

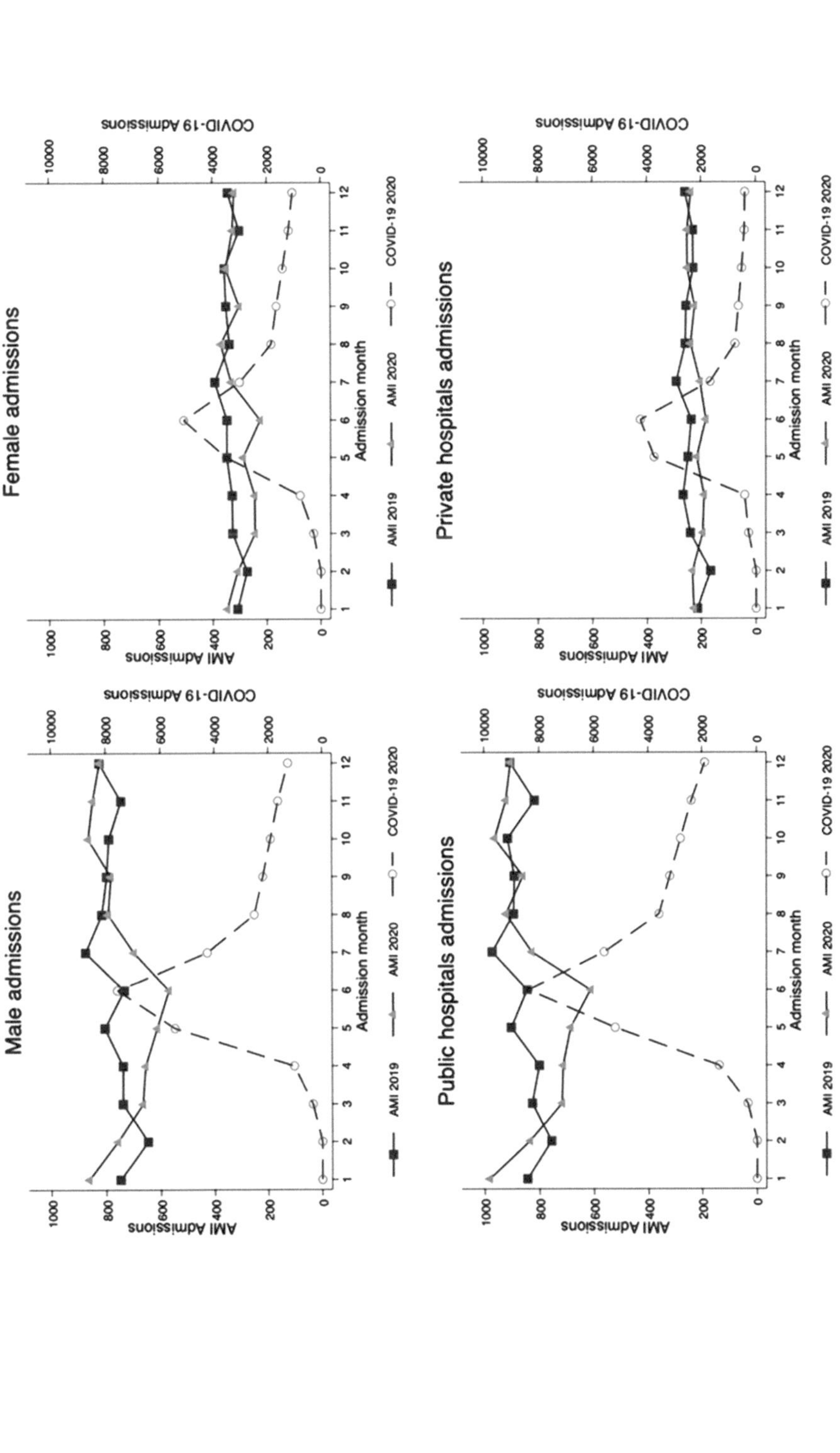

Fig. 7.6 Hospital admission due to AMI according to sex and health provider, Chile 2019–2020

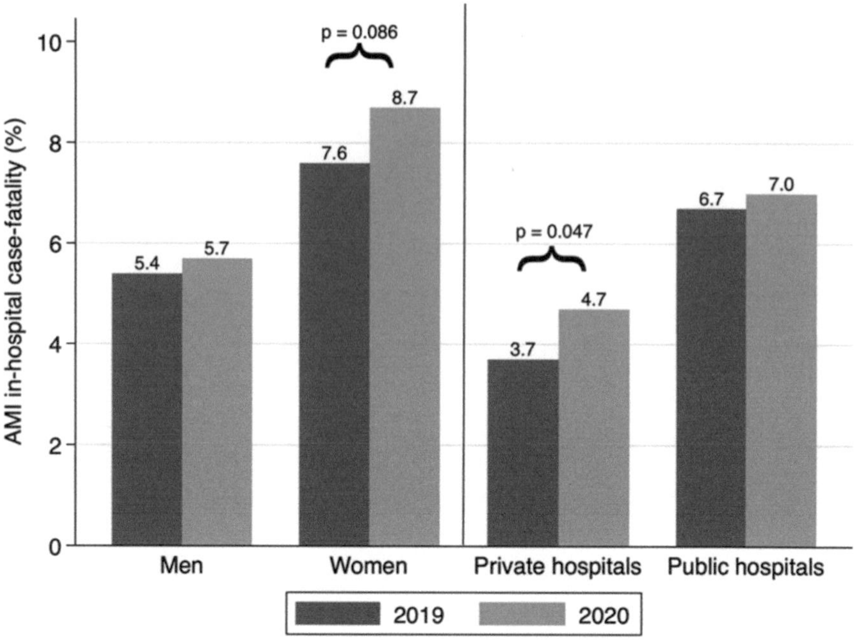

Fig. 7.7 In-hospital case fatality in AMI patients, according to sex and health provider in Chile 2019–2020

Ensuring that patients in secondary prevention continue their treatment, especially those with established cardiovascular disease, is a critical concern. Additionally, data from the Chilean Ministry of Health indicate a nearly 60% decrease in control for patients with cardiovascular risk factors or those in secondary prevention in 2020 compared to 2018 and 2019 [43].

Regarding *cardiovascular risk factors* control during the pandemic in Chile, different scenarios were observed. More than half of tobacco users sought to quit smoking and only 17% increased their consumption. Additionally, a decrease in smoking initiation was observed in young populations. Physical activity was heavily altered due to quarantines and its mobility restrictions; sedentarism, associated with an increase in screen time, was more prevalent. When analyzing weight variations 26% of men and 38% of women gained weight during the first half year of the pandemic, while 54% of men and 48% of women reduced their body weight. Alcohol consumption was also haltered during the first year, decreasing by 42%. People referred that lack of opportunities (social activites) were the main cause of this reduction, highlighting the effect of access regulations. Goals for Type 2 Diabetes achievements were also affected: program admission was reduced by 40%, total number of patients in control by 14% and compensation rate was reduced by 24%. For hypertensioin admissions to GES program decreased by 26%, total number of patients in control by 24%, and compensation rated was 18% lower than the previous 3 years [43].

Access to medical care was also affected, especially during the first year of the pandemic. Fear of contagion and interruptions of medical care access were the main explanations to stop seeking for health care in primary care. This resulted in a 72% reduction in cardiovascular disease screening, a 46% drecrease in admissions to the cardiovascular diseases program, and a 60% reduction in CD controls, in 2020, compared to the previous 3 years. However, telemedicine proved to be very useful in addressing the situation. In 2021, a detriment was also observed but of a lesser magnitude. Annual hypertension emergency room and hospital admissions were also reduced by 15 and 13%, respectively. For stroke, ER consultations decreased by 10% and hospital admissions by 8.6% [43].

Health Expenditures

According to the Ministry of Finance of Chile, the total health expenditure in Chile increased during the Pandemic. The total health expenditure in the previous year, i.e., 2019 was 13,516,849,573 Chilean pesos, representing 9.3% of GDP (Gross domestic product). Comparing 2019, during the most affected pandemic years, i.e., 2020, 2021, and 2022, the total heath expenditure in Chile increased by 14.8%, 24.1%, and 16.0%, respectively. It is notwworthy that during those years, the investment in new infrastructure was severely halted [46].

7.3 Lessons and Challenges for Future Pandemics and Prevention of Cardiovascular Diseases

It is supposed that viruses will continue generating new variants in the future, mostly RNA viruses derived from animal reservoirs. Consequently, the herd immunity will be less effective in stopping their diffusion. Probably social and scientific advances in controlling pandemic emergences will make them milder, with less lethality.

The SARS-CoV-2 impact will probably be similar to the actual influenza problem, supposedly influenced by the use of vaccines and antivirals.

It is supposed that according to the worldwide COVID-19 experience, the scientific world will cooperate (WHO, Universities, and state/private institutions) and will rapidly identify any emergent agent and define the possibility that it constitutes a Public Health Emergency of International Concern (PHEIC).

Vaccines candidate preparation will start in many places taking advantages of the new technology developed against the COVID-19 pandemic. Also, a genomic network surveillance will be set up to predict and prevent pandemic emergence risks.

Governments will dictate public health measures to "control the diffusion" of epidemics as it has been described in many countries in relation to COVID-19. Strengthen the primary care network with strategies that incorporate telemedicine to control patients with risk factors such as high blood pressure and diabetes.

In relation to cardiovascular diseases, it will represent both a challenge and an opportunity to reshape the care model for cardiovascular patients, emphasizing the need for an integrated approach across different levels of care. This entails active involvement of community nursing and the incorporation of diverse telemedicine modalities to restore continuity in managing these patients [44, 45].

International organizations and local authorities have advocated for the implementation of telemedicine services, encompassing remote patient care, triage, and telephone monitoring.

The emphasis on risk stratification is crucial, directing priority towards those most vulnerable, considering both their biological and social profiles. This approach ensures a closer and more vigilant monitoring of individuals at heightened risk, aligning with the objective of bringing the health system closer to the community. The overarching focus on equity should be the main goal, recognizing that the impact of the pandemic has disproportionately affected individuals with fewer resources.

Besides reshaping healthcare policies towards addressing health inequities such as Universal Health Coverage, certainly, preparing for future pandemics involves a comprehensive set of strategies to enhance global resilience and response capabilities. Here are key strategies that could be considered, among others:

- Integration of a network of public-private healthcare providers.
- Strengthening primary health care to ensure the continuity of rapid diagnosis, control, and treatment, mostly in high-risk patients (such as diabetics and patients with previous major cardiovascular events).
- Reinforce collaboration between health authorities and the scientific community (Health and Science secretaries, Universities, Research institutions) to get effective management of the pandemic and improve the prevention and treatment measures, like rapid diagnosis, effective vaccine access, intensive care units increments, and others.
- To educate the population on the importance of seeking prompt medical attention in the presence symptoms despite mobility restrictions.
- Strengthen the TTI strategy, mainly in relation to traceability. An important challenge is the incorporation of effective digital contact tracing technology using mobile phones.

References

1. Yuval N. Harari. Sapienship: a brief history of humankind. https://www.ynharari.com/book/sapiens-2/.
2. LePan N, Routley N, Schell H. Visualizing the history of pandemics. 2020. https://www.visualcapitalist.com/history-of-pandemics-deadliest/.
3. Lewis D, Kozlov M, Lenharo M. COVID-origins data from Wuhan market published: what scientists think. Nature. 2023;616(7956):225–6. https://doi.org/10.1038/d41586-023-00998-y.

4. Avendaño LF, Ferrés M, Luchsinger V, Spencer E. Virología clínica. 2nd ed. Santiago: Mediterráneo; 2018.
5. Zambon M, Potter PH. Chapter 16. Influenza. In: Zuckerman AJ, Banatvala JE, Schoub BD, Griffiths PD, Mortimer P, editors. Principles and practice of clinical virology. 6th ed. Wiley; 2009.
6. Klain R. Perspective. Politics and pandemics. N Engl J Med. 2018;379(23):2191–3. https://doi.org/10.1056/NEGMp1813905.
7. Murray JL, Piot P. The potential future of the COVID-19 pandemic will SARS-CoV-2 become a recurrent seasonal infection? JAMA. 2021;325(13):1249–50. https://doi.org/10.1001/jama.2021.2828.
8. Baric RS. Emergence of a highly fit SARS-CoV-2 variant. N Engl J Med. 2020;383(27):2684–6. https://doi.org/10.1056/NEJMcibr2032888.
9. Imperial College COVID-19 Response Team. Report 9: impact of non-pharmaceutical interventions (NPIs) to reduce COVID-19 mortality and healthcare demand. 2020. https://doi.org/10.25561/77482.
10. Krause PR, Gruber MF. Emergency use authorization of Covid vaccines—safety and efficacy follow-up considerations. N Engl J Med. 2020;383:e107. https://doi.org/10.1056/NEJMp2031373.
11. Kupferschmidt K, Wadman M; WHO. Director-General Tedros Adhanom Ghebreyesus today declared an end to the COVID-19 Public Health Emergency of International Concern. https://doi.org/10.1126/science.adi5890.
12. INE. 2023. https://www.ine.gob.cl/estadisticas/sociales/censos-de-poblacion-y-vivienda.
13. MINSAL. 2023. https://www.minsal.cl/wp-content/uploads/2022/01/Informe-Mortalidad-Prematura-y-AVPP-por-C%C3%A1ncer-2009-2018.pdf.
14. Canals M. Learning from the COVID-19 pandemic: concepts for good decision-making. Letter to Editor. Rev Med Chile. 2020;148:415–20.
15. Canals M. Conceptos para una Buena toma de decisiones en la pandemia COVID-19 en Chile. Punto de vista. Rev Chil Infectol. 2020;37(2):170–2.
16. Li Y, Undurraga EA, Zubizarreta J. Effectiveness of localized lockdowns in the COVID-19 pandemic. Am J Epidemiol. 2022;191(5):812–24.
17. Ministerio de Hacienda. COVID-19: evolución, efectos y políticas adoptadas en Chile y el mundo. 2023. https://www.dipres.gob.cl/598/articles-266625_doc_pdf.pdf.
18. Canals M, Canals A. Resumen analítico de la experiencia chilena de la pandemia COVID-19, 2020-2022. Cuad Méd Soc. 2022;62(23):5. https://doi.org/10.56116/cms.v62.n3.2022.374.
19. Jara A, Undurraga EA, González C, Paredes F, Fontecilla T, Jara G, et al. Effectiveness of an inactivated SARS-CoV-2 vaccine in Chile. N Engl J Med. 2021;385:875. https://doi.org/10.1056/NEJMoa2107715.
20. Sauré D, O'Ryan M, Torres JP, Zuñiga M, Santelices E, Basso LS. Dynamic IgG seropositivity after rollout of CoronaVac and BNT162b2 COVID-19 vaccines in Chile: a sentinel surveillance study 40. Lancet Infect Dis. 2022;22:56–63.
21. Acevedo ML, Gaete-Argel A, Alonso-Palomares L, et al. Differential neutralizing antibody responses elicited by CoronaVac and BNT162b2 against SARS-CoV-2 lambda in Chile. Nat Microbiol. 2022;7:524–9. https://doi.org/10.1038/s41564-022-01092-1.
22. Canals M, Canals A, Cuadrado C. Incidence moments: a simple method for study the memory and short term forecast of the COVID-19 incidence time-series. Epidemiol Methods. 2022;11(s1):20210029. https://doi.org/10.1515/em-2021-0029.
23. Siches I, Vega J, Chomalí M, Yarza B, Estay R, Goyenechea M, et al. El impacto de COVID en el sistema de salud y propuestas para la reactivación. COLMED; 2020.
24. Cuadrado C, Vidal F, Pacheco J, Flores-Alvarado S. Cancer care access in Chile's vulnerable populations during the COVID-19 pandemic. Am J Public Health. 2022;112(S6):S591–601. https://doi.org/10.2105/AJPH.2021.306587.
25. Canals M, et al. Epidemic trends, public health response and health system capacity: the Chilean experience in COVID-19 epidemic. Rev Panam Salud Publica. 2020;44:e99. https://doi.org/10.26633/RPSP.2020.99.

26. Pérez P, Navarrete P. Informe Unidad de Gestión Centralizada de Camas (UGCC), enero 2014—diciembre 2017. Ministerio de Salud, Gobierno de Chile; 2018. p. 1–31.
27. Mena GE, Martinez PP, Mahmud AS, Marquet PA, Buckee CO, Santillana M. Socioeconomic status determines COVID-19 incidence and related mortality in Santiago, Chile. Science. 2021;372:934.
28. Canals M. En el tercer año pandémico en Chile: evolución epidemiológica y sanitaria. Bol Acad Chilena Med. 2022;LIX:259–66.
29. Ito K, Piantham C, Nishiura H. Relative instantaneous reproduction number of omicron SARS-CoV-2 variant with respect to the Delta variant in Denmark. J Med Virol. 2022;94:2265–8.
30. De Filippo O, D'Ascenzo F, Angelini F, Bocchino PB, Conrotto F, Saglietto A, et al. Reduced rate of hospital admissions for ACS during COVID-19 outbreak in northern Italy. N Engl J Med. 2020;383(1):88–9. https://doi.org/10.1056/NEJMc2009166.
31. Mafham MM, Spata E, Goldacre R, Gaic D, Curnow P, Bray M, et al. COVID-19 pandemic and admission rates for and management of acute coronary syndromes in England. Lancet. 2020;396(10248):381–9. https://doi.org/10.1016/S0140-6736(20)31356-8.
32. Solomon MD, McNulty EJ, Rana JS, Leong TK, Lee C, Sung SH, et al. The Covid-19 pandemic and the incidence of acute myocardial infarction. NEJM. 2020;383:691. https://doi.org/10.1056/NEJMc2015630.
33. Baum A, Schwartz MD. Admissions to veteran affairs hospitals for emergency conditions during the COVID-19 pandemic. JAMA. 2020;324(1):96–9. https://doi.org/10.1001/jama.2020.99729.
34. Rudilosso S, Laredo C, Vera V, Vargas M, Renú A, Llull L, et al. Acute stroke care is at risk in the era of COVID-19. Experience at a comprehensive stroke center in Barcelona. Stroke. 2020;51:1991–5. https://doi.org/10.1161/STROKEAHA.120.030329.
35. Hoyer C, Ebert A, Huttner HB, Puetz V, Kallmünzed B, Barlinn K, et al. Acute stroke in times of the COVID-19 pandemic. A Multicenter study. Stroke. 2020;51:2224–7. https://doi.org/10.1161/STROKEAHA.120.030395.
36. Zhao J, Li H, Kung D, Fisher M, Shen Y, Liu R. Impact of the COVID-19 epidemic on stroke care and potential solutions. Stroke. 2020;51:1996–2001. https://doi.org/10.1161/STROKEAHA.120.030225.
37. Marijon E, Karam N, Jost D, Perrot D, Frattini B, Derkenne C, et al. Out-of-hospital cardiac arrest during the COVID-19 pandemic in Paris, France: a population-based, observational study. Lancet Public Health. 2020;5:e437. https://doi.org/10.1016/S2468-2667(20)30117-1.
38. Baldi E, Sechi GM, Mare C, Canevari F, Brancaglione A, Primi R, et al. Out-of-hospital cardiac arrest during the Covid-19 outbreak in Italy. N Engl J Med. 2020;383(5):496–8. https://doi.org/10.1056/NEJMc2010418.
39. Toro L, Parra A, Miriam A. Epidemia de COVID-19 en Chile: impacto en atenciones de Servicios de Urgencia y Patologías Específicas. Rev Med Chile. 2020;148:557–64.
40. Santelices E, Luis SJ. Descripción Y Análisis Del Sistema De Red De Urgencia (Rdu) En Chile. Recomendaciones Desde Una Mirada Sistémica. Rev Méd Clín Las Condes. 2017;28(2):186–98. https://doi.org/10.1016/j.rmclc.2017.04.005.
41. Alonso F, Nazzal C, Cerecera F, Ojeda J. Reducing health inequalities: comparison of survival after acute myocardial infarction according to health provider in Chile. Int J Health Serv. 2018;49:127.
42. Chomali M, Guell M, Hervé B, Angulo M, Huerta C, Gutiérrez C, et al. Impacto de la Primera Ola Pandémica de COVID-19 en el Personal de Salud en un Hospital Privado. Rev Med Clin Condes. 2021;32(1):90–104. https://www.elsevier.es/es-revista-revista-medica-clinica-las-condes-202-articulo-impacto-de-la-primera-ola-S0716864020301012.

43. Ministerio de Salud Subsecretaría de Salud Pública. Impacto de la Pandemia por COVID-19 en las Enfermedades no Transmisibles en Chile. https://redcronicas.minsal.cl/wp-content/uploads/2022/02/2022.03.07_INFORME-IMPACTO-COVIDEN-LAS-ENT-FINAL-1.pdf
44. Lau D, McAlister FA. Implications of the COVID-19 pandemic for cardiovascular disease and risk-factor management. Can J Cardiol. 2021;37(5):722–32. https://pubmed.ncbi.nlm.nih.gov/33212203/.
45. World Health Organization. Health topics. Rapid assessment of service delivery for NCDs during the COVID-19 pandemic. 2020. https://www.who.int/publications/m/item/rapid-assessment-of-service-delivery-for-ncds-during-the-covid-19-pandemic
46. Dirección de Presupuestos de Chile. Serie Histórica Años 2019–2023, Información De Ejecución Presupuestaria, Ministerio de Salud. https://www.dipres.gob.cl/597/articles-318964_doc_pdf.pdf. Accessed 17 Jan 2024.

Chapter 8
Cardiovascular Disease Prevention in Latin America: Comparative Outcomes According to Socioeconomic Status

Fernando Lanas, Pamela Serón, and Cheryld Muttel

8.1 Latin America, Cardiovascular Diseases and Its Risk Factors

Latin America has more than 40 countries and territories from Mexico to Cape Horn, with an area of 21,069,500 km^2 (7,880,000 sq. mi), which can be subdivided based on geographic location in South America, Central America, the Caribbean, and Mexico. The region brings together countries whose predominant languages are Latin, mainly Spanish and Portuguese although French, English, and Dutch are also spoken in the territories located on the Caribbean Sea. According to the International Monetary Fund [1], in 2022, the estimated total population of Latin America and the Caribbean will be approximately 645.6 million inhabitants; about 434 million people live in the southern part of the American continent, while Central America and the Caribbean are home to 82 million inhabitants. During the last decades, marked human and social development have occurred so the population has better access to education, health services, primary health care, and immunizations and, along with this, the prevention and control of numerous infectious diseases in several Latin American countries. Consequently, an epidemiological transition has been observed with a marked increase in the adult population.

According to the Economic Commission for Latin America and the Caribbean (ECLAC) [2], population aging is one of the main demographic phenomena in Latin America and the Caribbean. In 2022, 88.6 million people over 60 years old lived in the region, representing 13.4% of the total population, a proportion that will reach 16.5% in 2030. Likewise, life expectancy for both sexes has increased from 48.6 years in 1950 to 75.1 years in 2019. Despite the decline of 2.9 years in 2021 compared to 2019 due to the impact of the coronavirus disease (COVID-19)

F. Lanas (✉) · P. Serón · C. Muttel
Facultad de Medicina, Universidad de La Frontera, Temuco, Chile
e-mail: fernando.lanas@ufrontera.cl; pamela.seron@ufrontera.cl

T. Romero et al. (eds.), *Global Challenges in Cardiovascular Prevention in Populations with Low Socioeconomic Status*,
https://doi.org/10.1007/978-3-031-79051-5_8

pandemic, life expectancy is expected to continue to increase in the future and reach 77.2 years in 2030. All of the above has resulted in an increase in cardiovascular risk factors and an increase in morbidity and mortality rates related to both stroke and myocardial infarction.

Cardiovascular disease (CVD) is the leading burden of morbidity and mortality in the world. Likewise, according to the World Health Organization (WHO) [3], CVD continues to be the leading cause of mortality and burden of disease and disability in the Region of the Americas. In the latest report from the WHO [3], in 2019, two million people died from CVDs. However, the age-standardized mortality rate decreased from 203.3 deaths (95% II: 176.0–227.1) per 100,000 inhabitants in 2000–137.2 deaths (95% II: 110.3–165.5) per 100,000 inhabitants in 2019. However, age-standardized mortality rates from CVD vary substantially between countries, from 428.7 deaths per 100,000 inhabitants in Haiti to 73.5 deaths per 100,000 inhabitants in Peru; the countries with the highest rates are Haiti, Guyana, Suriname, the Dominican Republic, and Honduras. Regarding Disability Adjusted Life Years (DALYs), for the same year, CVD caused 40.8 million DALYs and 36.4 million years of life lost due to premature death. It has been observed that in the last two decades, the number of years of life lived with disabilities has almost doubled.

Ischemic heart disease and stroke are the two leading causes of mortality and disability from CVD. Considering that the most important risk factors in all countries are high blood pressure and dyslipidemia [4], screening and treatment of these conditions are the main strategies to follow for the primary prevention of CVD. Likewise, smoking cessation programs should be implemented, along with promoting physical activity and healthy eating habits. Other risk factors include overweight and obesity, whose rates have tripled in the region in the last 50 years, currently affecting 62.5% of the population, and diabetes mellitus, whose prevalence has also increased three times in the previous 30 years in Latin America [5], as had excessive alcohol intake, which is a factor that is often underestimated and contributes to CVD.

Another important risk factor in Latin America is Chagas disease, which mainly affects poor populations in Latin America. It has been postulated that positive serology would be an independent risk factor for cardiovascular events.

Showing that, for example, serology for Chagas is associated with a greater risk of death for patients with heart failure. However, little evidence relates positive serology for Chagas with cardiovascular events in asymptomatic subjects [6].

Regarding the economic indicator Gross Domestic Product (GDP), Puerto Rico and the Bahamas had the highest GDP per capita in Latin America and the Caribbean in 2022, with an average GDP generated per person greater than 30,000 US dollars. Excluding Caribbean countries and territories, Uruguay recorded Latin America's highest GDP per capita in 2022, with an income of more than $20,000 per person; in turn, the lowest GDP per capita in the region was that of Haiti, with less than 1,800 US dollars in current prices [7].

Although the risk factors for CVD are known, the various strategies to control them are limited by economic reasons that, for example, determine differences in access to a healthy diet. According to multiple sources such as the International Fund for Agricultural Development (IFAD), the WHO, and the World Food Program (WFP), a large proportion of the population in Latin America and the Caribbean is limited in maintaining a healthy diet due to the cost of such foods in their place of residence. It is estimated that, in 2020, nearly nine out of ten people in Haiti could not access a healthy diet due to economic reasons, making it the most affected country within a selected group of nations in the region.

This puts the situation in Latin America and the Caribbean into perspective, and according to recent reports from the World Bank, growth projections for 2023 are 2%. The growth forecast for 2024 is 2.3%, indicating that the region has regressed to low pre-pandemic growth levels. The region will also suffer from global adverse effects, such as declining commodity prices, rising interest rates in Group of Seven (G7) countries, and China's unstable recovery. Household income losses due to the pandemic have not been fully recovered, especially for the middle class. The average poverty rate is now above pre-pandemic levels, at 30.3%. Overall, employment has returned to 2019 levels, including for women, but real wages remain stagnant and often below 2019 levels. Less-educated workers and older adults are the furthest behind in the recovery, while informality has mainly remained stable since 2019. On the other hand, currently, the region is going through the worst migration crisis in its history. In addition to traditional flows from Central America and Mexico to the United States, Venezuela and Haiti have recently experienced significant outflows of people. Around 7.5 million Venezuelans have left their country since 2015, while 1.7 million Haitians are abroad, adding to the two million internally displaced people.

8.1.1 Health Care in Indigenous Groups

It is estimated that more than 400 different indigenous groups live in the Latin American and Caribbean region, approximately 10% of the total population, in just five countries: Bolivia, Guatemala, Peru, Ecuador, and Mexico live 89% of them, between 5 and 13 million indigenous citizens [8]. Language is an essential factor that identifies and allows the differentiation of the indigenous groups. There are approximately 400 different indigenous languages across Latin America, and, as a World Bank report suggests, each country has 7–200 languages. Uruguay is the only country on the continent that is monolingual in Spanish. Language is fundamental to the health of indigenous people as a means for transmitting knowledge within cultures and health systems.

Regarding health determinants, people living within natural ecosystems are exposed to many health hazards their environment produces. In the past, health risks were related to primary access to food, water, and shelter and, in many cases, risks from predators. However, over the years, the colonization of the indigenous regions has led to the development of new diseases and different disease patterns, also determined by the ethnic origin of the populations, so that despite the variations in the trajectory of inclusion of different ethnic groups, they continue to be disadvantaged both in terms of their well-being and their access to opportunities [9]. Existing studies suggest that in most Latin American countries, indigenous peoples have higher rates of mortality and morbidity than their non-indigenous counterparts. In some cases, indigeneity may be a surrogate indicator of poverty. Regarding disease patterns within and among indigenous peoples, these depend intensely on the degrees of contact with society, so a series of health outcomes in indigenous communities in the region are related to their social environment and linked to acculturation.

The indigenous communities most integrated into society, in general, are more vulnerable to the so-called modern diseases and the diseases of poverty; this vulnerability can be linked to exposure to diseases and poor living conditions. For example, in 2002, in an indigenous community in Venezuela, researchers reported severe rates of alcohol consumption (86.5% of all men and 7.5% of all women were heavy alcohol users). This would have been directly related to the fact that the consumption of corn liquor had gradually been replaced by the consumption of commercial beer and rum at more frequent intervals and with negative social consequences [10]. Other studies have recorded an increase in cardiovascular risk factors, such as obesity and hypertension, related to changes in diet, lifestyle, and blood pressure [11, 12], related to changes in nutrition and the transition from a nomadic life to a sedentary urban one [13, 14].

In general, 43% of the indigenous population and 25% of Afro-descendants in the region are poor, and many indigenous peoples of Latin America still live in isolated environments with precarious sanitary and environmental conditions. Therefore, an important aspect that should be considered is the geographic segregation each group faces. For example, although more than 80% of Afro-descendants in the region live in cities, most of them are relegated to poor neighborhoods and marginal neighborhoods. So today, despite the traditional paradigms that link indigenous peoples with the rural population, the reality today is very different since almost half of them live in marginalized urban areas, which implies differences in access to health services and care, which is emerging as an essential determinant of health in the indigenous population of the region [9].

8.2 Impact of Socioeconomic Disparities on Risk Factors and Cardiovascular Disease in Latin America

The multinational PURE cohort has reported that individuals from wealthier nations have a higher risk of cardiovascular events, assessed by the INTERHEART risk score. However, the incidence of cardiovascular events and 1-year lethality is higher in low- and middle-income countries (LMIC) [15]. Additionally, within affluent countries, it is the socioeconomically disadvantaged segments of the population that face the highest risk of developing CVD [16].

Socioeconomic disparities in Latin America significantly impact risk factors [17]. While some risk factors have decreased, such as smoking, other risk factors, such as obesity, diabetes, or physical inactivity, are increasing and continue to contribute to the burden of CVD, disproportionately affecting the socially disadvantaged [18]. Recent evidence demonstrated a link between socioeconomic status and atherosclerosis-related biological pathways involving inflammation, platelet activation, and blood pressure [19].

Also, socioeconomic disparities impact CVD incidence and prognosis; the relative contribution of socioeconomic position to CVD prevalence in Latin American countries varies widely from 9.4% to 23.4% [17, 20]. While some countries have seen a decrease in CVD mortality, others have noticed an increase, particularly in Central American and Caribbean countries [21]. Countries with greater incidence of cardiovascular disease and mortality in Latin America are those with higher levels of poverty, lower education levels, limited access to healthcare services, and less favorable socioeconomic conditions, leading to a higher prevalence of risk factors such as hypertension, high cholesterol, and diabetes [22]. Thus, countries with less mortality from cardiovascular disease are Chile, Uruguay, and Peru, with a standardized rate per 100,000 inhabitants of 94.6, 106.5, and 93.4, respectively, compared to countries with higher levels of poverty and socioeconomic disparities as Mexico, Ecuador, or Paraguay (198.5, 167.5, and 155.5 death per 100,000, respectively) [23]. In a report of the PURE Study [24] comparing data from four countries, the incidence of CVD (per 1000 person-years) only modestly varied between countries, with the highest incidence in Brazil (3.86) and the lowest in Argentina (3.07). However, there was a more significant variation in mortality rates (per 1000 person-years) between countries, with the highest in Argentina (5.98) and the lowest in Chile (4.07). In this study, deaths were higher in rural than urban areas regardless of the country [24]. These findings suggest that there are complex interactions between socioeconomic factors, access to healthcare services, and the prevalence of cardiovascular disease and its risk factors in Latin America.

Inequality in access to education is the most frequently reported factor and likely the most significantly associated with cardiovascular disease and its risk factors. The SALURBAL project, for example, which included survey data from cities in Argentina, Brazil, Chile, Colombia, El Salvador, Guatemala, Mexico, and Peru, reported frequencies of hypertension by socioeconomic status. In women, a higher level of education was associated with a lower likelihood of hypertension. However, living in suburban areas with higher education was linked to a higher likelihood of hypertension in both genders. The association between city-level education and hypertension varied across countries, with an inverse pattern observed in Peru (higher city-level education was associated with lower odds of hypertension). Additionally, the inverse relationship between individual-level education and hypertension became stronger (in women) or emerged (in men) as city or suburban education levels increased [25].

While disparities are shown between countries, they can also be observed within countries. Within countries, socioeconomic inequality based on income and education contributes to increased CVD risk factors. In Argentina, the fourth National Risk Factor Survey showed that the prevalence of diabetes, hypertension, and high cholesterol, defined by step methodology proposed by the WHO (Step 1: self-report;

Step 2: physical measurements; Step 3: biochemical determinations), was related to the level of education. The prevalence of diabetes was 29.2% (95% CI: 19.1–39.3) in those with incomplete primary education, compared to 12.8% (95% CI: 10.3–15.2) and 7.7% (95% CI: 6.2–9.3) in those who had completed primary or advanced secondary education and those who completed secondary education, respectively. Meanwhile, the prevalence of hypertension was 65.2% (95% CI: 60.7–69.7) in those with incomplete primary education, compared to 53.5% (95% CI: 51.2–55.8) and 40.1% (95% CI: 38.3–42) in those who had completed primary or advanced secondary education and those who completed secondary education, respectively. Cholesterol was also higher in people with incomplete primary education, with a prevalence of 53.3% (95% CI: 41.4–65.2) compared to 39.8% (95% CI: 35–44.6) and 37.9% (95% CI: 34.6–41.2) prevalence in those with incomplete secondary education and complete secondary education respectively. Additionally, 79.7% (95% CI: 76.5–82.8) of the population with incomplete primary education in this national survey were overweight and obese by anthropometrics measurements, while 70.6% (95% CI: 68.3–72.8) and 61.5% (95% CI: 59.8–63.2) were overweight or obese when they had finished secondary education or had even started higher education, respectively. In the case of tobacco, although no relation was found with educational level, there was a gradient according to income quintiles with 24.7% (95% CI: 22.7–26.7) of those in the first quintile are smokers, and 20.3% (95% CI: 18.6–21.9) are in the fifth income quintile [26].

In Brazil, the National Health Survey found that factors such as advanced age, being male, white race/color, lower education levels, not having health insurance, and self-assessing health as regular or poor were associated with a higher prevalence of cardiovascular disease [27]. Also, it has been reported that slum inhabitants in Brazil have higher rates of behavioral cardiovascular disease risk factors [28]. The "Pesquisa Nacional de Saúde"(PNS) 2014–2015 reported a prevalence of total cholesterol ≥200 mg/dL of 32.7% (95% CI: 31.5–34.1) in the general population; low high-density lipoprotein cholesterol (HDLc) of 31.8% (95% CI: 30.5–33.1), and high low-density lipoprotein cholesterol (LDLc) of 18.6% (95% CI: 17.5–19.7). A greater level of education was related to a lower prevalence of high total cholesterol, high LDLc, and low HDLc [29]. In the ELSA study, hypertension was reduced among individuals holding postgraduate degrees (28.4%), in contrast to those lacking a complete secondary education (44%). Additionally, a lower prevalence of hypertension was observed in individuals with a per capita family income surpassing USD 1000.00 (30.7%) compared to those with an income below USD 500.00 (40.9%) [30]. About diabetes, the prevalence has been reported higher among illiterate individuals or those with incomplete elementary education and those with incomplete secondary education [9.61% (PR 1.42, 95% CI: 1.13–1.77) and 5.36% (PR 1.59, 95% CI: 1.23–2.06), respectively], while in those with higher education, the prevalence is 4.18% [31]. Also, in the ELSA cohort, the highest percentages of overweight and obesity were observed among low education levels (35.0%), and overweight increased with low per capita income and fewer years of schooling [32]. Finally, the prevalence of tobacco use among adults in Brazil is lower in populations with higher education, being 17.6% (95% CI: 16.8–18.4) among those without education or with incomplete primary education, 15.5% (95% CI: 14.3–16.6) among those with complete primary education and incomplete secondary education, 9.6% (95% CI: 8.9–10.2) among individuals with complete secondary education and incomplete college education, and 7.1% (95% CI: 6.3–7.8) among those with complete college education [33].

In Colombia, similar patterns were observed, with lower socioeconomic status, lower education levels, and limited access to healthcare services contributing to higher rates of cardiovascular disease and its risk factors among older individuals. Specifically, the risk of CVD mortality has been reported to be higher in less economically and socially privileged municipalities [34]. Also, educational level is the most critical determinant of hypertension awareness, treatment, and control. Specifically, hypertension prevalence is 25% higher among those with the lowest educational level [35].

In Chile, a higher educational level is associated with fewer risk factors such as diabetes, hypertension, or obesity [36]. For example, obesity in people with less than 8 years of education is 43.2% compared to 29.8% and 27% in people with 8–12 years and 12 years or more of schooling, respectively. The same is observed for hypertension and diabetes, both of which are more than twice as prevalent in groups with less than 8 years of education, with 57% of people with suspected hypertension and 25.3% with suspected diabetes. The prevalence of low HDLc is also different according to years of education, being significantly lower in those with more than 12 years of schooling (36%) compared to those with less than 8 years (48.5%) or between 8 and 12 years of schooling (50.3%). Tobacco use is higher as people have more education, with a prevalence of 18% for those with less than 8 years of schooling, 35% for those with 8–12 years of education, and 38.9% for those with 12 or more years of schooling. This survey also assessed cardiovascular risk and showed that high cardiovascular risk was 51% in people with less than 8 years of education, compared to 14.2% in people with 12 or more years of education [36].

The National Health and Nutrition Survey findings in Ecuador indicate a direct correlation between educational attainment, residential location, ethnicity, and economic quintile. This reaffirms the existing disparities in access to education, exerting a substantial influence on the health and nutritional well-being of the population and consequently contributing to the prevalence of chronic non-communicable diseases such as CVD [37].

In Mexico, ENSANUT 2022 reported a prevalence of diagnosed and total diabetes was higher at lower levels of education. A higher percentage of non-diagnosis was also found in people with low socioeconomic status and no health insurance [38]. The prevalence of adults with a diagnosis of hypertension and controlled blood pressure is also different according to the level of education, being 26% (95% CI: 18.4–35.8) among those who have not completed primary education, 31.9% (95% CI: 28.1–35.9) among those with primary or secondary education and 39.8% (95% CI: 32.7–47.3) among those with more than secondary education [39]. The prevalence of obesity was lower in people with a bachelor's degree (32.0% [95% CI: 28.6–35.7]) than in those with a secondary or high school education (38.9% [95% CI: 36.6–41.2]). Also, it was observed that adults with a bachelor's degree or more were less likely to have obesity as measured by body mass index (BMI) (0.7 [95% CI: 0.5, 0.9]) and central obesity (0.5 [95% CI: 0.4, 0.7]) than adults with a primary school education or less [40].

The available evidence from various studies in Latin America demonstrates that socioeconomic disparities, particularly in access to education, play a crucial role in the prevalence of risk factors and CVD. However, caution should be taken when interpreting this evidence as most of it comes from national surveys that report prevalence according to educational level or other variables representing socioeconomic status but do not study associations through models that adjust for other co-variables such as age, which can potentially be confounding, for example, in the Argentina survey it is explicit that people in the lowest educational strata are older people. Only the reports from Brazil and Colombia mention that a multivariate analysis adjusting for co-variables was performed. Despite this shortcoming, the consistency between the findings of the different studies at the national level in Latin America strengthens the conclusion that socioeconomic disparities, represented mainly by the educational status of individuals and communities, determine cardiovascular risk and CVD. Addressing these disparities and improving access to education and healthcare services is essential in mitigating the burden of CVD in the region.

8.3 Initiatives for Cardiovascular Prevention in Latin America

Several initiatives have been implemented in Latin America to control risk factors. WHO programs addressing the control of smoking, obesity, and hypertension are the ones that have been widely applied in different countries in the regions and will be described in detail. Some relevant clinical trials with strategies that have not yet been widely implemented will also be mentioned. Governments have moved towards offering Universal Health Coverage (UHC) to their population. However, in the implementation of different strategies, it is critical to consider the environmental, racial, social, and economic conditions of the population [41].

8.3.1 Smoking

In 2001, the Pan American Health Organization (PAHO) Member States signed a resolution urging all countries of the Americas to protect nonsmokers through a smoke-free environment (SFE) in all workplaces and public places as soon as possible: the Framework Convention on Tobacco Control (FCTC). This resolution also included a mandate for the PAHO Secretariat to develop a plan of action under the name "Smoke-Free Americas" and to support countries to adopt and implement SFE through capacity-building actions aimed at policymakers and local tobacco control advocates [42]. In 2005, the FCTC entered into force, which in its Article 8 requires States Parties to "adopt and implement effective measures providing for protection from exposure to tobacco smoke in indoor workplaces, public transport, indoor public places, and, as appropriate, other public places" [43]. In addition, in 2007, WHO presented a policy package to help countries fulfill obligations under the FCTC. It included six effective tobacco control policies, known as MPOWER, an acronym for **M**onitor tobacco use; **P**rotect people from tobacco smoke; **O**ffer help to quit tobacco use; **W**arn about the dangers of tobacco; **E**nforce bans on tobacco advertising and promotion; and **R**aise taxes on tobacco products [44].

Progressive, sustained, and synergistic implementation of FCTC measures has contributed to a regional reduction in smoking prevalence of more than 50% over 15 years [45]. In 2005, Uruguay became the first country to adopt a 100% smoke-free policy by decree; Colombia, in 2008, and Peru, in 2010, adopted similar measures. According to the 2021, WHO report on the global tobacco epidemic, SFE, jointly with health warning labels, was the most implemented measure by American countries in alignment with the FCTC and WHO criteria [46]. Almost 20 years after launching the "Smoke-Free Americas" initiative, in December 2020, South America became the first subregion in the Americas to accomplish 100% smoke-free environments. Latin American countries have achieved these 100% SFE policies through laws, decrees, resolutions, or a combination. In addition, Brazil, with Mauritius, Netherlands, and Turkey, is setting new global standards for tobacco control, adopting all six MPOWER measures at the highest possible level [47]. With sustained commitment, most of the regions should continue reducing the smoking prevalence to below 12.9% by 2025 [48].

However, despite these advances, tobacco use remains a leading preventable risk factor for disease, disability, and premature death in Latin America, accounting for 10% of all deaths [48]. Additionally, some countries have more robust provisions than others, and the lack of enforcement weakens the implementation of comprehensive smoke-free laws in the subregion. New and emerging tobacco and nicotine products pose a severe threat to smoke-free measures. Tobacco and related industries market e-cigarettes and other new and emerging nicotine and tobacco products as alternatives. These products include nicotine pouches, e-shishas, e-pipes, e-cigars, and supplementary products to conventional cigarettes that can be used in indoor public areas, even where smoking bans exist [46].

Latin America needs to strengthen its existing measures of tobacco control aiming at their full implementation: (1) substantial increases in tobacco taxes to reach international standards; (2) complete implementation and enforcement of smoke-free environments; (3) plain packaging; and (4) complete bans on tobacco advertising, promotion, and sponsorship [49].

8.3.2 Obesity

To face the severe health threat derived from obesity in Latin America, PAHO launched 2015 the Latin American Action Plan for Prevention of Child and Adolescent Obesity [50]. They acknowledge that the individual's food preferences, purchasing decisions, and eating behaviors are shaped by price, marketing, availability, and affordability and that these factors are, in turn, influenced by upstream policies and regulations on trade and agriculture. The document also mentions the need to promote coordination between ministries and public institutions, primarily in the sectors of education, agriculture, finance, trade, transportation, and urban planning, as well as with local city authorities, to achieve national consensus and synergize actions to halt the progression of the obesity epidemic among children [50]. The action plan has five aspects:

1. **Primary health care and breastfeeding promotion.** Breastfeeding is one of the most effective ways to ensure child health and survival. In 2012, the World Health Assembly approved the global nutrition target of increasing the rate of exclusive breastfeeding in the first 6 months of age to at least 50% by 2025. However, in the Region of the Americas, the prevalence of exclusive breastfeeding in infants under 6 months of age is 32.3%, a rate that has not improved in two decades [51].
2. **Healthy eating improvement of school nutrition and physical activity environments.** Programs directly providing healthy foods effectively reduce obesity [52]. Student feeding programs that adapt their nutritional guidelines to tackle obesity are supported by the World Food Program and the Food and Agricultural Organization (FAO) (Global Food Research Program UNC 2021) [53]. Nearly 85 million children receive some school meal at zero cost or reduced price annually [54].
3. **Fiscal policies and regulation of food marketing and labeling.** Market-based food interventions, including taxes on junk food, nutrition labeling, and marketing restrictions, decrease the consumption of targeted foods. They include policies designed to change the relative prices of different foods in the market via taxes or subsidies. Chile and Mexico were among the earliest countries to implement a tax on sugar-sweetened beverages. Panama, Ecuador, and Peru shortly followed [55]. Studies showed a positive effect on reducing consumption, purchase, and sale and decreased purchases of non-essential energy-dense foods. However, nutritional education in vulnerable groups is essential to understand their interpretation better [56]. Chile enacted a Food Labeling law in 2016 that includes a new front warning labeling on food, which consists of a black octagon with white edges placed on the front of the food or beverage package, with the message high in calories, sodium, sugars, or saturated fats [57]. An evaluation of sugar-sweetened beverage purchases after implementing Chile's law found that purchases declined by nearly 24% in the first 18 months although Chile's law combines marketing and labeling policies [58].

   Marketing of less healthy food has been widely implemented. Chile, for example, restricted the sale of junk food in educational establishments, followed by Uruguay, Peru, and Brazil [59]. However, subsidies for increasing healthy food consumption have been less popular among policymakers. Interventions are also necessary to improve natural and whole foods production, storage, and distribution systems. The family farming initiative is one example of those interventions.

4. **Other multisector actions.** The provision of urban spaces for physical activity, such as parks, implementation of "open streets" programs, and establishment of rapid public transportation systems are initiatives that promote physical activity policies and programs focused on increasing accessibility and promoting physical activity, which is crucial for nutritional health. One area of expansion has been cycling infrastructure. A recent study showed a massive increase in the construction of bike paths in major cities across Latin America. However, green space investments are not distributed equitably.
5. **Surveillance, research, and evaluation.** The review identified 115 PAHO policies/interventions (43% implemented after signing the proposed plan in 2014). Nearly all (18/19) countries implemented food guidelines or school feeding programs, but fiscal and marketing policies were less commonly implemented (6/19). Through the review, 44 valuations of PAHO policies were identified, of which 23% were qualitative and 77% quantitative. The results of these evaluations were in general positive (e.g., decrease in sugar-sweetened beverages consumption following tax implementation), but no studies evaluated the outcome of reduced obesity.

8.3.3 Hypertension

Strategies to improve hypertension controls have been developed in the last decade. In 2013, the US Centers for Disease Control and Prevention (US CDC) and PAHO launched the Standardized Hypertension Treatment Project [60]. Inspired by the success achieved by Canada [61] and Kaiser Permanente in the United States [62]. The use of standardized treatment protocols, a core set of high-quality, affordable medicines, patient registries for cohort monitoring, and team-based care. At the end of 2015, the Standardized Hypertension Treatment Project was successfully piloted in Barbados and a year later, it was introduced in parallel in Colombia, Cuba, and Chile [63].

To support governments in strengthening the prevention and control of CVDs, in 2016, WHO and the US CDC launched the Global Hearts Initiative. HEARTS technical package aims to improve the management of CVDs in primary health care. In 2016, the WHO and other partners launched the Global Hearts Initiative [64]. The HEARTS in the Americas Initiative, spearheaded by PAHO, is the regional adaptation of the WHO HEARTS technical package [65], a new model that shifts the focus of hypertension and CVD secondary prevention management, including diabetes, from the secondary or tertiary level of care to the primary care setting.

The WHO HEARTS technical package details components of a successful national hypertension control program. HEARTS is an acronym for **H**: Healthy lifestyle, including diet and exercise recommendations **E**: Evidence-based, simple hypertension treatment protocol, with a linear stepwise algorithm for medication use, defined drugs, and doses at each step. Specific medicines and doses were selected from WHO-recommended antihypertensive medication classes; **A**: Access to quality, affordable hypertension medicines, and blood pressure monitoring with validated automated digital oscillometric devices; **R**: Risk-based hypertension management, with risk and blood pressure thresholds to define HTN diagnosis and treatment goals defined at the national level. **T:** Team-based, patient-centered HTN care, multidisciplinary, often supervised by a physician and including trained and licensed nonphysician staff. Task allocation depends on local regulations, customs, and preferences. S: Systems are used to monitor progress in controlling blood pressure at the individual patient level and for improving outcomes at the healthcare facility level.

HEARTS recommends that each country develop a national protocol through a consensus process that engages local stakeholders, including healthcare professionals, scientists, pharmacy and health system managers, and ministries of health [66].

By 2022, HEARTS hypertension control programs treated 12.2 million patients in 32 participants LMICs in 165,000 primary care facilities. Hypertension control was 38% (median 48%; range 5–86%). In four HEARTS countries using the same digital health information system, facility-based control improved from 18% at baseline to 46% in 48 months. At the population level, the median estimated population-based hypertension control was 11.0% of all hypertension patients (range 2.0–34.7%) [67]. The Global Hearts experience of implementing WHO HEARTS demonstrates the feasibility of controlling hypertension in LMICs primary care settings [67]. As of 2022, 12 countries in the Latin America and Caribbean region implemented a protocol using initial two-drug combinations [68]. After 5 years, the program's success demonstrates that hypertension control is feasible and affordable in LMICs and can be scaled and sustained with government leadership and support [69].

8.3.4 Clinical Trials

A comprehensive model of care led by NPHWs, involving primary care physicians and family that was informed by local context, substantially improved blood pressure control and CVD risk. This strategy is effective and pragmatic and has the potential to substantially reduce CVD compared with current strategies that are typically physician-based.

The Heart Outcomes Prevention and Evaluation 4, conducted in Colombia and Malaysia, evaluated a multifaceted intervention package that includes (1) detection, treatment, and control of cardiovascular risk factors by nonphysician health workers in the community who use tablet-based simplified management algorithms, decision support, and counseling programs; (2) free dispensation of combination antihypertensive and cholesterol-lowering medications, supervised by local physicians; and (3) support from a participant-nominated treatment supporter (either a friend or family member) [70]. At the 12-month follow-up, the reduction in Framingham Risk Score was −6.40% in the control group and −11.17% in the intervention group, and an absolute 11.45 mm Hg reduction in systolic blood pressure, and a 0.41 mmol/L reduction in LDL with the intervention group (both $p < 0{\cdot}0001$).

Change in blood pressure control status (<140 mm Hg) was 69% in the intervention group versus 30% in the control group [71].

The Hypertension Control Program in Argentina was a cluster randomized trial testing a multicomponent intervention that targeted the healthcare system, providers, and family groups among low-income patients in Argentina—including a community health worker-led home intervention (health coaching, home BP monitoring, and BP audit and feedback), a physician intervention, and a text-messaging intervention. The community health workers are trained in motivational interviewing techniques, measuring blood pressure, facilitating behavioral change, and providing management skills to improve medication adherence and lifestyle modifications [72]. This comprehensive intervention has been demonstrated to reduce blood pressure and improve hypertension control effectively. The proportion of patients with controlled hypertension increased from 17.0% at baseline to 72.9% at 18 months in the intervention group and from 17.6% to 52.2% in the usual care group; the difference in the increase was 20.6% (95% CI: 15.4–25.9%; $P < 0.001$ [73]. The multicomponent intervention was effective in increasing fruit and vegetable intake and physical activity with no effect on alcohol consumption, smoking, addition of salt, or body weight among low-income families in Argentina [74] and was also cost-effective [75].

8.3.5 *Universal Health Coverage*

Universal health coverage (UHC) means that all people have access to the full range of quality health services they need, when and where they need them, without financial hardship. Achieving UHC is one of the targets the nations of the world set when they adopted the 2030 Sustainable Development Goals (SDGs) in 2015. The UHC service coverage index worldwide increased from 45 to 68 between 2000 and 2021. However, recent progress in increasing coverage has slowed compared to pre-2015 gains, rising only three index points between 2015 and 2021 [76].

Since the 1980s, many Latin American countries began reforms to reduce inequalities in health access and outcomes focused on expanding universal health coverage, especially for poor citizens, with an approach to universal health coverage based on principles of equity, solidarity, and collective action to overcome social inequalities. In most countries, government financing enabled the introduction of supply-side interventions to expand insurance coverage for uninsured citizens. During the 2000s, several countries in the region improved healthcare coverage for informal workers by expanding the treatments available to them and making explicit the healthcare benefits to which the entire population was entitled [77].

The effect of those health reforms in Latin America was that effective health coverage improved between 1990 and 2012 in all Latin American countries but one [78]. However, the median expenditure in the region has not changed much over the past 20 years and is about 6.64% of GDP, much lower than the median 8.97% of OECD country expenditure. Out-of-pocket expenditures have fallen over the past

20 years, but they are still high at 28.62% for the median country, far more than the 17.25% for OECD countries, reflecting inadequate default coverage [9]. On average, 29.3% of people in countries of the Americas reported forgoing needed care due to access barriers, including long waiting times, inappropriate hours of operation, cumbersome administrative requirements, and financial, language, and geographic barriers. People in the poorest quintile were likelier to experience those barriers [79].

A recent telephone survey was conducted in Colombia, Mexico, Peru, and Uruguay. The authors found that although access to care was high, only a third of respondents reported having a high-quality source of care, and only 25% of those with mental health needs had their needs met. Two-thirds of adults could access relevant preventive care, and 42% of older adults were screened for cardiovascular disease. Telehealth access, communication, and autonomy in most recent visits, reasonable waiting times, and receiving preventive health checks showed inequalities favoring people with a high income [80].

To achieve UHC in Latin America, PAHO has proposed (1) Expanding equitable access to comprehensive, quality, people- and community-centered health services, (2) Strengthening stewardship and governance, (3) Increasing and improving financing with equity and efficiency, and advancing towards eliminating direct payments that constitute a barrier to access at the point of service, and (4) Strengthening multisectoral coordination to address the social determinants of health that ensure the sustainability of universal coverage [81].

References

1. Fondo Monetario Internacional. https://www.imf.org/external/datamapper/LP@WEO/CBQ/CMQ/SMQ/MEX.
2. Comisión Económica para América Latina y el Caribe (CEPAL). Envejecimiento en América Latina y el Caribe: inclusión y derechos de las personas mayores. 2022 (LC/CRE). https://www.cepal.org/es/publicaciones/48567-envejecimiento-america-latina-caribe-inclusion-derechos-personas-mayores.
3. WHO. World health statistics 2023: Monitoring health for the SDGs, sustainable development goals. The World health statistics report 2023. p. 119.
4. Ruilope LM, Chagas AC, Brandão AA, Gómez-Berroterán R, Alcalá JJ, Paris JVCJ. Hypertension in Latin America: current perspectives on trends and characteristics. Hipertens Riesgo Vasc. 2017;34(1):50–6. https://doi.org/10.1016/j.hipert.2016.11.005.
5. World Hear tFederation. World heart report 2023: confronting the world's number one killer. Geneva: World Heart Federation; 2023.
6. Linetzky B, Konfino J, Castellana N, De Maio F, Bahit MC, Orlandini ADR. Risk of cardiovascular events associated with positive serology for Chagas: a systematic review. Int J Epidemiol. 2012;41(5):1356–66. https://doi.org/10.1093/ije/dys125.
7. Bank W. Indicadores de desarrollo Mundial. 2022; databank.bancomundial.org
8. Montenegro RA, Stephens C. Indigenous health in Latin America and the Caribbean. Lancet. 2006;367(9525):1859–69. https://doi.org/10.1016/S0140-6736(06)68808-9.
9. Inter American Development Bank. The inequality crisis: Latin America and the Caribbean at the crossroads. Washington, DC: Inter American Development Bank; 2020. https://publications.iadb.org/en/the-inequality-crisis-latin-america-and-the-caribbean-at-the-crossroads.

10. Seale JP, Shellenberger S, Rodriguez C, Seale JD, Alvarado M. Alcohol use and cultural change in an indigenous population: a case study from Venezuela. Alcohol Alcohol. 2002;37:603–8. https://doi.org/10.1093/alcalc/37.6.603.
11. Tavares EF, Vieira-Filho JP, Andriolo A, Sanudo A, Gimeno SG, Franco LJ. Metabolic profi le and cardiovascular risk patterns of an Indian tribe living in the Amazon region of Brazil. Hum Biol. 2003;75:31–46. https://doi.org/10.1353/hub.2003.0028.
12. Filozof C, Gonzalez C, Sereday M, Mazza C, Braguinsky J. Obesity prevalence and trends in Latin-American countries. Obes Rev. 2001;2:99–106.
13. Santos RV. Physical growth and nutritional status of Brazilian Indian populations. Cad Saude Publica. 1993;9(suppl 1):46–57. https://doi.org/10.1046/j.1467-789x.2001.00029.x.
14. Hollenberg NK, Martinez G, McCullough M, Meinking T, Passan D, Preston M, et al. Aging, acculturation, salt intake, and hypertension in the Kuna of Panama. Hypertension. 1997;29(1 Pt 2):171–6. https://doi.org/10.1161/01.hyp.29.1.171.
15. Rosengren A, Smyth A, Rangarajan S, Ramasundarahettige C, Bangdiwala SI, AlHabib KF, et al. Socioeconomic status and risk of cardiovascular disease in 20 low-income, middle-income, and high-income countries: the prospective urban rural epidemiologic (PURE) study. Lancet Glob Health. 2019;7(6):e748–60. https://doi.org/10.1016/S2214-109X(19)30045-2.
16. Chang CL, Marmot MG, Farley TM, Poulter NR. The influence of economic development on the association between education and the risk of acute myocardial infarction and stroke. J Clin Epidemiol. 2002;55(8):741–7. https://doi.org/10.1016/s0895-4356(02)00413-4.
17. Zhang J, Fang Y, Yao Y, Zhao Y, Yue D, Sung M, Jin Y, Zheng Z-J. Disparities in cardiovascular disease prevalence among middle-aged and older adults: roles of socioeconomic position, social connection, and behavioral and physiological risk factors. Front Cardiovasc Med. 2022;9:972683. https://doi.org/10.3389/fcvm.2022.972683.
18. Rivera-Andrade A, Luna MA. Trends and heterogeneity of cardiovascular disease and risk factors across Latin American and Caribbean countries. Prog Cardiovasc Dis. 2014;57(3):276–85. https://doi.org/10.1016/j.pcad.2014.09.004.
19. Shafi BH, Bøttcher M, Ejupi A, Jensen G, Osler M, Lange T, Prescott E. Socioeconomic disparity in cardiovascular disease: possible biological pathways based on a proteomic approach. Atherosclerosis. 2022;352:62–8. https://doi.org/10.1016/j.atherosclerosis.2022.05.020.
20. Perner MS, Alazraqui M, Amorim LD. Social inequalities between neighborhoods and cardiovascular disease: a multilevel analysis in a Latin American city. Ciênc Saúde Colet. 2022;27(7):2597–608. https://doi.org/10.1590/1413-81232022277.21662021.
21. Sosa-Liprandi Á, Sosa Liprandi MI, Alexánderson E, Avezum Á, Lanas F, López-Jaramillo JP, et al. Clinical impact of the polypill for cardiovascular prevention in Latin America: a consensus statement of the Inter-American Society of Cardiology. Glob Heart. 2019;14(1):3–16.e1. https://doi.org/10.1016/j.gheart.2018.10.001.
22. Lanas F, Seron P, Lanas A. Cardiovascular disease in Latin America: the growing epidemic. Prog Cardiovasc Dis. 2014;57(3):262–7. https://doi.org/10.1016/j.pcad.2014.07.007.
23. WHO Mortality Database. https://www.who.int/data/data-collection-tools/who-mortality-database. Accessed 10 Aug 2023.
24. Lopez-Jaramillo P, Joseph P, Lopez-Lopez JP, Lanas F, Avezum A, Diaz R, et al. Risk factors, cardiovascular disease, and mortality in South America: a PURE substudy. Eur Heart J. 2022;43(30):2841–51. https://doi.org/10.1093/eurheartj/ehac113.
25. Coelho DM, de Souza Andrade AC, Silva UM, Lazo M, Slesinski SC, Quistberg A, et al. Gender differences in the association of individual and contextual socioeconomic status with hypertension in 230 Latin American cities from the SALURBAL study: a multilevel analysis. BMC Public Health. 2023;23(1):1532. https://doi.org/10.1186/s12889-023-16480-3.
26. 4° Encuesta Nacional de Factores De Riesgo. Dirección Nacional de Promoción de la Salud y Control de Enfermedades Crónicas No Transmisibles. Informe Definitivo. https://bancos.salud.gob.ar/sites/default/files/2020-01/4ta-encuesta-nacional-factores-riesgo_2019_informe-definitivo.pdf. Accessed 5 Jan 2024.
27. Gomes CS, Gonçalves RPF, Silva AGD, Sá ACMGN, Alves FTA, Ribeiro ALP, Malta DC. Factors associated with cardiovascular disease in the Brazilian adult population:

National Health Survey, 2019. Rev Bras Epidemiol. 2021;24(suppl 2):e210013. https://doi.org/10.1590/1980-549720210013.supl.2.
28. Chan JJL, Tran-Nhu L, Pitcairn CFM, Laverty AA, Mrejen M, Pescarini JM, Hone TV. Inequalities in the prevalence of cardiovascular disease risk factors in Brazilian slum populations: a cross-sectional study. PLOS Glob Public Health. 2022;2(9):e0000990. https://doi.org/10.1371/journal.pgph.0000990.
29. Malta DC, Szwarcwald CL, Machado ÍE, Pereira CA, Figueiredo AW, Sá ACMGN, et al. Prevalence of altered total cholesterol and fractions in the Brazilian adult population: National Health Survey. Rev Bras Epidemiol. 2019;22(Suppl 2):E190005.SUPL.2. https://doi.org/10.1590/1980-549720190005.
30. Chor D, Ribeiro ALP, Sá Carvalho M, Duncan BB, Lotufo PA, Nobre AA, et al. Prevalence, awareness, treatment and influence of socioeconomic variables on control of high blood pressure: results of the ELSA-Brasil study. PLoS One. 2015;10(6):e0127382. https://doi.org/10.1371/journal.pone.0127382.
31. Malta DC, Bernal RT, Souza MF, Szwarcwald CL, Lima MG, Barros MB. Social inequalities in the prevalence of self-reported chronic non-communicable diseases in Brazil: National Health Survey 2013. Int J Equity Health. 2016;15(1):153. https://doi.org/10.1186/s12939-016-0427-4.
32. Matos SMA, Duncan BB, Bensenor IM, Mill JG, Giatti L, Molina MDCB, et al. Incidence of excess body weight and annual weight gain in women and men: results from the ELSA-Brasil cohort. Am J Hum Biol. 2021;34(3):e23606. https://doi.org/10.1002/ajhb.23606.
33. Oliveira GMM, Brant LCC, Polanczyk CA, Malta DC, Biolo A, Nascimento BR, et al. Cardiovascular statistics—Brazil 2021. Arq Bras Cardiol. 2022;118(1):115–373. English, Portuguese. https://doi.org/10.36660/abc.20211012.
34. Pérez-Flórez M, Achcar JA. Desigualdades socioeconómicas en la mortalidad por enfermedades cardiovasculares: Región Pacifico de Colombia, 2002-2015 [Socioeconomic inequalities in mortality due to cardiovascular diseases: Pacific Region of Colombia, 2002–2015]. Ciênc Saúde Colet. 2021;26(suppl 3):5201–14. https://doi.org/10.1590/1413-812320212611.3.02562020.
35. Camacho PA, Gomez-Arbelaez D, Molina DI, Sanchez G, Arcos E, Narvaez C, et al. Social disparities explain differences in hypertension prevalence, detection and control in Colombia. J Hypertens. 2016;34(12):2344–52. https://doi.org/10.1097/HJH.0000000000001115.
36. inisterio de Salud de Chile. Encuesta Nacional de salud 1016-16. https://www.minsal.cl/wp-content/uploads/2017/11/ENS-2016-17_PRIMEROS-RESULTADOS.pdf.
37. Freire WB, Ramírez-Luzuriaga MJ, Belmont P, Mendieta MJ, Silva-Jaramillo MK, Romero N, et al. Tomo I: Encuesta Nacional de Salud y Nutrición de la población ecuatoriana de cero a 59 años. ENSANUT-ECU 2012. Quito-Ecuador: Ministerio de Salud Pública/Instituto Nacional de Estadísticas y Censos; 2014.
38. Basto-Abreu A, López-Olmedo N, Rojas-Martínez R, Aguilar-Salinas CA, Moreno-Banda GL, Carnalla M, Rivera JA, et al. Prevalencia de prediabetes y diabetes en México: Ensanut 2022. Salud Publica Mex. 2023;65:s163–8. Spanish. https://doi.org/10.21149/14832.
39. Campos-Nonato I, Oviedo-Solís C, Vargas-Meza J, Ramírez-Villalobos D, Medina-García C, Gómez-Álvarez E, et al. Prevalencia, tratamiento y control de la hipertensión arterial en adultos mexicanos: resultados de la Ensanut 2022. Salud Publica Mex. 2023;65:s169–80. https://doi.org/10.21149/14779.
40. Campos-Nonato I, Galván-Valencia Ó, Hernández-Barrera L, Oviedo-Solís C, Barquera S. Prevalencia de obesidad y factores de riesgo asociados en adultos mexicanos: resultados de la Ensanut 2022. Salud Publica Mex. 2023;65:s238–47. https://doi.org/10.21149/14809.
41. Ramos E, Andreis M, Beam C, Bissessar R, Chen D, Cordido M, et al. Equity and prevention of cardiovascular diseases in Latin America and the Caribbean. Glob Heart. 2022;17(1):35. https://doi.org/10.5334/gh.1123.
42. Pan American Health Organization. Framework Convention on Tobacco Control. 43rd Directing Council of the Pan American Health Organization, 53rd Session of the Regional Committee of WHO for the Americas; 2001 Sep 24–28; Washington, DC. (Resolution CD43.R12 2001). Washington, DC: PAHO; 2001. [cited 2021 Oct 31]. https://iris.paho.org/bitstream/handle/.10665.2/1442/cd43.r12-e.pdf.

43. World Health Organization. WHO framework convention on tobacco control. Geneva: WHO; 2003. updated reprint 2004, 2005 [cited 2022 Mar 7]. https://apps.who.int/iris/handle/10665/42811.
44. World Health Organization. MPOWER: a policy package to reverse the tobacco epidemic. Geneva: WHO; 2008. https://www.afro.who.int/publications/mpower-policy-package-reverse-tobacco-epidemic.
45. WHO. WHO report on the Global Tobacco Epidemic: offer help to quit tobacco use. Geneva: World Health Organization; 2019. https://www.who.int/publications/i/item/WHO-NMH-PND-2019.5.
46. WHO report on the global tobacco epidemic 2021: addressing new and emerging products. Geneva: World Health Organization; 2021. Licence: CC BY-NC-SA 3.0 IGO. https://www.who.int/publications/i/item/9789240032095.
47. Severini G, Sandoval RC, Sóñora G, Sosa P, Gutkowski P, Severini L, et al. Towards a smoke-free world? South America became the first 100% smoke-free subregion in the Americas. Rev Panam Salud Publica. 2022;46:e103. https://doi.org/10.26633/RPSP.2022.103.
48. Pan American Health Organization. Report on tobacco control in the region of the Americas. Washington, DC: PAHO; 2018. https://iris.paho.org/handle/10665.2/49237
49. Pichon-Riviere A, Bardach A, Rodríguez Cairoli F, et al. Health, economic and social burden of tobacco in Latin America and the expected gains of fully implementing taxes, plain packaging, advertising bans and smoke-free environments control measures: a modelling study. Tob Control. 2024;33(5):611–21. https://doi.org/10.1136/tc-2022-057618.
50. Latin American Action Plan for Prevention of Child and Adolescent Obesity PAHO. Plan of action for the prevention of obesity in children and adolescents. https://www.paho.org/hq/dmdocuments/2015/Obesity-Plan-Of-Action-Child-Eng-2015.pdf.
51. Infant exclusive breastfeeding in the Region of the Americas: results from national population-based surveys. ENLACE data portal. Department of Noncommunicable Diseases and Mental Health, Pan American Health Organization; 2022. https://www.paho.org/en/enlace/exclusive-breastfeeding-infant-under-six-months-age.
52. Melo G, Aguilar-Farias N, López Barrera E, Chomalí L, Moz-Christofoletti MA, Salgado JC, Swensson LJ, Caro JC. Structural responses to the obesity epidemic in Latin America: what are the next steps for food and physical activity policies? Lancet Reg Health Am. 2023;21:100486. https://doi.org/10.1016/j.lana.2023.100486.
53. Berdegué J, Fuentealba R. Latin America: the state of smallholders in agriculture. 2014. https://doi.org/10.1093/acprof:oso/9780199689347.003.0005.
54. FAO. The state of food security and nutrition in the world 2021; 2021. https://doi.org/10.4060/CB4474EN).
55. The Global Food Research Program. Sugar. The Global Food Research Program. 2022. https://www.globalfoodresearchprogram.org/wp-content/uploads/2022/02/Sugary_Drink_Tax_maps_2022_02.pdf.
56. Ríos-Reyna C, Díaz-Ramírez G, Castillo-Ruíz O, Pardo-Buitimea NY, Alemán-Castillo SE. Políticas y estrategias para combatir la obesidad en Latinoamérica. Rev Med Inst Mex Seguro Soc. 2022;60(6):666–74.
57. Rodríguez OL, Pizarro QT. Ley de Etiquetado y Publicidad de Alimentos: Chile innovando en nutrición pública una vez más. Rev Chil Pediatr. 2018;89(5):579–81. https://doi.org/10.4067/S0370-41062018005000806.
58. Taillie LS, Reyes M, Colchero MA, Popkin B, Corvalán C. An evaluation of Chile's law of food labeling and advertising on sugar-sweetened beverage purchases from 2015 to 2017: a before and after study. PLoS Med. 2020;17(2):1–22., e1003015. https://doi.org/10.1371/journal.pmed.1003015.
59. The Global Food Research Program. Regulations. 2022. https://www.globalfoodresearchprogram.org/wp-content/uploads/2022/02/Sugary_Drink_Tax_maps_2022_02.pdf.
60. Patel P, Ordunez P, DiPette D, Escobar MC, Hassell T, Wyss F, et al. Standardized hypertension treatment and prevention network. Improved blood pressure control to reduce cardiov

disease morbidity and mortality: the standardized hypertension treatment and prevention project. J Clin Hypertens (Greenwich). 2016;18(12):1284–94. https://doi.org/10.1111/jch.12861.
61. Campbell NR, Chen G. Canadian efforts to prevent and control hypertension. Can J Cardiol. 2010;26 Suppl C(Suppl C):14C–7C. https://doi.org/10.1016/s0828-282x(10)71076-x.
62. Jaffe MG, Lee GA, Young JD, Sidney S, Go AS. Improved blood pressure control associated with a large-scale hypertension program. JAMA. 2013;310(7):699–705. https://doi.org/10.1001/jama.2013.108769.
63. Ordunez P, Campbell NRC, Giraldo Arcila GP, Angell SY, Lombardi C, Brettler JW, et al. HEARTS in the Americas: innovations for improving hypertension and cardiovascular disease risk management in primary care. Rev Panam Salud Publica. 2022;46:e96. https://doi.org/10.26633/RPSP.2022.96.
64. World Health Organization. Global Hearts Initiative. https://www.who.int/news/item/15-09-2016-global-heartsinitiative. Accessed March 2022.
65. Campbell NRC, Ordunez P, Giraldo G, Rodriguez Morales YA, Lombardi C, Khan T, et al. WHO HEARTS: a global program to reduce cardiovascular disease burden: experience implementing in the Americas and opportunities in Canada. Can J Cardiol. 2021;37(5):744–55. https://doi.org/10.1016/j.cjca.2020.12.004.
66. Valdés González Y, Campbell NRC, Pons Barrera E, Calderón Martínez M, Pérez Carrera A, Morales Rigau JM, et al. Implementation of a community-based hypertension control program in Matanzas, Cuba. J Clin Hypertens (Greenwich). 2020;22(2):142–9. https://doi.org/10.1111/jch.13814.
67. Moran AE, Gupta R. Global Hearts initiative collaborators. Implementation of global hearts hypertension control programs in 32 low- and middle-income countries: JACC international. J Am Coll Cardiol. 2023;82(19):1868–84. https://doi.org/10.1016/j.jacc.2023.08.043.
68. Pan American Health Organization. Innovative care for chronic conditions: organizing and delivering high quality care for chronic noncommunicable diseases in the Americas. Washington, DC: PAHO; 2013. https://iris.paho.org/handle/10665.2/18639?show=full
69. Chivardi C, Hutchinson B, Molina V, et al. Assessing costs of a hypertension program in primary care: evidence from the HEARTS program in Mexico. Rev Panam Salud Publica. 2022;46:e144. https://doi.org/10.26633/RPSP.2022.144.
70. Schwalm JR, McCready T, Lamelas P, Musa H, Lopez-Jaramillo P, Yusoff K, et al. Rationale and design of a cluster randomized trial of a multifaceted intervention in people with hypertension: the heart outcomes prevention and evaluation 4 (HOPE-4) study. Am Heart J. 2018;203:57–66. https://doi.org/10.1016/j.ahj.2018.06.004.
71. Schwalm JD, McCready T, Lopez-Jaramillo P, Yusoff K, Attaran A, Lamelas P, et al. Community-based comprehensive intervention to reduce cardiovascular risk in hypertension (HOPE 4): a cluster-randomised controlled trial. Lancet. 2019;394(10205):1231–42. https://doi.org/10.1016/S0140-6736(19)31949-X.
72. Mills KT, Rubinstein A, Irazola V, Chen J, Beratarrechea A, Poggio R, et al. Comprehensive approach for hypertension control in low-income populations: rationale and study design for the hypertension control program in Argentina. Am J Med Sci. 2014;348(2):139–45. https://doi.org/10.1097/MAJ.0000000000000298.
73. He J, Irazola V, Mills KT, Poggio R, Beratarrechea A, Dolan J, et al. Effect of a community health worker-led multicomponent intervention on blood pressure control in low-income patients in Argentina: a randomized clinical trial. JAMA. 2017;318(11):1016–25. https://doi.org/10.1001/jama.2017.11358.
74. Poggio R, Melendi SE, Beratarrechea A, Gibbons L, Mills KT, Chen CS, et al. Cluster randomized trial for hypertension control: effect on lifestyles and body weight. Am J Prev Med. 2019;57(4):438–46. https://doi.org/10.1016/j.amepre.2019.05.011.
75. Zhang Y, Yin L, Mills K, Chen J, He J, Palacios A, Riviere AP, Irazola V, Augustovski F, Shi L. Cost-effectiveness of a multicomponent intervention for hypertension control in low-income settings in Argentina. JAMA Netw Open. 2021;4(9):e2122559. https://doi.org/10.1001/jamanetworkopen.2021.22559.

76. Universal Health Coverage (UHC)-Key. Facts. https://www.who.int/news-room/fact-sheets/detail/universal-health-coverage-(uhc).
77. Cotlear D, Gómez-Dantés O, Knaul F, Atun R, Barreto IC, Cetrángolo O, et al. Overcoming social segregation in healthcare in Latin America. Lancet. 2015;385(9974):1248–59.
78. Wagstaff A, Dmytraczenko T, Almeida G, Buisman L, Hoang-Vu Eozenou P, et al. Assessing Latin America's progress toward achieving universal health coverage. Health Aff (Millwood). 2015;34(10):1704–12. https://doi.org/10.1377/hlthaff.2014.1453.
79. Báscolo E, Houghton N, Del Riego A. Leveraging household survey data to measure barriers to health services access in the Americas. Rev Panam Salud Publica. 2020;44:e100. https://doi.org/10.26633/RPSP.2020.100.
80. Roberti J, Leslie HH, Doubova SV, Ranilla JM, Mazzoni A, Espinoza L, et al. Inequalities in health system coverage and quality: a cross-sectional survey of four Latin American countries. Lancet Glob Health. 2024;12(1):e145–55. https://doi.org/10.1016/S2214-109X(23)00488-6.
81. PAHO. Universal Health. https://www.paho.org/en/topics/universal-health.

Chapter 9
Tackling the Challenge of the Epidemic of Cardiovascular Diseases: A Case of Sub-Saharan Africa

Elijah N. Ogola and Yubrine M. Gachemba

9.1 Introduction

SSA is now facing a double burden of disease where patients are suffering from non-communicable diseases such as coronary heart disease, hypertension, kidney disease, and diabetes while still grappling with communicable diseases [1]. Due to this double burden, CVD prevention and treatment has been overlooked for a very long time, allowing the rates to continue to rise unchecked.

Due to adoption of western lifestyles, the rates of CVD risk factors, such as diabetes, are expected to increase by 50%. Because of this, 80% of CVD deaths worldwide take place in developing countries like those in SSA [2]. CVD is emerging as a leading cause of mortality overtaking communicable diseases [3]. It is therefore imperative that concerted efforts are taken to combat the looming epidemic.

9.2 The Unique Challenges in SSA

Globally, CVD deaths have steadily increased by over a third from just over 12 million in 1990 to 18.6 million in 2019. More than 80% of these cases were in low- and middle-income countries (LMICs) [4]. Risk factors for the development of CVD are similar throughout the world [5]. SSA is witnessing a marked increase in major CVD risk factors, such as hypertension, diabetes, overweight and obesity, physical inactivity, tobacco use, and the dyslipidemia. This is mainly driven by an increase

E. N. Ogola (✉)
University of Nairobi, Nairobi, Kenya
e-mail: elijah.ogola@uonbi.ac.ke

Y. M. Gachemba
Aberdeen Royal Infirmary, University of Aberdeen School of Medicine, Aberdeen, UK

T. Romero et al. (eds.), *Global Challenges in Cardiovascular Prevention in Populations with Low Socioeconomic Status*,
https://doi.org/10.1007/978-3-031-79051-5_9

in urbanization leading to behavioral and dietary changes like increase in salt and alcohol consumption [6, 7].

In SSA, CVDs are the largest contributor to the total NCD burden, accounting for 38.3% of NCD deaths and 22.9 million DALYs [8, 9]. CVD deaths have jumped from the sixth to the second leading cause of death in sub-Saharan Africa (SSA) between 1990 and 2019 [7]. More than half of CVD deaths in Africa are categorized as premature mortalities, occurring between the ages of 30 and 70 years [10]. The rise in traditional CVD risk factors largely leads to a rise in atherosclerotic cardiovascular disease (ASCVD). However, there remains a large burden of endemic CVD in Africa that are largely neglected. These include conditions such as rheumatic valve disease, various cardiomyopathies, for example, peripartum cardiomyopathy and endomyocardial fibrosis (EMF), and pericardial disease, often HIV-associated tuberculous pericarditis. These neglected cardiac diseases impose a major burden upon the patients, their families, the health systems, and the societies as a whole [7].

On average, Africa still has low health expenditure (averaged at 103 US$ per capita in 2016), with several countries still below the minimum recommended $44 per capita. Compounded by the lack of universal health coverage in most SSA countries, there is a resultant high out-of-pocket cost for citizens of SSA, causing impoverishment and inequity in health care access [7].

Variations in the levels of risk factors for CVDs in SAA, such as high sodium intake, low potassium intake, obesity, alcohol consumption, physical inactivity, and unhealthy diet, might explain some of the regional heterogeneity in CVD prevalence in SSA [11].

The WHO Global Action Plan for the prevention and Control of NCDs [12] set targets for a 25% decrease in premature CVD mortality by 2025 and a third reduction for premature NCD mortality by 2030, covered in the sustainable development goals (SDGs). Even in the context of ASCVD, the drivers of mortality and morbidity in SSA are considerably different compared to high-income countries (HICs). Ischemic heart disease (IHD) has been identified as the leading cause of cardiovascular mortality globally (nearly 50% of all CVD deaths), but on the other hand, stroke (specifically hypertensive stroke), has been the greatest contributor to ASCVD mortality in Africa [13].

There have been regional efforts to address Africa specific challenges mostly spearheaded by the Pan-African Society of Cardiology (PASCAR). Among these is the PASCAR roadmap on the control of hypertension which aims to achieve a 25% reduction in hypertension prevalence in Africa by 2025 [6]. Another significant initiative was the Addis Ababa communique on the eradication of rheumatic heart disease [14]. This led to the World Health Assembly passing a resolution in 2018 on the eradication of RHD, which emphasizes political commitment to tackle RHD as a matter of priority with the emphasis on the need for technical guidance on the design of RHD control programs that can be integrated within primary health care and universal health coverage systems in SSA [15].

Hypertension deserves special mention being the leading cause of global mortality and morbidity [16]. Hypertension prevalence is exponentially rising in SSA [6].

It is dubbed the "silent killer," and many patients in SSA present for the first time to health care facilities with fatal complications. This "silent killer" is responsible for more than half of total CVD-related deaths, being the main driver to IHD, heart failure, and stroke burden on the continent [17, 18].

A prospective study in Tanzania showed that hypertension-related deaths accounted for 33.9% of all NCD deaths and 15.3% of total mortality [19]. Benefits of adequately controlled blood pressure are well-known and cannot be overemphasized [20]. Africa not only has the highest age-adjusted prevalence but also one of the regions with a rising age-adjusted prevalence [13]. Of importance is the large burden of undiagnosed, untreated, and uncontrolled hypertension in SSA [13, 21]. The poor awareness rates are due to poor screening systems for hypertension. A national NCD risk factor survey in Kenya showed that about two thirds of adults have never had a BP measurement. Even among treated cases, poor control is common [22]. The need for hypertension control in Africa is undoubtedly one of the highest priorities as the region aims to lower the CVD burden of disease.

9.3 Gender Inequalities in CVD Care

There is evidence of sex differences in the risk and occurrence of CVDs in SSA, which has not been adequately addressed [23]. A review of the evidence from Ghana, Nigeria, South Africa, and Tanzania indicates a poor health system response to the increasing risk of CVDs with no discussion on the risk associated with sex and gender [24]. While sex-based studies, especially in NCDs, are gaining more advocacy globally, there is a sex and gender research gap and data paucity in the African context.

Understanding the mechanisms that contribute to worsening risk factor profiles in young women to reduce future CVD morbidity and mortality in SSA is paramount. Data is required to recognize the prevalence of traditional ASCVD risk factors, and their differential impact in SSA women, as well as their unique emerging, non-traditional risk factors, so as to contribute to new understanding of mechanisms leading to worse outcomes for women.

Evidence [25] shows that awareness of CVD as the primary cause of mortality in women has been slowly increasing. For instance in 1997, only 30% of American women surveyed were aware that CVD was the leading cause of death in women and this increased to 54% in 2009 and has subsequently plateaued when last surveyed in 2012 [25].Noteworthy available evidence indicates that women are less likely to receive preventive treatment or guidance, such as lipid-lowering therapy, aspirin (ASA), and therapeutic lifestyle changes, than are men at similar ASCVD risk, and when medications are prescribed, treatment is less likely to be aggressive or to achieve optimal effects [26].

The Women's Ischemia Syndrome Evaluation (WISE) [27] implicated abnormal coronary reactivity, microvascular dysfunction, and plaque erosion/distal microembolization as causative to female-specific IHD pathophysiology. Women with IHD have a persistent suboptimal treatment pattern, higher mortality, and poorer CVD outcomes compared with men.

The few trained cardiologists in SSA have traditionally been trained to equate IHD with angiographically defined obstructive CAD; failure to recognize unique aspects of IHD in women has contributed to less aggressive lifestyle and medical preventive interventions in women relative to men and may contribute to the observed sex-based mortality gap. With more data from SSA women a paradigm shift beyond solely an anatomic description of obstructive CAD is needed to translate into earlier IHD risk detection and treatment for SSA women. These unique challenges of CVD in women have not been studied in SSA, which is a major evidence gap.

Biological variances among women and men are called sex differences and are frequently reproducible in animal models. Sex differences in CVD risk and events have been investigated but their association with sociocultural gender has not received the same attention. Unfortunately, sex and gender are often used interchangeably and incorrectly in scientific writing, obscuring the relationships and insights that would otherwise be revealed. While sex and gender are distinct concepts, they are also interrelated and intersect and therefore are not mutually exclusive.

A general acceptance and use of agreed upon definitions may go some way in resolving this confusion. The body is at once both biological and social, and thus physical health is simultaneously influenced by both sex (the biological) and gender (the social) [28].

Sex-stratified analysis lacks considerations of the influences of gender and may not present a complete description of CVD health/events, directly impacting the design and implementation of interventions designed to meet the targets for Sustainable Development Goal 3 and achieve a 30% reduction in premature mortality due to cardiovascular diseases and other NCDs [23].

Cardiac disease is a leading cause of non-obstetric maternal death worldwide, but little is known about its burden in sub-Saharan Africa [29]. The growing population in SSA comes with more pregnancies and labor. This poses remarkable physiological and hemodynamic stress and portends significant negative consequences on both maternal and fetal outcomes [30]. Globally, 1–4% of pregnancies are complicated by maternal CVDs (excluding systemic arterial hypertension). On its own, hypertension occurs in up to 10% of all pregnancies, while pre-eclampsia complicates 2–8% of all pregnancies and is responsible for the highest maternal mortality in SSA [7].

Challenges still exist in the management of patients with heart disease in pregnancy in SSA. African women in general are under social pressure to bear children and will take the risk despite the severity of disease. Improving outcomes of pregnant mothers with CVD requires a well-tailored, integrated, and context-specific approach that engages the patient (understanding the patient needs) and involves a multidisciplinary team headed by a pregnancy heart team [31].

Currently half way between 2015 and 2030, current projections indicate that in SSA, overall progress is not enough to achieve SDG 3.4 by 2030. There is limited awareness and access to preconception counselling, with many women seeking health care after or at the end of the first trimester while on chronic cardiac medications and anticoagulation therapy which are contraindicated in pregnancy [7].

The rising prevalence of overweight/obesity in young population of females in SSA is very worrisome as it is associated with increasing risks of hypertension and diabetes that are known risk factors of CVD mortality and morbidity. In order to impact the rising epidemic of hypertension in women in SSA, gender factors need to be considered in the interventions aimed at the prevention and control of hypertension. For example, the CREOLE (Comparison of Three Combination Therapies in Lowering Blood Pressure in Black Africans) Trial done across 10 sites across sub-Saharan Africa found clinically important differences in the therapeutic response to antihypertensive combination therapy among African women compared with African men [32].

Therefore, it is important to consider the gender-related risk factors while implementing preventive programs and creating effective health policies. There is definitely need for future research that is directed in exploring the association of other important gender-related factors and their role in CVDs in SSA.

9.4 Social Disparities and CVD in SSA

Although CVD mortality rates have almost halved over recent decades in developed economies it continues to rise in LMIC like SSA [13] and thus, there is no room for complacency in the efforts required to address the major challenges that CVD continues to play in individual lives, communities, and society as a whole in SSA.

Furthermore, CVD is one of the conditions most strongly associated with health inequalities, even within individual countries and regions. If you live in SSA's most deprived areas, you are almost four times more likely to die prematurely than those in the least deprived areas somewhere else in the globe [33].

Data from industrialized countries [34] has suggested a positive association of obesity with low-income and deprived neighborhoods. This contradiction has been demonstrated to be due to heightened deprivation and exposure to poor-quality foods, which are the default choice due to low income among the poor in Western countries. In sharp contrast in Africa, a possible explanation for the higher prevalence of obesity and malnutrition in affluent and urban populations in Africa may be explained by the increasing evolvement of urbanization within the African continent [35].

The majority of SSA countries are undergoing swift changes in their social and economic environments, accompanied with concomitant changes in food-consumption patterns. The consequence of urbanization in SSA, which is often connected with the adoption of a lifestyle commonly referred to as "westernization," is the increased intake of energy-dense foods and high-calorie sugary meals and drinks associated with less energy-demanding jobs, complemented by increased sedentary lifestyles and the adoption of detrimental eating habits. All of these factors above may have contributed to the higher prevalence of obesity noticed in the urban and affluent populations of African countries [36]. This creates the unique situation where "undernutrition" and "over nutrition" exist side by side.

9.5 Lack of Patient and Public Involvement and Engagement

In the SSAs, sustainable primary prevention of cardiovascular disease is associated with the engagement of facilitators that support it and hindered by barriers that undermine the support of a healthy lifestyle at the community and family level.

SSA countries do not have the benefit of integrated primary health care (PHC) programs for prevention, early detection, and treatment of CVD compared to high-income settings. As a result, individuals in low- and middle-income countries are often detected late in the course of the disease resulting in increased mortality and morbidity. They die younger from CVD and other NCDs while in their most productive years with major consequences to the society [37].

For instance, in 2013, an estimated one million premature deaths were attributed to CVD in sub-Saharan Africa, constituting 5.5% of all global CVD-related deaths and 11.3% of all deaths [35].

Preventing and managing CVD in low-resource and urban poor settings in SSA countries should consider perceptions and understanding of risk factors for CVD in these countries, and the interrelationships among them while accounting for cultural and contextual issues of the citizens involved.

Locally generated evidence on awareness and opportunities for CVD care is a good place to start, coupled with effective risk communication through health care providers. Screening for and treatment of CVD must address issues such as prohibitive cost of health care without overlooking social determinants of disease and health, mainly poverty and illiteracy, which are important social determinants of CVD in low-resource settings.

9.6 Poor Health Care Systems in SSA

The epidemiological transition in SSA has created enormous public health challenges, by leading to a double burden of disease. The double burden of communicable and chronic NCDs has long-term public health impact as it exerts considerable strain on health care systems. Failure to address the problem will impose significant burden for the health sector and the economy of sub-Saharan African countries.

SSA countries, similar to most developing countries, often do not have the public health infrastructure and finances to address both communicable and poverty-related illness and behavior/chronic-related illnesses. In addition, health care funding, especially from donor agencies, is disproportionately directed at communicable diseases at the expense of NCDs [38].

The involvement of SSA governments on both national levels and local jurisdictions is necessary to curb the emerging epidemic on CVD in SSA. Lack of awareness of the rising burden CVDs by policy makers leads to lack of prioritization of NCD programs. Advocacy towards prioritizing NCD programs is therefore necessary.

Despite the high cardiovascular risk burden, it is important to note that health care systems in many parts of SSA are designed to treat acute communicable diseases, rather than chronic NCDs such as CVDs, in part due to resources. As a result, the health care system is ill equipped for the management of CVDs.

Some important issues such as lack of protocols for CVDs, evaluation and monitoring, little or non-existent referral systems, inadequate health facilities, and absence of multidisciplinary approach to care teams also make CVD care difficult [39].

9.7 Poor Resources and Low Prioritization of CVD in SSA

NCD prevention and control is of low but increasing priority in SSA; challenges to addressing this burden relate to huge numbers with NCDs (especially hypertension) requiring care, overall resource constraints and wider systemic issues, including poorly supported primary care services and access barriers. In addition to securing and strengthening political will and commitment and directing more resources and attention towards this area, there is a need for constructive engagement to shape future SSA governments involvement and commitments to lowering the burden of CVD in SSA [40].

Health systems in many sub-Saharan African countries remain fragile, fragmented, under-resourced, and limited for mounting an effective response to the double burden of communicable diseases and NCDs [41].

Notably the migration of skilled health workers from sub-Saharan African countries has significantly increased. Despite the growing problem of health worker migration for the effective functioning of health care systems, there is a remarkable paucity and incompleteness of data on this subject and its contribution to CVD in SSA underscoring the real extent of migration from, and within, Africa, so as to develop effective forecasting or remedial policies.

Increasingly, fragility is recognized as a multi-dimensional phenomenon reflective of country and historical context, the vulnerabilities of the health system in SSA countries and the population itself, as well as breakdowns in interactions between populations and health systems. For example, violence and prolonged conflict, political and economic instability, marginalization and inequality, weak and distorted national governance structures and processes and substantive environmental threats including climate change and natural disasters undermine, and even reverse, the advances in health and well-being in SSA [42].

Most of the time there is lack of contextual data from SSA, hindering priority setting. Reliance on donor-funded initiatives programs gives the donors undue influence in setting the agenda leading to skewed priorities.

Moving forward, investment in cost-effective ways for the prevention and treatment of risk factors for CVD is paramount [40].

Systematic screening, improving access to medication, and implementing standardized guideline-directed clinical management is vital to control efforts. CVD research output from Africa is rising but remains low and out of proportion to the rising burden of CVD on the continent, despite some progress over the past 50 years. The extent of collaboration within Africa is much lower than the level of collaboration with non-African countries [7].

Advocating for strategies to improve the quantity and impact of cardiovascular research, including increased resources to train cardiovascular health professionals and researchers, build infrastructures, and fund research on CVD priorities for SSA cannot be overemphasized.

Creating and expanding collaborative research networks within Africa will be pivotal to improve global cardiovascular health [6]. Lack of systematic surveillance data covering vital statistics such as causes of mortality within countries hinders disease burden estimates and consequently affects monitoring and evaluation of interventions.

Therefore, there is a large gap to fill for general access to CVD care, and the contributory factors include [12]:

Low health budget allocation—Most SSA countries have insufficient health financing systems with high out of pocket expenditures. Almost half of all African countries still have out-of-pocket expenditures of above 40% [43].

In general, health spending in still very low in Africa, with the Central, Western, and Eastern African regions documented to have the lowest worldwide. In addition, there is a huge reliance on donor funding among several African countries and relatively less government health service expenditure on primary care with donor funding mostly directed towards communicable diseases.

The lack of universal health coverage and consequently high out-of-pocket expenditure often results in catastrophic health spending for citizens of SSA.

Inadequate access and long-term affordability of evidenced-based CVD medications, including important drugs for CVD prevention [37].

Lack of centers of excellence not only to offer advanced care and training, but also to spearhead advanced home grown research and innovation [37].

Low education and health literacy levels, affects health choices made, including health-seeking behavior partly contributing to challenges described such as the late presentation of CVDs and subsequently poor prognosis [7].

There is a paucity of cost-effective, integrated, and evidenced-based approaches for CVD prevention targeted at whole populations and supported by effective policies and government commitment.

9.8 Solutions

Prevention of CVD in SSA should be strengthened across the whole spectrum, from primordial, primary, secondary to tertiary prevention levels. For example, the Strategic Plan from the AHA for 2020 [44], articulated the goal "by 2020 to improve the cardiovascular health of all Americans by 20%," while reducing deaths from CVD and stroke by 20%." To achieve these goals, the AHA outlined a series of steps, many of which depend on lifestyle modalities with an overall strategy based on three pillars: (a) primordial prevention, (b) evidence that risk factors for CVD develop early in life, and (c) balancing individualized risk approaches with population level approaches.

SSA countries need to identify and implement cost-effective, preventive strategies targeting both high risk and the general population. Integration and strengthening of primary health care services is an important strategy. This should be in the backdrop of preventive efforts such as the adoption of the FCTC for tobacco control, introducing sugar tax for processed foods, and implementing population-based interventions that promote healthy lifestyles that have proven effective in several settings.

This will therefore require sustained advocacy by in-country stakeholders such as cardiovascular specialists, patient organizations, civil society, policy makers, and implementers to prioritize these policies in order to improve CVD outcomes.

Most critically in the context of SSA, hypertension prevention deserves concerted efforts given its contribution to CVD. Universal and periodic screening, diagnosis, and guideline-directed treatment through strengthening and integration into primary care facilities, task-shifting, and universal availability of effective drugs should be prioritized in SSA countries.

9.9 Improvement of Access

Access to Affordable care: Reducing out-of-pocket expenditure and implementing health financing plans with the objective of increasing equitable and effective access to CVD care is of critical importance [1].

Strengthening PHC: Health reforms in SSA countries to promote progress towards UHC will involve country commitments to increasing revenue generation and overall government expenditure on health, employing a whole system approach. SSA governments need to increase health expenditure by allocating at least 15% of their national budgets to the health sector, including a minimum of US$ 44 per capita for health funding [45].

Task shifting: Task shifting of cardiovascular care strategies like screening, lifestyle modification counselling, routine, uncomplicated, follow-ups, specialized care linkage, and coordination of NCD support groups will assist in closing the current gap in staffing shortages [46].

Management protocols and clear referral pathways: To optimize the impact of task shifting, both simplified management protocols and well-defined referral pathways have to be put in place.

Motivating the workforce: Incentivizing the workforce with the aim of retaining knowledgeable and skilled medical personnel within SSA countries is crucial and will actually build a strong chain of CVD care advocates [47].

Integration of chronic care model in the management of cardiovascular diseases: Borrowing from well-studied *Chronic Care Models*, has been proposed as a solution to improve the integrated management of CVD in SSA. This model identifies six essential elements: community resources and policies, health care organization, self-management support, delivery system design, decision support, and clinical information systems. For example, the untapped capacity of chronic care models for HIV/AIDS care in SSA should be viewed as a model for CVD care. Lessons learnt from the implementation of care models for HIV/AIDS and tuberculosis in SSA could be effectively applied to improve care models for CVD care in SSA [48].

9.10 Increase Research Output

High-quality epidemiological and implementation research, as well as dedicated investments towards strengthening vital statistical data and systematic surveillance, will inform cardiovascular care practice in SSA and contribute towards identifying and evaluating sustainable interventions in various settings, track progress, and strengthen policy development and adoption.

9.11 Improve Training of Human Resource for Cardiovascular Care

Priorities to improve cardiovascular care training should include establishing in-country cardiology training centers and strengthening existing training centers through bench marking and fostering collaboration with strong external cardiology training institutions. Not to forget the training of the allied medical cadres that are critical to the delivery care especially in an environment with a net deficit of health care workers.

9.12 Conclusion

There is a growing burden of CVD in SSA. This is as a result of increasing and unchecked risk factors with considerable heterogeneity in risk trends across the different countries leading to explosive rates of CVD-related morbidity and mortality in the region.

Despite the sustained efforts to combat CVDs on the continent by the different advocacy groups such as WHO, PASCAR, and the World Heart Federation, the adoption of effective policies is lagging in many SSA states. Overall, available evidence suggests applying preventive strategies targeting the whole population aiming at targeting major risk factors and collectively contributing towards reaching the set targets by 2030.

Intensified and tailored regional efforts need to be channeled to lower blood pressure and other risk factors that should be coupled with continued surveillance and reliable data collection and monitoring of programs. The promotion of efforts of global, regional, and local experts needs to be encouraged to contribute towards increased advocacy for CVDs.

Efforts towards identifying innovative ways to improve access and service provision at a primary health care level, and investing towards universal health coverage, cost-effective preventive approaches that are easily adaptable and prioritizing research are important areas of focus.

Countries in SSA need to work together to support delivery of these important ambitions, including research and shared commitments and by highlighting how the whole SSA region can each collaborate with each other in the prevention of CVD, which we know still negatively impact lives of millions of people, often living in our more deprived communities.

With commitment by SSA countries, individually and collectively, to strengthen health systems, adopt and implement key metrics targeting CVD awareness, prevention and management, significant strides are possible towards changing the current trajectory of CVD burden in SSA leading to the improvement of cardiovascular and overall health of the population of SSA.

Acknowledgments We wish to express our sincere gratitude to the following for their contribution towards the success of this document: Pan African Society of Cardiology and the Kenya Cardiac Society and individuals who have worked tirelessly and very patiently to ensure completion of this document.

We also wish to thank Professor Tomas E. Romero and the editors for inviting us to contribute to this novel project.

We are thankful to our individual families for the unwavering support, patience, and love they accorded us towards this course.

To all our friends and colleagues who supported us immeasurably, we are grateful.

Glossary

Gender Male or female sex when considered with respect to cultural or social differences rather than biological ones.

Low- and middle-income countries (LMIC) Defined by the world bank as having a gross national income (GNI) per capita of US$ 1045 or less (low income), or between US$ 1046 and 12,745 (middle income).

Non-communicable diseases Diseases that are not spread by infection or through other people but are typically caused by unhealthy behaviors.

Sub-Saharan Africa (SSA) The region of Africa that lies south of the Sahara.

References

1. Amegah AK. Tackling the growing burden of cardiovascular diseases in Sub-Saharan Africa. Circulation. 2018;138(22):2449–51. https://doi.org/10.1161/CIRCULATIONAHA.118.037367.
2. Ikem I, Sumpio BE. Cardiovascular disease: the new epidemic in sub-Saharan Africa. Vascular. 2011;19(6):301–7. https://doi.org/10.1258/vasc.2011.ra0049.
3. Cappuccio FP, Miller MA. Cardiovascular disease and hypertension in sub-Saharan Africa: burden, risk and interventions. Intern Emerg Med. 2016;11(3):299–305. https://doi.org/10.1007/s11739-016-1423-9.
4. Bowry ADK, Lewey J, Dugani SB, Choudhry NK. The burden of cardiovascular disease in low- and middle-income countries: epidemiology and management. Can J Cardiol. 2015;31(9):1151–9. https://doi.org/10.1016/j.cjca.2015.06.028.
5. Yusuf PS, Hawken S, Ôunpuu S, Dans T, Avezum A, Lanas F, McQueen M, Budaj A, Pais P, Varigos J, Lisheng L. Effect of potentially modifiable risk factors associated with myocardial infarction in 52 countries (the INTERHEART study): case-control study. Lancet. 2004;364(9438):937–52. https://doi.org/10.1016/S0140-6736(04)17018-9.
6. Dzudie A, Rayner B, Ojji D, Schutte AE, Twagirumukiza M, Damasceno A, Ba SA, Kane A, Kramoh E, Kacou JB, Onwubere B, Cornick R, Sliwa K, Anisiuba B, Mocumbi AO, Ogola E, Awad M, Nel G, Otieno H, et al. Roadmap to achieve 25% hypertension control in Africa by 2025. Cardiovasc J Afr. 2017;28(4):262–72. https://doi.org/10.5830/CVJA-2017-040.
7. Minja NW, Nakagaayi D, Aliku T, Zhang W, Ssinabulya I, Nabaale J, Amutuhaire W, de Loizaga SR, Ndagire E, Rwebembera J, Okello E, Kayima J. Cardiovascular diseases in Africa in the twenty-first century: gaps and priorities going forward. Front Cardiovasc Med. 2022;9:1008335. https://doi.org/10.3389/fcvm.2022.1008335.
8. Mocumbi AO, Ferreira MB. Neglected cardiovascular diseases in Africa. J Am Coll Cardiol. 2010;55(7):680–7. https://doi.org/10.1016/j.jacc.2009.09.041.
9. Akumiah FK, Yakubu A-S, Ahadzi D, Tuglo LS, Mishra S, Mohapatra RK, Doku A. Cardiovascular care in Africa—cost crisis and the urgent need for contextual health service solutions. Global Heart. 2023;18(1):47. https://doi.org/10.5334/gh.1259.
10. Sun J, Qiao Y, Zhao M, Magnussen CG, Xi B. Global, regional, and national burden of cardiovascular diseases in youths and young adults aged 15–39 years in 204 countries/territories, 1990–2019: a systematic analysis of global burden of disease study 2019. BMC Med. 2023;21(1):222. https://doi.org/10.1186/s12916-023-02925-4.
11. Mudie K, Jin MM, Tan, Kendall L, Addo J, Dos-Santos-Silva I, Quint J, Smeeth L, Cook S, Nitsch D, Natamba B, Gomez-Olive FX, Ako A, Perel P. Non-communicable diseases in sub-Saharan Africa: a scoping review of large cohort studies. J Glob Health. 2019;9(2):20409. https://doi.org/10.7189/jogh.09.020409.
12. Banatvala N, Akselrod S, Bovet P, Mendis S. The WHO global action plan for the prevention and control of NCDs 2013–2030. Noncommunicable Diseases; 2023. p. 234–239. https://doi.org/10.4324/9781003306689-36.
13. Yuyun MF, Sliwa K, Kengne AP, Mocumbi AO, Bukhman G. Cardiovascular diseases in sub-Saharan Africa compared to high-income countries: an epidemiological perspective. Glob Heart. 2020;15(1):15. https://doi.org/10.5334/gh.403.
14. Watkins D, Zuhlke L, Engel M, Daniels R, Francis V, Shaboodien G, Kango M, Abul-Fadl A, Adeoye A, Ali S, Al-Kebsi M, Bode-Thomas F, Bukhman G, Damasceno A, Goshu DY, Elghamrawy A, Gitura B, Haileamlak A, Hailu A, Hugo-Hamman C, Justus S, Karthikeyan G, Kennedy N, Lwabi P, Mamo Y, Mntla P, Sutton C, Mocumbi AO, Mondo C, Mtaja A, Musuku J, Mucumbitsi J, Murango L, Nel G, Ogendo S, Ogola E, Ojji D, Olunuga TO, Redi MM, Rusingiza KE, Sani M, Sheta S, Shongwe S, van Dam J, Gamra H, Carapetis J, Lennon D, Mayosi BM. Seven key actions to eradicate rheumatic heart disease in Africa: the Addis Ababa communiqué. Cardiovasc J Afr. 2016;27(3):184–7. https://doi.org/10.5830/CVJA-2015-090. Epub 2016 Jan 12. PMID: 26815006; PMCID: PMC5125265

15. Abrams J, Watkins DA, Abdullahi LH, Zühlke LJ, Engel ME. Integrating the prevention and control of rheumatic heart disease into country health systems: a systematic review and meta-analysis. Glob Heart. 2020;15(1):62. https://doi.org/10.5334/gh.874.
16. GBD 2019 Diseases and Injuries Collaborators. Global burden of 369 diseases and injuries in 204 countries and territories, 1990–2019: a systematic analysis for the global burden of disease study 2019. Lancet (London, England). 2020;396(10258):1204–22. https://doi.org/10.1016/S0140-6736(20)30925-9.
17. Damasceno A, Mayosi BM, Sani M, Ogah OS, Mondo C, Ojji D, Dzudie A, Kouam CK, Suliman A, Schrueder N, Yonga G, Ba SA, Maru F, Alemayehu B, Edwards C, Davison BA, Cotter G, Sliwa K. The causes, treatment, and outcome of acute heart failure in 1006 Africans from 9 countries. Arch Intern Med. 2012;172(18):1386–94. https://doi.org/10.1001/archinternmed.2012.3310.
18. Ebireri J, Aderemi AV, Omoregbe N, Adeloye D. Interventions addressing risk factors of ischaemic heart disease in sub-Saharan Africa: a systematic review. BMJ Open. 2016;6(7):e011881. https://doi.org/10.1136/bmjopen-2016-011881.
19. Peck RN, Green E, Mtabaji J, Majinge C, Smart LR, Downs JA, Fitzgerald DW. Hypertension-related diseases as a common cause of hospital mortality in Tanzania: a 3-year prospective study. J Hypertens. 2013;31(9):1806–11. https://doi.org/10.1097/HJH.0b013e328362bad7.
20. Brunström M, Carlberg B. Association of blood pressure lowering with mortality and cardiovascular disease across blood pressure levels: a systematic review and meta-analysis. JAMA Intern Med. 2018;178(1):28–36. https://doi.org/10.1001/jamainternmed.2017.6015.
21. Ataklte F, Erqou S, Kaptoge S, Taye B, Echouffo-Tcheugui JB, Kengne AP. Burden of undiagnosed hypertension in Sub-Saharan Africa: a systematic review and meta-analysis. Hypertension. 2015;65(2):291–8. https://doi.org/10.1161/HYPERTENSIONAHA.114.04394.
22. Ogola EN, Mbau L, Gachemba YM, Gitura BM, Barasa FA, Nguchu H, Beaney T, Xia X, Poulter NR. May measurement month 2019: an analysis of blood pressure screening results from Kenya. Eur Heart J Suppl. 2021;23(Suppl B):B86–8. https://doi.org/10.1093/eurheartj/suab040.
23. Dev R, Favour-Ofili D, Raparelli V, Behlouli H, Azizi Z, Kublickiene K, Kautzky-Willer A, Herrero MT, Pilote L, Norris CM. Sex and gender influence on cardiovascular health in Sub-Saharan Africa: findings from Ghana, Gambia, Mali, Guinea, and Botswana. Glob Heart. 2022;17(1):63. https://doi.org/10.5334/gh.1146.
24. Sommer I, Griebler U, Mahlknecht P, Thaler K, Bouskill K, Gartlehner G, Mendis S. Socioeconomic inequalities in non-communicable diseases and their risk factors: an overview of systematic reviews. BMC Public Health. 2015;15(1):914. https://doi.org/10.1186/s12889-015-2227-y.
25. Garcia M, Mulvagh SL, Bairey Merz CN, Buring JE, Manson JE. Cardiovascular disease in women. Circ Res. 2016;118(8):1273–93. https://doi.org/10.1161/CIRCRESAHA.116.307547.
26. Roeters van Lennep JE, Tokgözoğlu LS, Badimon L, Dumanski SM, Gulati M, Hess CN, Holven KB, Kavousi M, Kayıkçıoğlu M, Lutgens E, Michos ED, Prescott E, Stock JK, Tybjaerg-Hansen A, Wermer MJH, Benn M. Women, lipids, and atherosclerotic cardiovascular disease: a call to action from the European Atherosclerosis Society. Eur Heart J. 2023;44(39):4157–73. https://doi.org/10.1093/eurheartj/ehad472.
27. Bairey Merz CN, Kelsey SF, Pepine CJ, Reichek N, Reis SE, Rogers WJ, Sharaf BL, Sopko G. The Women's ischemia syndrome evaluation (WISE) study: protocol design, methodology and feasibility report. J Am Coll Cardiol. 1999;33(6):1453–61. https://doi.org/10.1016/S0735-1097(99)00082-0.
28. Day S, Mason R, Lagosky S, Rochon PA. Integrating and evaluating sex and gender in health research. Health Res Policy Syst. 2016;14(1):75. https://doi.org/10.1186/s12961-016-0147-7.
29. Lumsden R, Barasa F, Park LP, Ochieng CB, Alera JM, Millar HC, Bloomfield GS, Christoffersen-Deb A. High burden of cardiac disease in pregnancy at a National Referral Hospital in Western Kenya. Glob Heart. 2020;15(1):10. https://doi.org/10.5334/gh.404.
30. Diao M, Kane A, Ndiaye MB, Mbaye A, Bodian M, Dia MM, Sarr M, Kane A, Monsuez J-J, Ba SA. Pregnancy in women with heart disease in sub-Saharan Africa. Arch Cardiovasc Dis. 2011;104(6):370–4. https://doi.org/10.1016/j.acvd.2011.04.001.

31. Kotit S, Yacoub M. Cardiovascular adverse events in pregnancy: a global perspective. Glob Cardiol Sci Pract. 2021;2021(1):e202105. https://doi.org/10.21542/gcsp.2021.5.
32. Ojji DB, Shedul GL, Sani M, Ogah OS, Dzudie A, Barasa F, Mondo C, Ingabire PM, Jones ESW, Rayner B, Albertino D, Ogola E, Smythe W, Hickman N, Francis V, Shahiemah P, Shedul G, Aje A, Sliwa K, Stewart S. A differential response to antihypertensive therapy in African men and women: insights from the CREOLE trial. Am J Hypertens. 2022;35(6):551–60. https://doi.org/10.1093/ajh/hpac014.
33. Kreatsoulas C, Anand SS. The impact of social determinants on cardiovascular disease. Can J Cardiol. 2010;26 Suppl C(Suppl C):8C–13C. https://doi.org/10.1016/s0828-282x(10)71075-8.
34. Adeboye B, Bermano G, Rolland C. Obesity and its health impact in Africa: a systematic review. Cardiovasc J Afr. 2012;23(9):512–21. https://doi.org/10.5830/CVJA-2012-040.
35. Keates AK, Mocumbi AO, Ntsekhe M, Sliwa K, Stewart S. Cardiovascular disease in Africa: epidemiological profile and challenges. Nat Rev Cardiol. 2017;14(5):273–93. https://doi.org/10.1038/nrcardio.2017.19.
36. Azomahou TT, Diene B, Gosselin-Pali A. Transition and persistence in the double burden of malnutrition and overweight or obesity: evidence from South Africa. Food Policy. 2022;113:102303. https://doi.org/10.1016/j.foodpol.2022.102303.
37. Douglas M, Kgatla N, Sodi T, Musinguzi G, Mothiba T, Skaal L, Makgahlela M, Bastiaens H. Facilitators and barriers in prevention of cardiovascular disease in Limpopo, South Africa: a qualitative study conducted with primary health care managers. BMC Cardiovasc Disord. 2021;21(1):492. https://doi.org/10.1186/s12872-021-02290-1.
38. Adeniji FIP, Obembe TA. Cardiovascular disease and its implication for higher catastrophic health expenditures among households in Sub-Saharan Africa. J Health Econ Outcomes Res. 2023;10(1):59–67. https://doi.org/10.36469/001c.70252.
39. Kruk ME, Gage AD, Arsenault C, Jordan K, Leslie HH, Roder-DeWan S, Adeyi O, Barker P, Daelmans B, Doubova SV, English M, García-Elorrio E, Guanais F, Gureje O, Hirschhorn LR, Jiang L, Kelley E, Lemango ET, Liljestrand J, et al. High-quality health systems in the sustainable development goals era: time for a revolution. Lancet Glob Health. 2018;6(11):e1196–252. https://doi.org/10.1016/S2214-109X(18)30386-3.
40. Witter S, Zou G, Diaconu K, Senesi RGB, Idriss A, Walley J, Wurie HR. Opportunities and challenges for delivering non-communicable disease management and services in fragile and post-conflict settings: perceptions of policy-makers and health providers in Sierra Leone. Confl Heal. 2020;14:3. https://doi.org/10.1186/s13031-019-0248-3.
41. Azevedo MJ. The state of health system(s) in Africa: challenges and opportunities. In: Historical perspectives on the state of health and health systems in Africa, volume II: the modern era; 2017. p. 1–73. https://doi.org/10.1007/978-3-319-32564-4_1.
42. Diaconu K, Falconer J, Vidal N, O'May F, Azasi E, Elimian K, Bou-Orm I, Sarb C, Witter S, Ager A. Understanding fragility: implications for global health research and practice. Health Policy Plan. 2020;35(2):235–43. https://doi.org/10.1093/heapol/czz142.
43. Karamagi HC, Njuguna D, Kidane SN, Djossou H, Kipruto HK, Seydi AB-W, Nabyonga-Orem J, Muhongerwa DK, Frimpong KA, Nganda BM. Financing health system elements in Africa: a scoping review. PLoS One. 2023;18(9):e0291371. https://doi.org/10.1371/journal.pone.0291371.
44. Rippe JM. Lifestyle strategies for risk factor reduction, prevention, and treatment of cardiovascular disease. Am J Lifestyle Med. 2019;13(2):204–12. https://doi.org/10.1177/1559827618812395.
45. Oladosu AO, Chanimbe T, Anaduaka US. Effect of public health expenditure on health outcomes in Nigeria and Ghana. Health Policy Open. 2022;3:100072. https://doi.org/10.1016/j.hpopen.2022.100072.
46. Ogedegbe G, Gyamfi J, Plange-Rhule J, Surkis A, Rosenthal DM, Airhihenbuwa C, Iwelunmor J, Cooper R. Task shifting interventions for cardiovascular risk reduction in low-income and middle-income countries: a systematic review of randomised controlled trials. BMJ Open. 2014;4(10):e005983. https://doi.org/10.1136/bmjopen-2014-005983.

47. Thompson SC, Nedkoff L, Katzenellenbogen J, Hussain MA, Sanfilippo F. Challenges in managing acute cardiovascular diseases and follow up care in rural areas: a narrative review. Int J Environ Res Public Health. 2019;16(24):5126. https://doi.org/10.3390/ijerph16245126.
48. Otieno P, Agyemang C, Wao H, Wambiya E, Ng'oda M, Mwanga D, Oguta J, Kibe P, Asiki G. Effectiveness of integrated chronic care models for cardiometabolic multimorbidity in sub-Saharan Africa: a systematic review and meta-analysis. BMJ Open. 2023;13(6):e073652. https://doi.org/10.1136/bmjopen-2023-073652.

Chapter 10
Socio-economic Factors and Cardiovascular Outcomes in Japan: Is Unrestricted Access to Healthcare Resources Enough?

Neiko Ozasa and Toshiko Yoshida

10.1 Cardiovascular Disease Prevention in Japan, an Economic Superpower: The Limitations of Medical Care

To prevent and treat cardiovascular diseases, it is important to improve lifestyle and social environment related to nutrition and diet, physical activity and exercise, sleep and rest, moderation of alcohol consumption and smoking, and dental and oral health [1, 2]. In Japan, medical insurance covers nutritional guidance by physicians, nurses, and dietitians for patients with diabetes, dyslipidemia, and hypertension as primary prevention of cardiovascular diseases. Cardiac rehabilitation is also covered by medical insurance as a secondary prevention for cardiovascular diseases and is provided to patients with myocardial infarction, angina pectoris, heart failure, postoperative cardiac surgery, arteriosclerosis obliterans, aortic disease, and post-transcatheter aortic valve implantation (TAVI). The patients are provided with comprehensive and specialized guidance for lifestyle improvement by a multidisciplinary team of doctors, nurses, dietitians, physical therapists, exercise instructors, occupational therapists, psychologists, etc. [2, 3].

However, these interventions, which are covered by medical insurance established by the government, also incur a co-payment of 10–30%, depending on the

N. Ozasa (✉)
Department of Cardiovascular Medicine, Kyoto University, Graduate School of Medicine, Kyoto, Japan

Department of Cardiology, Kansai Heart Center, Takanohara Central Hospital, Nara, Japan
e-mail: nei126@kuhp.kyoto-u.ac.jp

T. Yoshida
St. Luke's International University, College of Nursing, Graduate School of Nursing Science, Chuo City, Japan
e-mail: tyoshidas@slcn.ac.jp

T. Romero et al. (eds.), *Global Challenges in Cardiovascular Prevention in Populations with Low Socioeconomic Status*,
https://doi.org/10.1007/978-3-031-79051-5_10

type of medical insurance. Japan has a "universal health insurance system" that requires all citizens to have some form of medical insurance, but if a person is unable to pay the co-payments or purchase medical insurance due to poverty, there is a system of public assistance available. Under the public assistance, medical care is paid for in kind, and there is no co-payment of medical expenses. Therefore, it can be said that only patients who have the financial ability to pay the co-payments of medical insurance or those who are approved for public assistance can receive lifestyle guidance for the prevention of cardiovascular diseases as part of medical care in Japan.

10.2 Growing Income Inequality and Health Inequities

Japan is known as the "world's third largest economy," has "a universal healthcare system unlike any other in the world," and is actively engaged in research on highly advanced medical care. In reality, however, wealth in Japan is concentrated in the hands of big capital and a few wealthy people, and poverty is a social problem. According to the Organization for Economic Co-operation and Development (OECD), wage growth over the past 20 years has increased in each country: 38.9% in Sweden, 27.7% in France, 18.8% in Germany, and 15.3% in the United States. In contrast, the rate of increase in Japan was −9.9%, a decrease of 9.9%. Average annual wage is the lowest among the seven industrialized countries and lower than the OECD average. One-fourth of the working population in Japan is called the "working poor," or those earning less than two million yen a year. When the poverty rate is defined as the ratio of the number of people (in a given age group) whose income falls below the poverty line; taken as half the median household income of the total population, Japan's poverty rate ranks tenth among OECD countries. (Inequality—Poverty rate—OECD Data, Viewed December 28, 2023).

As poverty spreads, the number of people without medical insurance is increasing due to their inability to raise the costs to purchase medical insurance, and as of 2022, approximately half a million households were uninsured [4]. The uninsured are less able to access healthcare and tend not to see a doctor until their illness becomes severe. These patients may also have difficulty accessing cardiac rehabilitation after a myocardial infarction or other cardiovascular events.

Low-income individuals, especially the older, are more likely to have an increased risk of developing disease, as they often have poor nutritional and dietary balance and few exercise habits. The medical insurance system for the older aged 75 and over has been changed in October 2022. The new system requires patients to pay 20–30% of the total cost, depending on their income, instead of the 10% that was previously required. These amendments to the healthcare insurance system for the aged have resulted in an increase in the number of patients who were required to pay two to three times more than the total cost, even if they were only required to pay 10% before the revision. There are concerns that older patients who are forced to pay the increased co-payments may be discouraged from receiving medical examinations, resulting in more severe illnesses and further escalation of medical costs.

10.3 Dealing with the Living Poorness Person

In addition to cash assistance, public assistance provides medical care and nursing care in kind to those in financial need. As of 2023, the number of households receiving public assistance has nearly doubled from 20 years ago to 2.02 million (Fig. 10.1). Medical care accounts for 50% of the payments to public assistance recipients, indicating a high need for medical care. However, another problem is that many households do not receive welfare benefits even though they are financially below the public assistance entitlement threshold, with the 2018 public assistance capture rate standing at 22.9%. The low capture rate is due to a variety of issues, including the complexity of the procedures for applying for and receiving public assistance and social prejudice [5].

Since 2008, Free/Low-Cost Medical Care (FLCMC) have been provided to enable living poorness person access medical care and nursing care [6], with a total of 6.84 million people using the FLCMC in 2022. On the other hand, this system is not fully recognized by general medical institutions and the general public in the community, and it is believed that there are many persons with poverty not able to use this system. The challenge is to create a system that enables more people to utilize the system.

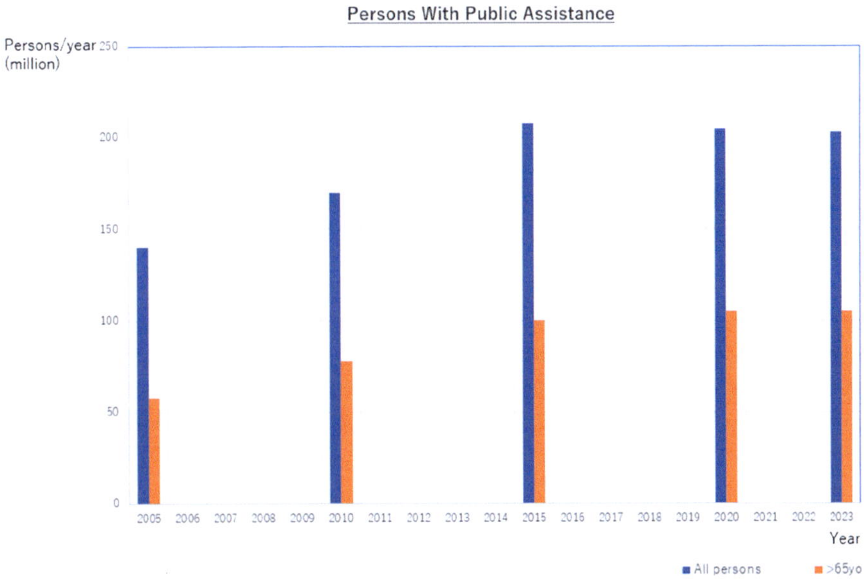

Fig. 10.1 Number of public assistance recipients (prepared by the author based on data released by the Ministry of Health, Labor and Welfare, Viewed December 28, 2023). The number of public assistance recipients has increased rapidly since the global financial crisis. Although the number has been decreasing in recent years, more than two million people are still receiving public assistance. The number of persons 65 years old and over continues to increase. Half of the total number of persons receiving public assistance are 65 years of age or older

10.4 Problem of Poverty Among Patients with Cardiovascular Diseases in Japan

There are few studies on poverty among patients with cardiovascular diseases in Japan. Because persons with poverty are less likely to make regular visits to medical institutions, the presence of poverty may not be noticed unless healthcare providers are aware of it. It is thought that by the time indigent patients, who are prone to medical inactivity, visit a medical institution, their disease is often severe.

We conducted a prospective, observational, multicenter study on heart failure, a terminal manifestation of cardiovascular diseases, among the indigent patients [7]. The KCHF study is an all-comers registry of consecutive patients who were admitted to 19 Kyoto University affiliated facilities distributed nationwide between October 2014 and March 2016 due to acute decompensated heart failure and received intravenous heart failure medications within 24 h. In this study, socioeconomic background was investigated, including status of public assistance [7]. In addition, adherence to medication and the presence or absence of a cohabitant were also investigated in detail. The results of this study showed that 3728 patients were included in the study, of which 218, or 5.8%, were public assistance recipients, that was approximately three times the recipient rate of 1.6% for the Japanese population at that time. The mean age of public assistance recipients was significantly younger than that of non-recipients (72.3 ± 12.2 vs. 78.0 ± 11.9 years), more current smokers (31 vs. 11%) and more chronic lung disease (21 vs. 13%) ($p < 0.001$). Medication adherence was low (27 vs. 16%), more people lived alone (56 vs. 19%), and employment rates were low (5.1 vs. 14%) ($p < 0.001$). Although there was no significant difference in mortality within 1 year of discharge from the hospital between those with and without public assistance, the heart failure rehospitalization rate after 180 days, adjusted for age and other factors, was significantly higher among those on public assistance ($p = 0.02$). Poverty is likely to lead to social isolation, reducing not only the ability to pay for expenses and time, but also the ability to recognize health needs, to accept and search for the need for medical assistance, and to reach needed medical care. The development of cardiovascular diseases, particularly symptomatic heart failure, contributes to the decline in these abilities. Furthermore, the poor prognosis among patients with public assistance in the current study suggests that they are likely not receiving early consultations and exacerbating their disease until they present to the emergency department with worsening heart failure.

10.5 Widening Health Inequities After the COVID-19 Pandemic, and Measures to Address the 2025 Problem

In Japan, the problems of poverty and inequality had been an issue even before the COronaVIrus Disease of 2019 (COVID-19) pandemic, but the decrease in local communication due to infection control measures further exacerbated the material and mental deprivation of the indigent patients. Opportunities to provide face-to-face information to the indigent patients, such as FLCMC introduced by social workers to their patients, have also decreased. Future studies are needed to address the health inequities that have become even more pronounced after the COVID-19 pandemic.

Japan's population is expected to continue aging, and by 2025, those aged 75 and over are expected to account for a quarter of the population. In order to maintain the accompanying medical and long-term care system, the Ministry of Health, Labor and Welfare announced in 2016 a policy to promote the establishment of the community-based integrated care system [8]. This system plans to establish regional comprehensive support centers throughout Japan and strengthen regional cooperation to support medical and nursing care for the older. At the present stage, however, most community comprehensive support centers are operated by the private sector under contract from the government, and there is no standardization of intervention methods among the centers. In operating Community General Support Centers, there is a need to enhance the training of front-line staff, as well as the education of the staff, so that necessary medical care and long-term care can be distributed appropriately in the future.

10.6 Social Determinants of Health Other Than Poverty and the Role of Healthcare Providers

In a model by Booske BC et al. based on data from four US states, the provision of healthcare and quality of healthcare affect only about 20% of health, social determinants of health (SDOH)—income, education, employment, family and social support, and community safety—40%, lifestyle factors that affect health 30%, and environmental factors such as clean water and air quality, climate change, and disasters account for 10% [9]. A well-known example of natural disasters and cardiovascular diseases is the increase in cardiovascular diseases among survivors of the 2011 Great East Japan Earthquake. Aoki et al. reported that the number of emergency room visits for heart failure, acute coronary syndrome, stroke, and cardiopulmonary arrest in the week following a major earthquake increased to about twice the previous level [10]. In major earthquakes, physical and psychological stress has a significant impact on disease, but other human factors, such as interference with the supply of medicines and medical care, also often cause disease exacerbation. With regard to social isolation and cardiovascular diseases, Takabayashi et al. reported on the KICKOFF study of 1253 acute heart failure patients admitted to 13 facilities in the Osaka area between April 2015 and August 2017, reported a significant association between living alone and 3-year heart failure hospitalization among male patients [11].

10.7 SDOH and Health Advocacy by Healthcare Providers

In routine medical care, healthcare providers tend to judge patients who do not show up for appointments or who tend to discontinue prescription medications as "nonadherent" or "unwilling" to receive treatment. However, SDOH may be hidden among such patients, and it is necessary for healthcare providers to view health inequities from the perspective of SDOH. However, if patients are unable to see a doctor or discontinue treatment because of social factors, it is difficult for the healthcare provider to address these social factors. In cardiovascular treatment especially in cardiac rehabilitation, where the goal of intervention is patients' self-management of their diseases, the decline in adherence, which is not a problem of the patient's own, cannot be ignored. The AHA SCIENTIFIC STATEMENT on SDOH in heart failure patients was published in 2020 [12]. This document includes a definition of SDOH, provider competencies, and SDOH assessment tools and addresses the following questions: (1) What models or frameworks guide healthcare providers to address? (2) What are the SDOH affecting the delivery of care and the interventions addressing them that affect the care and outcomes of patients with heart failure? (3) What are the opportunities for healthcare providers to address the SDOH affecting the care of patients with heart failure?

The Royal College of Physicians and Surgeons of Canada has identified seven roles for healthcare providers, one of which is that of the health advocate. The role of the health advocate is to "provide the non-medical care necessary for the health of patients," and to "work with those who make up the community, including patients in the area or specialty in which he or she practices, to make effective change at the organizational and institutional levels" [13].

10.8 Actions to Mitigate the Effect of SDOH

Several support tools for health advocates have been proposed for health providers in Japan. "Financial Support Tools for Medical and Nursing Staff" (https://www.hphnet.jp/study-data/5185/https://www.hpnhnet.jp/whats-new/5185/, Viewed December 8, 2024) for indigent patients, the "Guidelines for Supporting the Balance between Treatment and Work in the Workplace" (https://www.mhlw.go.jp/content/10900000/001179451.pdf https://www.mhlw.go.jp/content/11200000/001088186.pdf, Viewed December 8, 2024) for those seeking for employment, and several others have been proposed that can be utilized according to needs. However, these tools are not yet fully recognized by medical professionals in the cardiovascular field. It would be desirable for Japanese societies and organizations related to cardiovascular diseases and others need to encourage their further use.

On the other hand, the long-term care insurance system for the older, which has been in effect since 2000, has become widely accepted among medical professionals involved in cardiovascular care [14]. In the KCHF study and the KICKOFF study, 54% and 44% of patients were certified or scheduled to be certified for long-term care insurance at the time of discharge from the hospital, respectively [8, 15, 16]. As these studies are not randomized controlled trials (RCTs) planned to assess the efficacy of long-term care insurance so that they could not test the effect of long-term care insurance, the results of these studies demonstrated half of all patients with acute heart failure admissions required for care and support. For older patients with heart failure, it will be necessary to create a system to manage the disease during the stable phase, beyond the framework of lifestyle guidance and cardiac rehabilitation.

Telecardiac rehabilitation is about to be launched in Japan, but it should not exclude impoverished elderly heart failure patients, who are considered to have the poorest prognosis among heart failure patients. A system must be established to provide access and support disease management for these patients as well.

10.9 Conclusion

As Japan's population ages, there are many older patients with cardiovascular diseases who require nursing care and support. In addition, although not fully investigated, the number of people in need is increasing due to the growing income inequality in Japan, and heart failure patients are thought to be increasing among the older persons who are unable to find work. SODH such as climate change, including global warming, the increase in natural disasters such as earthquakes, and the increase in the number of single people and people living alone, as well as various other factors increase patients who are not able to access to medical care. Even in telemedicine, which is expected to increase in the near future in Japan, patients who are poor, elderly, or digitally illiterate may be left behind. Future Japanese healthcare needs to create a framework to accept patients facing SDOH.

Acknowledgment This work was supported by JSPS KAKENHI Grant Number JP 21K19669.

Glossary

Living poorness person A person who is in actual economic distress and is at risk of becoming unable to maintain a minimum standard of living.

Free/Low-Cost Medical Care (FLCMC) Free and Low-Cost Medical Services is a system that provides free or low-cost medical services so that people are not limited in their access to necessary medical care due to economic reasons.

Long-term care insurance system The public assistance system is a public welfare programs by the government that provides necessary protection to those in need and guarantees a minimum standard of living that is healthy and culturally acceptable.

SDOH (social determinants of health) The circumstances in which people are born, grow up, live, work, and age and the systems put in place to offer health care and services to a community.

References

1. Arnett DK, Blumenthal RS, Albert MA, et al. 2019 ACC/AHA guideline on the primary prevention of cardiovascular disease: a report of the American College of Cardiology/American Heart Association task force on clinical practice guidelines. Circulation. 2019;140(11):e596–646.
2. Makita S, Yasu T, Akashi YJ, et al. JCS/JACR 2021 guideline on rehabilitation in patients with cardiovascular disease. Circ J. 2022;87(1):155–235.
3. Virani SS, Newby LK, Arnold SV, et al. 2023 AHA/ACC/ACCP/ASPC/NLA/PCNA guideline for the management of patients with chronic coronary disease: a report of the American Heart Association/American College of Cardiology Joint Committee on clinical practice guidelines. Circulation. 2023;148(9):e9–e119.
4. Press Release, June 5, 2023. Ministry of Health, Labour and Welfare, Japan. https://www.mhlw.go.jp/content/12400000/001121231.pdf.
5. Kino S, Nishioka D, Ueno K, et al. Changes in social relationships by the initiation and termination of public assistance in the older Japanese population: a JAGES panel study. Soc Sci Med. 2022;293:114661.
6. Nishioka D, Tamaki C, Furuita N, et al. Changes in health-related quality of life among impoverished persons in the free/lowcost medical care program in Japan: evidence from a prospective cohort study. J Epidemiol. 2022;32(11):519–23.
7. Yaku H, Ozasa N, Morimoto T, et al.; KCHF Study Investigators. Demographics, management, and in-hospital outcome of hospitalized acute heart failure syndrome patients in contemporary real clinical practice in Japan—observations from the prospective, multicenter Kyoto congestive heart failure (KCHF) registry. Circ J. 2018;82(11):2811–19.
8. Song P, Tang W. The community-based integrated care system in Japan: health care and nursing care challenges posed by super-aged society. Biosci Trends. 2019;13(3):279–81.
9. Booske BC, Athens JK, Kindig DA, et al. Different perspectives for assigning weights to determinants of health. Madison: Population Health Institute, University of Wisconsin; 2010.
10. Aoki T, Fukumoto Y, Yasuda S, et al. The great East Japan earthquake disaster and cardiovascular diseases. Eur Heart J. 2012;33(22):2796–803.
11. Takabayashi K, Kitaguchi S, Iwatsu K, et al. Living alone and gender differences in rehospitalization for heart failure after discharge among acute heart failure patients. Int Heart J. 2020;61(6):1245–52.
12. White-Williams C, Rossi LP, Bittner VA, et al.; American Heart Association Council on Cardiovascular and Stroke Nursing; Council on Clinical Cardiology; and Council on Epidemiology and Prevention. Addressing social determinants of health in the care of patients with heart failure: a scientific statement from the American Heart Association. Circulation. 2020;141(22):e841–e863.
13. Tamiya N, Noguchi H, Nishi A, et al. Population ageing and wellbeing: lessons from Japan's long-term care insurance policy. Lancet. 2011;378(9797):1183–92.
14. Frank JR, Danoff D. The CanMEDS initiative: implementing an outcomes-based framework of physician competencies. Med Teach. 2007;29(7):642–7.
15. Nishimoto Y, Kato T, Morimoto T, et al. Public assistance in patients with acute heart failure: a report from the KCHF registry. ESC Heart Fail. 2022;9(3):1920–30.
16. Takabayashi K, Iwatsu K, Ikeda T, et al. Clinical characteristics and outcomes of heart failure patients with long-term care insurance—insights from the Kitakawachi clinical background and outcome of heart failure registry. Circ J. 2020;84(9):1528–35.

Chapter 11
Socioeconomic Status and Cardiovascular Disease Prevention in India

Ishita Gupta, Arun P. Jose, and Dorairaj Prabhakaran

11.1 Cardiovascular Diseases (CVDs) and Associated Risk Factors

Indians have a higher propensity of developing cardiovascular disease (CVD), experience CVD a decade earlier than their European counterparts, have a higher case fatality rate, and high premature mortality (nearly two-third of all CVD deaths) [1–4] leading to substantial loss of lives during their most productive ages. In India (2016), CVD alone was responsible for more than a quarter of total deaths (28.1%) and 14.1% of total Disability Adjusted Life Years (DALYs). This is considerably higher than the respective estimates of 15.2% and 6.9% in 1990 [5]. The state-level burden of disease study (GBD study group) reported that, as of 2016, all states in India have a predominance of non-communicable diseases (NCD) compared with communicable diseases, which was the case only in one state as early as 1990 [6]. This rapid transition and increase in disease burden has been driven by demographic transition (population growth and aging populations), advancements in medical care leading to greater life expectancy, and rapid urbanization.

Ischemic heart disease (IHD) and stroke were among the top CVD types in India contributing to 61.4% and 24.9% of total DALYs from CVDs, with the former being the largest contributor towards total deaths 17.8% (95% CI: 16.8%–18.5%) [6]. The Harvard School of Public Health and the World Economic Forum have estimated

I. Gupta · A. P. Jose
Centre for Chronic Disease Control, New Delhi, India
e-mail: ishita@ccdcindia.org; arunp.jose@ccdcindia.org

D. Prabhakaran (✉)
Centre for Chronic Disease Control, New Delhi, India

London School of Hygiene and Tropical Medicine, University of London, London, UK
e-mail: dprabhakaran@ccdcindia.org

T. Romero et al. (eds.), *Global Challenges in Cardiovascular Prevention in Populations with Low Socioeconomic Status*,
https://doi.org/10.1007/978-3-031-79051-5_11

that India will lose 2.17 trillion dollars before 2030 due to CVD alone [7]. It has been suggested that early life exposures among Indians (through the life-course) along with the changes that have happened alongside the epidemiological, demographic, nutritional, environmental, social-cultural, and economic transitions also put Indians at an increased risk of CVD and associated mortality [8]. As the transition progresses to more advanced stages, prevalence of NCDs including CVD gravitates towards the poor and vulnerable, affecting them even more than the rich which will further have a deleterious impact on the economic growth of the country. Such a loss has a huge bearing on our progress towards sustainable development goals [9] underscoring the importance of risk factors of CVD along with their social and economic determinants while formulating policy and planning implementation of CVD programs.

Risk Factors for CVD: Family history of CVD, tobacco use, physical inactivity, abnormal serum lipids, body weight, air pollution, hypertension, and diabetes are few of the known conventional CVD risk factors [10]. According to the ICMR-INDIAB study, a cross-sectional population-based survey of more than 1 lakh adults from 31 Indian states/UTs found that the prevalence of hypertension was 35.5%, dyslipidemia was 81.2%, and diabetes was 11.4% [11]. In addition to these individual-level risk factors that primarily include behavioral and metabolic factors, there is a set of upstream factors or social determinants of health that are important contributors of CVD as well as its risk factors [12].

Social Determinants of Health: According to the WHO, social determinants of health "are the conditions in which people are born, grow, work, live, and age, and the wider set of forces and systems shaping the conditions of daily life. These forces and systems include economic policies and systems, development agendas, social norms, social policies, and political systems" [13]. These include several socioeconomic and environmental factors that have a significant impact on both community and individual-level health. Socio-economic status (SES)/position is an important construct of the multi-dimensional social determinants of health. It refers to the social and economic factors that influence what positions individuals or groups hold within the structure of a society [14, 15] often characterized by income, education, occupation, physical assets, social position, caste, and so on. Nair et al. reported that while conventional risk factors are responsible for a large proportion of the CVD risk, several conditioning factors such as education, socio-economic status, and early life influences also contribute considerably [8]. This is further supported by the results of a meta-analysis with 1.7 million individuals that demonstrated an inverse association between socioeconomic position and premature all-cause as well as CVD-related mortality [16]. Thus, while the current practices continue to address individual/conventional risk factors (reducing tobacco and alcohol consumption, diet modification, and promoting physical activity), this approach alone may not be adequate due to the role of the social determinants that operate at a broader level and are responsible for shaping an individuals' health behavior and choices. Thus, it is imperative to address these upstream factors by broadening the scope of interventions and targeting families and communities for better health outcomes.

Pathways of SES and CVD: There are several pathways through which SES leads to CVD. In most LMICs during the early stages of epidemiological transition, CVD was more prevalent in affluent sections of the population who had the resources and economic stability to experiment with a change in lifestyle. As the risks associated with the new lifestyle (tobacco, unhealthy foods, and automated transport) became available and accessible for wider consumption, the impact of CVD became apparent in all socioeconomic groups [17]. As the transition evolves to more advanced stages, the educated and affluent segment utilizes resources to acquire better health-related information and resort to healthy lifestyle thus indicating a decline in the CVD events in this group. While, on the other hand, the risk factors and CVD burden gradually increased in the disadvantaged groups and spilled over to the rural areas having low education and awareness levels, served by a deficient health system [17].

While some models explain the role of early life factors which may or may not be influenced by the intervening life experiences to impact the occurrence of CVD [18, 19]. Others suggest a cumulative or additive effect of psychosocial and physiological experiences and environments during early and later life that accumulate to influence adult disease risk [20, 21]. As suggested by these models, often early life circumstances, shape adult social circumstances, which, in turn, influence CVD risk and mortality. Consistent with these observations, the life-course theory relies on a multidisciplinary approach to suggesting the role of early- and later-life biological, behavioral, social, and psychological exposures on an individual's health and how social inequities can be transmitted across generations [22].

11.2 An Overview of Socioeconomic Groups in India

The need to understand the role of socioeconomic determinants of CVD in India, home to a culturally and socially diverse population of 1.3 billion people (18% of the world's population) that have been shown to have a preponderance to CVD, becomes even more important to achieve global and national targets for CVD [23]. There are multiple, complex dimensions to socioeconomic status or position in India. Several indicators individually or combined have been proposed to characterize SES [24]. Each indicator reflects a differing but related aspect of an individual's position in society [25, 26]. For example, education represents achievement of milestones such as primary school, secondary school and beyond, and future earning potential. Occupation reflects social standing in society; however, homemakers, students, retired, and unemployed are often inadequately categorized. Monthly household income may be inconsistent as income can vary and/or is often under-reported due to bias and multiple sources of income. Household assets reflect current material wealth and may not capture generational wealth. Therefore, evaluating multiple SES indicators provides a more comprehensive representation of the social determinants of health and an opportunity to address the same [27, 28].

There are several scores or indices for the assessment of SES status in India. Some of which are solely based on a single measure assessment (including income or expenditure alone) while others are composite indices that are a combination of two or more measures (education and income and occupation, etc.). Rahman et al. report a total of 25 SES indices in their scoping review of more than 250 South Asian studies classified into asset-based wealth index, wealth index with education, indices based on income and expenditure, indices based on education and occupation, and other undescribed indices [29]. Some common indices used across Indian studies include: The Kuppuswamy Scale is a combination of material possession, education, occupation, and income [30]. Pareekh et al. further added caste and family type and created a new scale with a total of nine indicators [31]; and Tiwari et al. used housing, material possession, education, occupation, economic profile, cultivated land, and social profile in his scale [32]. These scales have been modified further in 2007 [33].

11.3 SES, CVD, and Its Risk Factors in India

Statistics based on the Central Bureau of Health Intelligence, National Health Profile 2022 suggest that the India's overall literacy rate was 73%, with urban areas reporting a 16% higher rate (84%) than rural (68%). An overall proportion of 21.9% people were below the poverty line [34]. As discussed previously, the occurrence of CVD and its risk factors varies by SES. While in developed countries those in the low socioeconomic group experience higher morbidity and mortality [35–37], in low-middle income countries such as India an initial predominance of CVD in the upper SES has been followed by increasing vulnerability of lower SES groups with the maturation of the transition.

Agarwal et al. with data obtained from a large, representative population (n = 38,457) in Himachal Pradesh, India observed that tobacco and alcohol consumption was higher among the low socioeconomic position population (as measured by education, household income, and household assets) [38]. Several other studies in the past are reflective of similar patterns of consumption of tobacco and alcohol. Data from 1983 individuals from villages in 18 states in India also reported a higher prevalence of tobacco and alcohol use in low socioeconomic position individuals [39]. When compared by education status, individuals with no education were more likely to be smokers (57.7% vs 39.5%, $p < 0.001$) and use alcohol (36.8% vs 25.5%, $p < 0.001$) compared to those with some level of education [40]. Greater prevalence of smoking and/or tobacco use (OR 3.27, 95% CI: 2.66–4.01) was observed when low education groups were compared to high education groups in urban settings [41]. The CARRS-Study, one of the largest population-based cohorts (>16,000 adults) in South Asia (>12,000 from two Indian cities, Delhi and Chennai) illustrates that tobacco smoking varied by education status with 17.0% (95% CI: 15.5–18.5) among primary, 12.2% (95% CI: 11.3–3.0) among secondary school education and 7.0% (95% CI: 5.8–8.2); $p < 0.001$) among graduates [42].

Similar trend was observed across the wealth quintile, with prevalence declining with an increase in wealth quintile.

The CARRS-Study also reported lower consumption of fruits/vegetables among those with lower level education (primary: 68.0%, 95% CI: 65.6–70.2 vs secondary: 60.3%, 95% CI: 58.6–62.0 vs graduate: 48.0%, 95% CI: 45.1–50.9; $p < 0.001$) and those belonging to lower wealth quintile [42]. The National Family Health Survey (NFHS-4), a large nationally representative periodic cross-sectional survey also confirms that less than half of the population consumes vegetables, legumes, or pulses every day [43]. This could be partly explained by healthier foods being priced higher than the unhealthier options making them less accessible [44–46]. Additionally, despite being an agrarian population with a higher consumption of plant-based foods [47], Indians experience a high CVD burden due to a transition in diet from coarse cereals to more refined ones (white rice, refined-flour), packaged and ready-to-eat food, a carbohydrate-rich diet which is gravy dense (high in saturated fats and salt) and often low in quality/quantity of protein, fruits and vegetables. Further, the vegetables are overcooked leading to loss of micronutrients [48–51].

The relationship of physical activity and SES is heterogeneous depending on the location and setting. A multicenter sentinel surveillance ($n > 19{,}000$) conducted among employees and their family members in ten medium-to-large industries (in urban, urban, and peri-urban regions) of India found that leisure-time physical activity was related to the educational status. A significantly higher proportion of men and women in the lower education groups reported lower leisure-time physical activity [17]. Likewise, in a population-based study ($n \sim 6000$ participants from 11 Indian cities) respondents with low education level had lower physical activity (1.15, 95% CI: 0.97–1.37) compared to higher education group [52]. According to the ICMR-INDIAB (2008–2010), a large cross-sectional survey with 14,227 adults from four regions in India, more than 50% participants were physically inactive which would translate to 392 million individuals at the country level [53]. This study also highlights that a significantly higher proportion of women (63.0% vs men 45.7%, $p < 0.001$) and participants from urban (65.0% vs. rural 50.0%, $p < 0.001$) areas were physically inactive. The average time spent doing moderate to vigorous intensity physical activity per day at work was higher compared to transport or recreation, with men spending significantly more time in physical activity at work [53]. The National Noncommunicable Disease Monitoring Survey reports similar findings and emphasizes the role of economic status in addition to education and rural/urban differences in the levels of physical activity [54]. Physical *inactivity* increased with increasing wealth status, with adults in the highest wealth quintile having insufficient physical activity twice higher than those in the lowest quintile (aOR 1.86, 95% CI: 1.32–2.60, $p < 0.001$) [54]. This could be attributed to time intensive and sedentary job profiles leaving less time for physical activity. The situation is further aggravated by lack of space due to rapid urbanization, inadequate foot path to walk or cycle and other limitations of the built environment infrastructure.

Although, studies indicate an increase in prevalence of obesity, hypertension, and diabetes among lower SES groups [52] it continues to remain higher among those belonging to higher socioeconomic positions. The National Family Health Survey ($n = 757,958$) (2015–2016) reported more than eight-fold higher odds of obesity among individuals in the highest quintile of income compared with those in the lowest quintile though the odds were lower when compared across education status [55]. Another nationally representative study of 1.3 million Indian adults with pooled data from two large household surveys in India: The District-Level Household Survey-4 (DLHS-4) and the second Annual Health Survey (AHS), reported higher probability of hypertension (rural: 4.2%, 95% CI: 3.7–4.6; urban: 3.01%, 95% CI: 2.38–3.65) and diabetes (rural: 2.8%, 95% CI: 2.5–3.1; urban: 3.47%, 95% CI: 3.03–3.91) among individuals of richest household wealth quintile compared to the poorest quintile. Although the prevalence of hypertension and diabetes tended to be higher in urban than rural areas, the relative differences across wealth quintiles in the probability of both conditions were higher in rural areas than in urban areas [56].

Despite the overlapping yet divergent gradient of conventional CVD risk factors across SES groups, the burden of CVD does seem to be disproportionately higher among those in the disadvantaged groups [57]. Studies conducted between the 1960s and 1990s suggested a direct relationship between income and CVD risk. However, recent research illustrates an inverse relationship between education and/or income with CVD [58–60]. One of the hospital-based case-control studies with 200 patients showed a significantly higher risk of acute myocardial infarction (AMI) among the low SES group compared to the high SES group (OR 0.32, $p = 0.005$ highest vs lowest; OR 0.75 middle vs lowest) [59]. Patients (350 cases, 700 controls) with no education had a higher relative risk of IHD 2.5 (95% CI: 1.0–6.0) compared to those with a graduate/professional level of education [60]. Results from 30-day follow-up data of more than 20,000 acute coronary syndrome (ACS) patients from the CREATE registry demonstrated a significantly higher mortality rate in the low SES group compared to the higher one (poor vs. rich patients: 8.2% vs 5.5%, $p < 0.0001$) [61]. When compared by education status, participants with <8 years of schooling were found to have a higher risk of AMI compared to those with higher education level in the INTERHEART Study [62]. Similarly, the PURE study, a prospective cohort of 155,722 participants without CVD from 21 countries (mostly LMICs) showed that low education level was associated with a higher hazard ratio of incident CVD (1.37, 95% CI:1.23–1.52) and associated mortality (1.55, 95% CI: 1.39–1.74) and was the single largest risk factor for CVD mortality (12·5%, 95% CI: 10.7%–14.3%) of the population attributable fraction [63].

It is worth noting that women are also at an increasing risk of CVD in India. Serial rounds of the NFHS data have shown that while the proportion of women consuming tobacco is less than men, an increasing trend of tobacco consumption has been observed among women [64]. Additionally, studies have shown an increasing prevalence of metabolic risk factors such as dyslipidemia, hypertension, diabetes, and obesity among Indian women, [65, 66] which has translated to a rapid increase in IHD and associated mortality among women (From 2007 to 2017: 0.32–0.62 million (+93.7%) compared to men (0.53–0.92 million, +73.6%) [67]. Lower education levels [66] among women along with individual social (stress, social stigma, family arrangements, social capital, etc.) and societal level (fewer job avenues, inequity, etc.) factors may be adding to this gender difference [68]. These factors may also be responsible for low awareness and access to treatment rates among women [67, 69].

11.4 Challenges and Possible Solutions

Since development is socially and regionally uneven in India, the role of SES and related factors in CVD risk and events simulates the same pattern. Lack of resources to access health-related information and services coupled with lower education status often contributes to social patterning of CVD and its risk factors thus marginalizing the disadvantaged groups [70–73]. This problem is further compounded by underdiagnosis and underreporting of CVD especially among the poor [74]. Literature suggests that economically underprivileged patients with CVD are less likely to receive evidence-based treatment because cardiac treatment often involves large out-of-pocket payments and catastrophic health expenditure on drugs/hospitalization over a long term and often no health insurance coverage [75]. An unprepared health system adds to the existing CVD-social gradient. The absence of efficient and quality care facilities in the form of sporadic presence of specialist-equipped centers in rural areas, not enough doctors and nurses (doctor–patient ratio, vacant posts in rural health facilities), drug supply chain issues and lack of low-cost evidence-based medicines further limit accessibility for disadvantaged people [76]. In addition to this, the large unorganized sector in the rural and urban slum areas makes provision of health insurance and health planning challenging.

CVD by its very nature demands lifestyle changes and lifelong therapy requiring regular follow-up and frequent drug titration. However, there are several social impediments for disadvantaged sections to manage the same.

Firstly, there are several s**ocial influences leading to physical inactivity** in India, which include lack of green spaces in urban areas, poor walkability index, air pollution, rise in sedentary jobs, and the move from a primarily agrarian to an industrial community over the last few decades. Secondly, **social influences leading to unhealthy diet** include an increase in availability of cheap processed ready-to-eat food, lack of time to prepare home-cooked meals [77, 78], an increase in trends of eating out or online food delivery, rise of trans-national food corporations that invest in cheaper foods with longer shelf-life and fast-food [77], increase in consumption of street foods, high consumption of sugar sweetened beverages (SSBs), high cost of fruits and seasonality of vegetables. Thirdly, there are **social factors influencing poor compliance to follow ups** such as poor health seeking behavior, poor access to care (in most instances individuals from rural regions must travel more than 100 km to access tertiary-level care), non-availability of specialists in rural areas, loss of daily wages while seeking care and inherent inequities reducing access to digital solutions such as telemedicine. Fourthly, there are **social and health system factors influencing poor drug titration** such as drug supply chain issues and therapeutic inertia among primary care physicians. Last but not least, s**ocial influences on medication adherence** like poor affordability, lack of drug availability in locality, education and health awareness and small drug refills in the public sector necessitating frequent visits also contribute to the high burden. Social adverse influences of gender on these cardiometabolic factors, access to treatment and adherence are more pronounced among women due to complex medication regime, lack of dispensable income available for accessing care, and other cultural factors [67].

As increasing disparities in CVDs are fundamentally driven by the wider upstream social determinants [79], addressing these via community and clinical interventions needs to be a global and national priority. A deeper understanding and due consideration of the social patterning of CVD can help develop, design, and implement contextually relevant efforts in India's resource-constrained health system. As one of the preliminary measures, we should emphasize on increasing the awareness of healthy diet, physical activity, and lifestyle among the population through a targeted and focused approach. National data on CVD risk factors, events, and related SES factors should be systematically collected and reported routinely to facilitate co-designing and scaling up of sustainable interventions [80]. This could be done by leveraging electronic health record (EHR)-based surveillance for valuable insights into the impact of SES and related factors on the overall CVD risk [81]. Further, the use of innovative models of care involving trained non-physician health workers (NPHWs), such as community health workers and pharmacists, with proven evidence in LMICs and India [82], implementing lifestyle change education and support at the worksite to deliver an intervention that acceptable, accessible, and overcomes barriers to lifestyle change (e.g., lack of time or resources) [83, 84] and rolling out mobile clinics and telehealth programs could be additional options worth exploring for their potential for sustainable delivery of CVD care addressing concerns of accessibility to evidence-based management.

These individual and community-based interventions need to be complemented by policies that promote cardiovascular health and prevent CVD morbidity and mortality, including "best-buys" for preventing NCDs [85]. This calls for a multifaceted approach, by targeted reductions in tobacco and alcohol usage through bans/taxes, promoting physical activity by better planning that takes into consideration neighborhoods that promote physical activity and promoting healthier dietary habits by imposing taxes or ban on unhealthy food items (processed, ready-to-eat food items, SSBs, trans-fat) through inter-sectoral collaboration with non-health sector entities. Several examples from across the globe highlight population level benefits of policy changes. Introduction of a tax on SSBs in Mexico led to a subsequent reduction in the purchase of the same [86]. Modeling studies suggest a 20% tax on SSB will show an estimated reduction in prevalence of overweight and obesity by 3% and incidence of type 2 diabetes mellitus by 2% [87]. Likewise, a tax on palm oil could potentially avert approximately 363,000 deaths from myocardial infarctions and strokes over a period of 10 years [88]. Several surveys in Finland show an increase in the level of physical activity through commitment to multisectoral policy, investment in community infrastructure [89]. Therefore, national policies should be aimed at ensuring affordable seasonal produce, offering subsidies to marginalized groups, and creating an environment conducive to healthy behaviors, such as ample green spaces for physical activity, along with tobacco control measures for reducing social disparities and ensuring equity [90].

References

1. Joshi P, Islam S, Pais P, Reddy S, Dorairaj P, Kazmi K, et al. Risk factors for early myocardial infarction in south Asians compared with individuals in other countries. JAMA. 2007;297(3):286–94.
2. Prabhakaran D, Jeemon P, Roy A. Cardiovascular diseases in India. Circulation. 2016;133(16):1605–20.
3. Prabhakaran D, Yusuf S, Mehta S, Pogue J, Avezum A, Budaj A, et al. Two-year outcomes in patients admitted with non-ST elevation acute coronary syndrome: results of the OASIS registry 1 and 2. Indian Heart J. 2005;57(3):217–25.
4. Yusuf S, Rangarajan S, Teo K, Islam S, Li W, Liu L, et al. Cardiovascular risk and events in 17 low-, middle-, and high-income countries. N Engl J Med. 2014;371(9):818–27.
5. Prabhakaran D, Jeemon P, Sharma M, Roth GA, Johnson C, Harikrishnan S, et al. The changing patterns of cardiovascular diseases and their risk factors in the states of India: the global burden of disease study 1990–2016. Lancet Glob Health. 2018;6(12):e1339–51.
6. Dandona L, Dandona R, Kumar GA, Shukla DK, Paul VK, Balakrishnan K, et al. Nations within a nation: variations in epidemiological transition across the states of India, 1990–2016 in the global burden of disease study. Lancet. 2017;390(10111):2437–60.
7. Bloom DE, Cafiero-Fonseca ET, Candeias V, Adashi E, Bloom L, Gurfein L, Jané-Llopis E, Lubet, A, Mitgang E, O'Brien JC, Saxena A. Economics of non-communicable diseases in India: the costs and returns on Investment of Interventions to promote healthy living and prevent, treat, and manage NCDs. 2014.
8. Nair M, Prabhakaran D. Why do south Asians have high risk for CAD? Glob Heart. 2012;7(4):307–14.
9. UN. Secretary-General. Progress towards the sustainable development goals: report of the secretary-general [internet]. New York; 2018 [cited 2023 Oct 27]. https://digitallibrary.un.org/record/1627573?ln=en.
10. Yusuf S, Hawken S, Ôunpuu S, Dans T, Avezum A, Lanas F, et al. Effect of potentially modifiable risk factors associated with myocardial infarction in 52 countries (the INTERHEART study): case-control study. Lancet. 2004;364(9438):937–52.
11. Anjana RM, Unnikrishnan R, Deepa M, Pradeepa R, Tandon N, Das AK, et al. Metabolic non-communicable disease health report of India: the ICMR-INDIAB national cross-sectional study (ICMR-INDIAB-17). Lancet Diabetes Endocrinol. 2023;11(7):474–89.
12. Bambra C, Gibson M, Sowden A, Wright K, Whitehead M, Petticrew M. Tackling the wider social determinants of health and health inequalities: evidence from systematic reviews. J Epidemiol Community Health (1978). 2010;64(4):284–91.
13. World Health Organization. What are the social determinants of health? [Internet]. Geneva; 2008 [cited 2023 Oct 30]. www.who.int/social_determinants/sdh_definition/en/.
14. Krieger N, Williams DR, Moss NE. Measuring social class in US public health research: concepts, methodologies, and guidelines. Annu Rev Public Health. 1997;18:341–78.
15. Lynch J, Kaplan G. Socioeconomic position. In: Berkman LF, Kawachi I, editors. Social epidemiology. 1st ed. Oxford: Oxford University Press; 2000. p. 13–35.
16. Stringhini S, Carmeli C, Jokela M, Avendaño M, Muennig P, Guida F, et al. Socioeconomic status and the 25 × 25 risk factors as determinants of premature mortality: a multicohort study and meta-analysis of 1.7 million men and women. Lancet. 2017;389(10075):1229–37.

17. Reddy KS, Prabhakaran D, Jeemon P, Thankappan KR, Joshi P, Chaturvedi V, et al. Educational status and cardiovascular risk profile in Indians. Proc Natl Acad Sci U S A. 2007;104(41):16263–8.
18. Power C, Hertzman C. Social and biological pathways linking early life and adult disease. Br Med Bull. 1997;53(1):210–21.
19. Hertzman C, Power C, Matthews S, Manor O. Using an interactive framework of society and lifecourse to explain self-rated health in early adulthood. Soc Sci Med. 2001;53(12):1575–85.
20. Davey Smith G. Life course approaches to inequalities in coronary heart disease. In: Stansfeld SA, Marmot MG, editors. Stress and the heart. London: BMJ Books; 2002. p. 20–49.
21. Marmot M. Relative contribution of early life and adult socioeconomic factors to adult morbidity in the Whitehall II study. J Epidemiol Community Health (1978). 2001;55(5):301–7.
22. Lynch J, Smith GD. A life course approach to chronic disease epidemiology. Annu Rev Public Health. 2005;26(1):1–35.
23. Office of the Registrar General and Census Commissioner India, Ministry of Home Affairs Government of India. Primary census abstract indicators search upto town/village level [Internet]. [cited 2023 Oct 30]. https://censusindia.gov.in/census.website/data/data-visualizations/PopulationSearch_PCA_Indicators.
24. Agarwal A. Social classification: the need to update in the present scenario. Indian J Community Med. 2008;33(1):50–1.
25. Galobardes B, Shaw M, Lawlor DA, Lynch JW, Davey Smith G. Indicators of socioeconomic position (part 1). J Epidemiol Community Health (1978). 2006;60(1):7–12.
26. Daly MC, Duncan GJ, McDonough P, Williams DR. Optimal indicators of socioeconomic status for health research. Am J Public Health. 2002;92(7):1151–7.
27. Adler NE, Newman K. Socioeconomic disparities in health: pathways and policies. Health Aff (Millwood). 2002;21(2):60–76.
28. Daniel H, Bornstein SS, Kane GC, Health and Public Policy Committee of the American College of Physicians, Carney JK, Gantzer HE, et al. Addressing social determinants to improve patient care and promote health equity: an American College of Physicians position paper. Ann Intern Med. 2018;168(8):577–8.
29. Saif-Ur-Rahman KM, Anwar I, Hasan MD, Hossain S, Shafique S, Haseen F, et al. Use of indices to measure socio-economic status (SES) in south-Asian urban health studies: a scoping review. Syst Rev. 2018;7(1):196.
30. Kuppuswami B. Manual of socioeconomic scale (urban). Delhi: Manasayan; 1981.
31. Pareekh U. Manual of socioeconomic status (rural). Delhi: Mansayan; 1981.
32. Tiwari SC, Kumar A, Kumar A. Development & standardization of a scale to measure socio-economic status in urban & rural communities in India. Indian J Med Res. 2005;122(4):309–14.
33. Majumder S. Socioeconomic status scales: revised Kuppuswamy, BG Prasad, and Udai Pareekh's scale updated for 2021. J Family Med Prim Care. 2021;10(11):3964–7.
34. Central Bureau of Health Intelligence. National Health Profile 2022. 16th ed. New Delhi: Ministry of Health and Family Welfare, Government of India; 2022. 1–449 p.
35. Sorlie PD, Backlund E, Keller JB. US mortality by economic, demographic, and social characteristics: the National Longitudinal Mortality Study. Am J Public Health. 1995;85(7):949–56.
36. Kaplan GA, Keil JE. Socioeconomic factors and cardiovascular disease: a review of the literature. Circulation. 1993;88(4 Pt 1):1973–98.
37. Rose G, Marmot MG. Social class and coronary heart disease. Br Heart J. 1981;45(1):13–9.
38. Agarwal A, Jindal D, Ajay VS, Kondal D, Mandal S, Ghosh S, et al. Association between socioeconomic position and cardiovascular disease risk factors in rural north India: the Solan surveillance study. PLoS One. 2019;14(7):e0217834.
39. Kinra S, Bowen LJ, Lyngdoh T, Prabhakaran D, Reddy KS, Ramakrishnan L, et al. Sociodemographic patterning of non-communicable disease risk factors in rural India: a cross sectional study. BMJ. 2010;341:c4974.
40. Zaman MJ, Patel A, Jan S, Hillis GS, Raju PK, Neal B, et al. Socio-economic distribution of cardiovascular risk factors and knowledge in rural India. Int J Epidemiol. 2012;41(5):1302–14.

41. Gupta R, Deedwania PC, Sharma K, Gupta A, Guptha S, Achari V, et al. Association of educational, occupational and socioeconomic status with cardiovascular risk factors in Asian Indians: a cross-sectional study. PLoS One. 2012;7(8):e44098.
42. Ali MK, Bhaskarapillai B, Shivashankar R, Mohan D, Fatmi ZA, Pradeepa R, et al. Socioeconomic status and cardiovascular risk in urban South Asia: the CARRS study. Eur J Prev Cardiol. 2016;23(4):408–19.
43. National Family Health Survey, India. 2015.
44. Kanungsukkasem U, Ng N, Van Minh H, Razzaque A, Ashraf A, Juvekar S, et al. Fruit and vegetable consumption in rural adults population in INDEPTH HDSS sites in Asia. Glob Health Action. 2009;2.
45. Ghosh J. Social policy in Indian development. In: Social policy in a development context. London: Palgrave Macmillan UK; 2004. p. 284–307.
46. Rao M, Afshin A, Singh G, Mozaffarian D. Do healthier foods and diet patterns cost more than less healthy options? A systematic review and meta-analysis. BMJ Open. 2013;3(12):e004277.
47. The state of food security and nutrition in the world 2023. Rome: FAO; IFAD; UNICEF; WFP; WHO; 2023.
48. Trichopoulou A, Martínez-González MA, Tong TY, Forouhi NG, Khandelwal S, Prabhakaran D, et al. Definitions and potential health benefits of the Mediterranean diet: views from experts around the world. BMC Med. 2014;12:112.
49. Misra A, Singhal N, Sivakumar B, Bhagat N, Jaiswal A, Khurana L. Nutrition transition in India: secular trends in dietary intake and their relationship to diet-related non-communicable diseases. J Diabetes. 2011;3(4):278–92.
50. Pan A, Lin X, Hemler E, Hu FB. Diet and cardiovascular disease: advances and challenges in population-based studies. Cell Metab. 2018;27(3):489–96.
51. Prabhakaran D, Jeemon P, Reddy KS. Commentary: poverty and cardiovascular disease in India: do we need more evidence for action? Int J Epidemiol. 2013;42(5):1431–5.
52. Gupta R, Gupta KD. Coronary heart disease in low socioeconomic status subjects in India: "an evolving epidemic". Indian Heart J. 2009;61(4):358–67.
53. Anjana RM, Pradeepa R, Das AK, Deepa M, Bhansali A, Joshi SR, et al. Physical activity and inactivity patterns in India—results from the ICMR-INDIAB study (Phase-1) [ICMR-INDIAB-5]. Int J Behav Nutr Phys Act. 2014;11(1):26.
54. Ramamoorthy T, Kulothungan V, Mathur P. Prevalence and correlates of insufficient physical activity among adults aged 18–69 years in India: findings from the National Noncommunicable Disease Monitoring Survey. J Phys Act Health. 2022;19(3):150–9.
55. Corsi DJ, Subramanian SV. Socioeconomic gradients and distribution of diabetes, hypertension, and obesity in India. JAMA Netw Open. 2019;2(4):e190411.
56. Geldsetzer P, Manne-Goehler J, Theilmann M, Davies JI, Awasthi A, Vollmer S, et al. Diabetes and hypertension in India: a nationally representative study of 1.3 million adults. JAMA Intern Med. 2018;178(3):363–72.
57. Gupta PC, Pednekar MS. Re: jumping the gun: the problematic discourse on socioeconomic status and cardiovascular health in India. Int J Epidemiol. 2014;43(1):276–8.
58. Chadha SL, Radhakrishnan S, Ramachandran K, Kaul U, Gopinath N. Epidemiological study of coronary heart disease in urban population of Delhi. Indian J Med Res. 1990;92:424–30.
59. Pais P, Pogue J, Gerstein H, Zachariah E, Savitha D, Jayprakash S, et al. Risk factors for acute myocardial infarction in Indians: a case-control study. Lancet. 1996;348(9024):358–63.
60. Rastogi T, Reddy KS, Vaz M, Spiegelman D, Prabhakaran D, Willett WC, et al. Diet and risk of ischemic heart disease in India. Am J Clin Nutr. 2004;79(4):582–92.
61. Xavier D, Pais P, Devereaux PJ, Xie C, Prabhakaran D, Reddy KS, et al. Treatment and outcomes of acute coronary syndromes in India (CREATE): a prospective analysis of registry data. Lancet [Internet]. 2008 [cited 2015 May 8];371(9622):1435–42. http://www.ncbi.nlm.nih.gov/pubmed/18440425.

62. Rosengren A, Subramanian SV, Islam S, Chow CK, Avezum A, Kazmi K, et al. Education and risk for acute myocardial infarction in 52 high, middle and low-income countries: INTERHEART case-control study. Heart. 2009;95(24):2014–22.
63. Yusuf S, Joseph P, Rangarajan S, Islam S, Mente A, Hystad P, et al. Modifiable risk factors, cardiovascular disease, and mortality in 155,722 individuals from 21 high-income, middle-income, and low-income countries (PURE): a prospective cohort study. Lancet. 2020;395(10226):795–808.
64. Bhan N, Srivastava S, Agrawal S, Subramanyam M, Millett C, Selvaraj S, et al. Are socioeconomic disparities in tobacco consumption increasing in India? A repeated cross-sectional multilevel analysis. BMJ Open. 2012;2(5):e001348.
65. Gupta R, Guptha S, Sharma KK, Gupta A, Deedwania P. Regional variations in cardiovascular risk factors in India: India heart watch. World J Cardiol [Internet]. 2012 [cited 2014 Sep 29];4(4):112–20. http://www.pubmedcentral.nih.gov/articlerender.fcgi?artid=3342579&tool=pmcentrez&rendertype=abstract.
66. Geldsetzer P, Manne-Goehler J, Theilmann M, Davies JI, Awasthi A, Danaei G, et al. Geographic and sociodemographic variation of cardiovascular disease risk in India: a cross-sectional study of 797,540 adults. PLoS Med. 2018;15(6):e1002581.
67. Kiran G, Mohan I, Kaur M, Ahuja S, Gupta S, Gupta R. Escalating ischemic heart disease burden among women in India: insights from GBD, NCDRisC and NFHS reports. Am J Prev Cardiol. 2020;2:100035.
68. O'Neil A, Scovelle AJ, Milner AJ, Kavanagh A. Gender/sex as a social determinant of cardiovascular risk. Circulation. 2018;137(8):854–64.
69. Magnani JW, Mujahid MS, Aronow HD, Cené CW, Dickson VV, Havranek E, et al. Health literacy and cardiovascular disease: fundamental relevance to primary and secondary prevention: a scientific statement from the American Heart Association. Circulation. 2018;138(2):e48.
70. Chadha SL, Gopinath N, Shekhawat S. Urban-rural differences in the prevalence of coronary heart disease and its risk factors in Delhi. Bull World Health Organ. 1997;75(1):31–8.
71. Singh RB, Ghosh S, Niaz AM, Gupta S, Bishnoi I, Sharma JP, et al. Epidemiologic study of diet and coronary risk factors in relation to central obesity and insulin levels in rural and urban populations of north India. Int J Cardiol. 1995;47(3):245–55.
72. Gupta R, Sharma AK, Prakash H. High prevalence of hypertension in rural and urban Indian populations. Transplant Proc. 2000;32(7):1840.
73. Prabhakaran D, Chaturvedi V, Shah P, Manhapra A, Jeemon P, Shah B, et al. Differences in the prevalence of metabolic syndrome in urban and rural India: a problem of urbanization. Chronic Illn. 2007;3(1):8–19.
74. Vellakkal S, Subramanian SV, Millett C, Basu S, Stuckler D, Ebrahim S. Socioeconomic inequalities in non-communicable diseases prevalence in India: disparities between self-reported diagnoses and standardized measures. PLoS One. 2013;8(7):e68219.
75. Huffman MD, Rao KD, Pichon-Riviere A, Zhao D, Harikrishnan S, Ramaiya K, et al. A cross-sectional study of the microeconomic impact of cardiovascular disease hospitalization in four low- and middle-income countries. PLoS One. 2011;6(6):e20821.
76. Deo MG. Doctor population ratio for India—the reality. Indian J Med Res. 2013;137(4):632–5.
77. Globalization and Health Knowledge Network RPapers. WHO Commission on Social Determinants of Health. Globalization, Food and Nutrition Transitions. Ottawa; 2007.
78. Chaturvedi S, Ramji S, Arora NK, Rewal S, Dasgupta R, Deshmukh V. Time-constrained mother and expanding market: emerging model of under-nutrition in India. BMC Public Health. 2016;16(1):632.
79. Powell-Wiley TM, Baumer Y, Baah FO, Baez AS, Farmer N, Mahlobo CT, et al. Social determinants of cardiovascular disease. Circ Res. 2022;130(5):782–99.
80. Aerts N, Van Royen K, Van Bogaert P, Peremans L, Bastiaens H. Understanding factors affecting implementation success and sustainability of a comprehensive prevention program for cardiovascular disease in primary health care: a qualitative process evaluation study combining RE-AIM and CFIR. Prim Health Care Res Dev. 2023;24:e17.

81. Magnani JW. Hypertension—A social disease in need of social solutions. Hypertension. 2023;80(7):1414–6.
82. Jafar TH, Hatcher J, Poulter N, Islam M, Hashmi S, Qadri Z, et al. Community-based interventions to promote blood pressure control in a developing country. Ann Intern Med. 2009;151(9):593.
83. Prabhakaran D, Jeemon P, Goenka S, Lakshmy R, Thankappan KR, Ahmed F, et al. Impact of a worksite intervention program on cardiovascular risk factors. J Am Coll Cardiol. 2009;53(18):1718–28.
84. Jeemon P, Prabhakaran D, Goenka S, Ramakrishnan L, Padmanabhan S, Huffman M, et al. Impact of comprehensive cardiovascular risk reduction programme on risk factor clustering associated with elevated blood pressure in an Indian industrial population. Indian J Med Res. 2012;135(4):485–93.
85. World Health Organization. Tackling NCDs "best buys" and other recommended interventions for the prevention and control of noncommunicable diseases; 2017.
86. Colchero MA, Molina M, Guerrero-López CM. After Mexico implemented a tax, purchases of sugar-sweetened beverages decreased and water increased: difference by place of residence, household composition, and income level. J Nutr. 2017;147(8):1552–7.
87. Basu S, Vellakkal S, Agrawal S, Stuckler D, Popkin B, Ebrahim S. Averting obesity and type 2 diabetes in India through sugar-sweetened beverage taxation: an economic-epidemiologic modeling study. PLoS Med. 2014;11(1):e1001582.
88. Basu S, Babiarz KS, Ebrahim S, Vellakkal S, Stuckler D, Goldhaber-Fiebert JD. Palm oil taxes and cardiovascular disease mortality in India: economic-epidemiologic model. BMJ. 2013;347:f6048.
89. Vuori I, Lankenau B, Pratt M. Physical activity policy and program development: the experience in Finland. Public Health Rep. 2004;119(3):331–45.
90. Miller V, Yusuf S, Chow CK, Dehghan M, Corsi DJ, Lock K, et al. Availability, affordability, and consumption of fruits and vegetables in 18 countries across income levels: findings from the prospective urban rural epidemiology (PURE) study. Lancet Glob Health. 2016;4(10):e695–703.

Chapter 12
Cardiovascular Disease Prevention, Management, and Outcomes in China

Doris Sau-fung Yu, Sophia Fen Ye, and Polly Wai-Chi Li

12.1 Epidemiology of CVD in China

Cardiovascular disease (CVD) is the primary contributor to global morbidity and mortality. China shares the same epidemiology. The age-standardized incidence and prevalence rate of CVD increased from 646 and 5848 per 100,000 persons in 1990 to 652.2 and 6177 per 100,000 in 2019, respectively [1]. Referring to the National CVD Report 2022, it was estimated that around 23% of the Chinese population (330 million people), were affected by CVD, with stroke and coronary heart disease being the most common types of CVD [2]. The incidence of stroke has seen a substantial increase by 86% since 1990, with the rate escalating to 276.7 per 100,000 population in 2019 [3].

In fact, when interpreting the epidemiological trend of CVD in China, consideration has to be given to the socio-demographic structure of the country. In particular, the increased life expectancy, rapid population ageing, and health inequalities due to regional disparities have play a part to contribute to the current landscape of CVD in China [4].

The Global Burden of Disease Study indicates that for every decade of age, the risk of CVD doubles [5]. According to the World Bank, the average life expectancy in China increased from years in 68 years in 1990 to 78 years in 2021 due to the improvement in health care and living standard [1]. This, on the other hand, is translated to a sharp increase in the CVD incidence. The extremely low fertility rate since the launch of the one-child policy in 1979 further shifts the demographic pattern towards the advanced age [6], and the United Nation projected that about 16.9% of

D. S.-f. Yu (✉) · S. F. Ye · P. W.-C. Li
School of Nursing, Li Ka Shing Faculty of Medicine, The University of Hong Kong, Pok Fu Lam, Hong Kong
e-mail: dyu1@hku.hk; yefen@connect.hku.hk; pwcli@hku.hk

T. Romero et al. (eds.), *Global Challenges in Cardiovascular Prevention in Populations with Low Socioeconomic Status*,
https://doi.org/10.1007/978-3-031-79051-5_12

the population will be at age 65 or above in 2030 [7]. Against this backdrop, a further rise in the epidemiological pattern of CVD in China would be anticipated.

Another socio-demographic characteristic which shapes the CVD epidemiology in China is about the regional disparities. China has the fourth-largest land area globally; there is considerable diversity in the socioeconomic development and geographic location which affect the CVD epidemiology. For example, the great variation in the per capital gross regional income between the eastern (e.g. Beijing and Jiangsu) and western (Cinjiang and Qinghai) China led to an unequal distribution of healthcare resource. The more remote and mountainous region in the west and central China also adds accessibility challenges on service delivery. For example, the utilization of medication for overall cardiovascular patients was greater in high- and middle-income and urban areas compared to low-income rural regions, suggesting inferior healthcare accessibility in the latter [8], reflecting disparities in healthcare accessibility. Another study conducted in 2016 found that only 36% of patients with acute myocardial infarction in rural areas received percutaneous coronary intervention, compared to 51% in urban areas [9]. The disparity in the CVD epidemiology in China was reported in a territory-wide survey covering 64 urban and 93 rural areas, in which the age-standardized mortality, prevalence, and incidence of stroke were higher in rural areas (117, 930, and 227 per 100,000) compared to urban areas (75, 168, and 789 per 100,000), respectively [10].

12.2 Impact of CVD in China

CVD is associated with detrimental health impact and economic loss in China. It is a leading cause of premature death in China, with survivors experiencing a lower life expectancy and poorer quality of life compared to those without the disease [11]. Living with CVD also cause high psychological morbidity such as anxiety and depression in China [12, 13], which further aggravates the mortality and morbidity, health deterioration (physical function, symptom burden, quality of life) and increases healthcare costs [14, 15]. The Global Burden of Disease Study 2019 estimated that there were more than 4.6 million CVD-related deaths in China, which accounts for 25% of global CVD-related death [1]. Furthermore, men had a higher age-standardized mortality rate (362 per 100,000) compared to women (220 per 100,000) in China [1]. The economic impact of CVD in China is massive and growing, with an estimated economic loss of $8.8 trillion at the national or regional level attributed to CVD between 2012 and 2030 [16]. As such, risk factor control, primary prevention, and effective CVD management are crucial to delimit the epidemiological growth.

12.3 Risk Factors of CVD in China

Lifestyle and environmental risk factors are the cornerstones shaping the development and progression of CVD. In China, the rapid urbanization casts an impact on the CVD risk profile. According to data from the National Bureau of Statistics of

China, the industrial value-added output increased by 2.4% year-on-year since 2020, despite the challenges posed by the COVID-19 pandemic [17]. Urbanization and industrialization have led to increased exposure to environmental pollutants and less healthy lifestyle changes with the risen income (disposable income: USD$ 2819 in 2014 vs. USD$ 4499 in 2020) [17, 18]. These changes are closely intertwined with the prevalence of CVD risk factors, such as hypertension, obesity, and diabetes [19]. Table 12.1 shows the prevalence of CVD risk factors and the disease manifestation and the mortality impact among regions of different income in China.

12.3.1 Unhealthy Diets

China had the highest age-standardized rates of CVD deaths associated with dietary factors [20]. Urbanization and the opening-up of China leads to a rapid nutrition transition from traditional diets rich in whole grains, fruits, and vegetables towards Western-style diets high in refined carbohydrates, fats, and sugars since the late 1980s [21]. Such dietary transition has greatly increased the risk profile for CVD including hypertension, obesity, and metabolic syndrome [22]. Children may be more affected by such dietary transition, as under the one-child policy, the only child usually received more resource and attention from parents, including food, which lead to overnutrition, obesity, and high blood pressure [23]. Increased consumption of processed foods, sugary beverages and high-sodium Chinese eating habit (e.g. pickled vegetables and soy sauce) further aggravates the CVD risk including hypertension [24] in China. According to the China Health and Nutrition Survey, the age-adjusted prevalence of overweight and obesity among adults increased from 24% and 4% in 1991 to 39% and 14% in 2011, respectively [21]. It is estimated that approximately two-thirds of Chinese adults would be affected by overweight/general obesity in 2030 [25]. Another study, indeed, reported that the average sodium intake in China was 5 g/day (9 g/day salt), which is far beyond the WHO recommended limit of 5 g/day salt in all provinces [26]. Tackling all the dietary risk for CVD control in China therefore need to take into consideration of the socio-cultural influence.

12.3.2 Physical Inactivity

Physical inactivity also contributes significantly to the CVD burden in China. Rapid urbanization and technological advancements (e.g. increased screen time) have led to increasingly sedentary lifestyles [27, 28]. More specifically, the concomitant social changes including increased access to higher educational institutions, improved housing infrastructure, advancements in sanitation, and heightened community economic well-being were consistently found to be account for 57% of the decline in total physical activity for men and nearly 40% for women from 1991 to 2006 [28]. According to a population-based study

Table 12.1 Prevalence of cardiovascular risk factors, cardiovascular disease, and mortality among different regions in China

City/province		Year Income[a] [99], (Chinese Yuan, CNY)	Hypertension[b] [40], (%)	Diabetes[c] [100], (%)	Obesity[d] [101], (%)	Smoking[e] [102], (%)	Prevalence[f] [103], (per 100,000)	Mortality[f] [103], (per 100,000)
Mainland (in average)		36,883	23.2	12.8[g]	5.2	25.2	6037	307.9
Higher income regions in mainland	Beijing	77,415	35.9	13.6	10.8	26.8	5914.6	209.2
	Shanghai	79,610	29.1	13.7	3.2	22.1	5075.5	129.4
	Zhejiang	60,303	23.2	11.2	2.9	23.8	5181.3	161.6
	Jiangsu	49,862	25.3	11.5	5.6	24.3	6470.8	196.1
	Tianjin	48,976	34.5	14.4	12.2	26.8	6455.6	305.2
	Guangdong	47,065	27.3	12.7	3.7	22.7	5980.3	239.6
	Fujian	43,118	23.9	17.3	2.5	24.1	5388.5	216.2
	Shandong	37,560	22.0	13.4	8.0	22.1	6037.3	314.2
	Liaoning	36,089	28.4	12.7	7.0	22.9	6661.3	336.8
	Inner Mongolia	35,921	19.7	19.9	5.7	29.3	6878.0	376.6
	Chongqing	35,666	20.6	16.0	3.2	28.4	6047.7	264.6
	Hunan	34,036	15.6	14.0	3.1	27.5	6103.5	350.3
	Hubei	32,914	18.1	10.6	2.9	26.3	5475.2	326.6
	Anhui	32,745	20.5	8.5	3.5	25.3	5846.9	336.5
	Jiangxi	32,419	17.3	12.1	2.8	25.0	5935.2	300.5
	Hainan	30,957	20.3	17.5	1.3	20.9	6326.7	296.0
	Hebei	30,867	23.3	14.4	7.3	25.0	6811.8	403.0
	Sichuan	30,679	23.6	15.6	4.4	27.1	5473.8	284.5
	Shaanxi	30,116	22.0	15.1	6.2	27.6	5365.0	385.1

City/province		Year Income[a] [99], (Chinese Yuan, CNY)	Hypertension[b] [40], (%)	Diabetes[c] [100], (%)	Obesity[d] [101], (%)	Smoking[e] [102], (%)	Prevalence[f] [103], (per 100,000)	Mortality[f] [103], (per 100,000)
Lower income regions in mainland	Shanxi	29,178	26.0	10.4	5.4	26.8	6460.5	358.5
	Ningxia	29,599	22.1	8.0	8.2	23.5	5929.0	364.8
	Heilongjiang	28,346	26.4	12.9	9.0	26.0	6668.8	429.7
	Henan	28,222	24.1	12.0	8.5	23.6	6378.4	407.5
	Guangxi	27,981	18.2	11.9	1.6	24.2	5460.2	341.8
	Jilin	27,975	26.2	13.4	6.5	27.8	6485.5	417.8
	Xinjiang	27,063	18.2	11.4	9.2	16.2	6335.6	435.4
	Qinghai	27,000	17.2	11.8	4.1	26.7	6361.2	432.9
	Yunnan	26,937	28.4	12.4	4.5	30.6	6130.8	338.3
	Tibet	26,675	25	6.5	6.1	18.4	6410.1	578.2
	Guizhou	25,508	23.6	6.2	3.8	34.6	6270.3	405.5
	Gansu	23,273	20.7	9.1	1.9	27.6	6023.3	339.9
Other regions								
	Hong Kong	376,719[h]	15[i,] [104]	8.5[j,] [104]	30.8[k,] [104]	9.5[l,] [105]	5269.3	99.4
	Macao	232,525[m]	34 [106]	7.8[n,] [107]	19.9 [108]	11.2 [109]	9007.0	145.9
	Taiwan	232,249[h]	25 [110]	4.9[o]	20.7[p]	11.2[o]	5952.2[o]	276.9[o]

[a]Per capita disposable income of households in 2022 (sort descending, 100 CNY ≈ 13.95 US Dollar as of January 7, 2024)

[b]Prevalence rate of hypertension (in Mainland) was weighted to represent the total population of Chinese aged 18 years or older based on Chinese census 2010 (A nationwide survey conducted from October 2012 to December 2015, $n = 451{,}755$)

[c]Age- and sex-adjusted prevalence rate (in Mainland) of diabetes was weighted represented the total population of Chinese aged 18 years or older (A nationwide survey conducted from October 2015 to December 2017, $n = 75{,}880$)

[d]Prevalence rate of obesity (in Mainland) was weighted to represent the total population of Chinese aged 18 years or older based on Chinese census 2010 (A nationwide survey conducted from October 2012 to December 2015, BMI ≥ 30 kg/m^2 according to the WHO classifications, $n = 441{,}306$)

[e]Prevalence rate of smoking (in Mainland) was standardized by age and gender according to the 2010 national census (A national survey conducted among individuals aged 15 years or older in 2013, $n = 229{,}676$)

(continued)

Table 12.1 (continued)

[f]Age-standardized valued (in China) from the 2016 Global Burden of Disease Study

[g]Estimates were weighted to reflect the age, sex, and urban-rural, distribution of provinces of the adults in Mainland of China, according to American Diabetes Association diagnostic criteria

[h]Per capita gross national income in 2022 (100 CNY ≈ 109 Hong Kong Dollar, 100 CNY ≈ 430 New Taiwan Dollar as of January 7, 2024)

[i]Age-standardized prevalence of raised blood pressure (systolic blood pressure ≥ 140 mmHg and/or diastolic blood pressure ≥ 90 mmHg disregarding of known history of hypertension) among individuals aged 18–84 who completed physical measurements ($n = 2072$) from 2020 to 2022

[j]Including individuals with self-reported doctor-diagnosed diabetes mellitus or those with no self-reported history but raised blood glucose or HbA1c by biochemical testing: fasting glucose ≥ 7.0 mmol/L or HbA1c ≥ 6.5% ($n = 505{,}000$; from 2020 to 2022)

[k]Age-standardized prevalence of overweight and obesity among individuals aged 18–84 years ($n = 2072$, from 2020 to 2022), according to WHO's BMI classification (i.e. overweight BMI ≥ 25.0 kg/m^2; obesity BMI ≥ 30.0 kg/m^2)

[l]Overall smoking prevalence in 2021

[m]Per capital gross domestic product in 2022 (100 CNY ≈ 112 Macanese Pataca as of January 7, 2024)

[n]Age-adjusted comparative diabetes prevalence (20–79 years old)

[o]See GBD compare for detail (2019, both sexes and age-standardized values): https://vizhub.healthdata.org/gbd-compare/

[p]See GBD compare for detail (2019, both sexes and age-standardized values, high body-mass index, BMI > 20–25 kg/m^2): https://vizhub.healthdata.org/gbd-compare/

(n = 645,903) in China, the age-adjusted prevalence of physical inactivity in Chinese adults increased from 18% in 2010 to 22% in 2018 [29]. This CVD risk factor, indeed, affects even more older adults for whom poor functional mobility and fear of fall further discourage physical activity. In the past two decades, a study identified a two–three folds increase in the time of watching television and a 24% reduction in exercise among the older Chinese individual. Given the increasing rates of urbanization and population ageing in China, the trends of increasing physical inactivity would be continued to threaten the cardiovascular health at the population level.

12.3.3 Smoking

Smoking is a significant risk factor of CVD, leading to atherosclerosis and an increased risk of coronary heart disease and stroke [30]. Despite governmental efforts to curb tobacco use, smoking prevalence remains high, particularly among men, with 64% of the male population are smokers and 2% among the women [31]. Several challenges, including high social acceptance of smoking, low awareness of the health risks, and the influence of the tobacco industry may explain such high smoking rate [32]. A territory-wide study, indeed, found that male in urban China starts smoking before aged 20 and was associated with a two-fold higher in ischemic heart disease and even mortality than the non-smoking counterpart [33].

12.3.4 Alcohol Consumption

Alcohol consumption, particularly heavy drinking, is a risk factor for CVD, contributing to hypertension, cardiomyopathy, and arrhythmias. The rapid economic growth in China leads to a drastic increase in alcohol consumption over the past decades. The WHO reported that the per capita alcohol consumption in China has increased significantly from 4.1 L in 2005 to 7.2 L of pure alcohol in 2016 (with an average daily intake of 27.9 g of pure alcohol per individual among drinkers) [34]. This rise has been particularly notable among men and younger age groups, reflecting changing social norms and increasing acceptance of drinking. In fact, accompanying China's documented surge in alcohol consumption is a noticeable shift in its drinking culture. This change indicates a burgeoning acceptance of alcohol consumption within contexts that were previously abstinent, such as work meetings [35]. In contemporary society, having drinks with work colleagues and clients is often viewed as crucial for career progression. Certain job postings even list a "high tolerance for alcohol" as a potential prerequisite for applicants [36]. Controlling this risk factor thereby needs to go beyond behavioural modification to influence the socio-cultural norm at the society level.

12.3.5 Psychosocial Stress

Rapid urbanization and the concomitant social change and economic transition also render psychological stress as a significant public health problem [37] which increases the risk of CVD in China [38–40]. An epidemiological study, involving a sample size of 32,552 participants, revealed that the prevalence of mental disorders (excluding dementia) in China is significant, with 17% of participants experienced some form of mental disorder at any point in their lives prior to the study [41]. Primary prevention of CVD needs to address the role adaptation and stress management of the population in China.

12.3.6 Environmental Factors

The environmental changes in China, notably air pollution and changes in temperature and humidity, along with rapid urbanization, present significant challenges for cardiovascular health. Air pollution is a significant environmental issue in China, primarily driven by industrial emissions, vehicle exhaust, and the burning of fossil fuels [42]. The main pollutants include particulate matter (e.g. PM2.5 and PM10), nitrogen oxides (NOx), sulphur dioxide (SO_2), and ozone (O_3) [43–45]. Studies have found a strong association between exposure to these pollutants and an increased risk of CVDs, including ischemic heart disease, stroke, and hypertension [43, 45, 46]. An interesting longitudinal cohort study (from year 2005–2017) found that those who were exposed to yearly average PM2.5 levels of 54 μg/m [3] or more were typically dwelling in urban areas with less physical activity (resulted from farming, etc.) than those exposed to a lower level of air pollution [43]. This implies the importance of considering the synergies between the territory-specific environmental and behavioural risk factors in CVD risk control.

12.4 Prevention and Management of CVD in China

To tackle the ever-escalating incidence and prevalence CVD, the Chinese Government has implemented various public health policies and initiatives to contain CVD through upstream health behaviour modification and risk factor control at primordial and primary prevention level, as well as improving the care of downstream management of CVD at secondary and tertiary level, and optimizing the health system policies to ensure proper medical treatment for the Chinese population.

12.4.1 Primordial and Primary CVD Prevention

The "Healthy China 2030" programme, launched by the Chinese government in 2016, signifies a national commitment to improve the health of its citizens by 2030. This initiative represents the country's first medium to long-term strategic plan specifically geared towards mitigating the risk factors implicated in non-communicable diseases including CVD (i.e. The Medium and Long-term Plan for Chronic Disease Prevention and Control (2017–2025)) [47, 48]. Noteworthy shift is embodied in this programme, transitioning from a focus on disease treatment to an emphasis on health promotion and management through avenues of education, policy reform, and environmental changes [47]. The government also promotes health education in schools, workplaces, and communities to raise awareness about the importance of a healthy diet, regular exercise, and the dangers of smoking and excessive alcohol consumption.

Promoting Nutritional Health

As part of ongoing efforts to monitor the health and nutrition status of its people, China has established a regular national nutrition survey. Since its inception, six rounds of this comprehensive survey have been conducted [49]. These surveys provide critical data to track the progress and effectiveness of health initiatives over time. The General Office of the State Council of the People's Republic of China introduced the National Nutrition Plan of Action (2017–2030) [50]. This strategic plan encompasses a variety of cross-disciplinary and cross-sector measures, all designed to improve the nutritional health of the Chinese population, including the development and implementation of guidelines for a balanced diet and for food companies to reduce the amount of salt, oil, and sugar in their products, and promoting nutritional education to improve dietary habits [51]. To address the urgent health concerns associated with unhealthy lifestyle, the Chinese Government initiated the "China Healthy Lifestyle for All" programme in 2007, with its day-to-day operation managed by the Chinese Center for Disease Control and Prevention (China CDC) [52] This initiative aimed to improve the public awareness on preventive health strategies, with particular emphasis on reducing the consumption of salt and oil [53]. A collaborative approach involving a diverse group of stakeholders was adopted to achieve the programme objectives. Health educational messages were disseminated via a wide range of media platforms, such as mass communication channels, academic programmes, outdoor advertisements, and printed materials. Apart from enhancing the public knowledge and awareness, the initiative also promoted the setup of healthier public policies, mobilization at the community level, peer-led education, and the establishment of environment conducive to health [53], under the supervision of the initiative of the National Health and Family Planning Commission, the Office of the National Patriotic Health Campaign Committee, and the China CDC [53].

Facilitating Physical Activity

The China's Government promotes physical activity through both hardware and software. In terms of hardware, much effort has been directed to increase the sports venues at the national level. In 2013, China carried out its Sixth National Sports Venues Census, which was the first of its kind carried out in 1974 [54, 55]. By the end of 2013, the density of these facilities stood at 12.45 venues per 10,000 residents, offering a per capita area of 1.46 m^2 [56]. Despite this growth, the availability of sports venues in China paled in comparison to countries like the United States and Japan [56]. Another drawback of this primary health initiative is about the accessibility of the sport venues. Over half of these venues (51.5%) are granted with full-time access, while 14.3% offered part-time access and 34.2% operated on a membership basis [56]. As for the software, territory-wide campaign is the core strategy. The Chinese Government has launched initiatives like the National Fitness Plan (2016–2020) [56], which sought to foster national fitness and physical health, aiming to increase the proportion of citizens regularly engaging in physical activity.

Tobacco Control

Though smoking is a highly prevalent public health problem in China, the Government in fact has ratified the Framework Convention on Tobacco Control of the World Health Organization as early as in 2005 [57]. To align with the declaration of The "Healthy China 2030" plan in reducing the adult smoking rate from 27.7% in 2015 to 20% by 2030, various measures have been implemented to reduce smoking and exposure to second-hand smoke through public smoking bans, restrictions on tobacco advertising, and increased taxes on tobacco products [58]. Territory-wide surveys were conducted to closely monitor the smoking rate in youth and second-hand smoking in a wide range of community facilities to inform policy making [59–61]. Efforts to protect people from second-hand smoke has led to the passing of 18 subnational legislations, but national laws have stalled [62]. The quality and accessibility of cessation services are being improved, and public awareness about the dangers of tobacco is being raised through media campaigns, despite the absence of pictorial health warnings. In 2014, the State Council released a national tobacco control guideline, the first of its kind, aiming to significantly curb tobacco consumption. The new regulations propose a smoking ban in all indoor and certain outdoor public places, a complete ban on tobacco advertising, large health warnings on tobacco packages, strict controls on selling tobacco to minors, and the promotion of smoke-free families [63]. The country is also attempting to enforce bans on tobacco advertising and promotion although legal loopholes and enforcement issues persist [64]. While cigarettes remain relatively affordable, there is recognition of the need to raise tobacco taxes in line with inflation and income.

Reduce Alcohol Consumption

As compared with tobacco cessation, the strategies for alcohol control are less obvious. On the other hand, tax reduction for alcohol in the past two decades triggered an increase in consumption [65]. The Health China 2030 initiative nevertheless advocates policies to restrict the sale of alcohol. However, these policies lack specificity, offering neither clear actions nor guidelines for consumption or restrictions on the alcohol industry [66].

Air Pollution

The Chinese Government launched an initiative—the Air Pollution Prevention and Control Action Plan (APPCAP), in 2013. This initiative represents China's first comprehensive and ambitious policy designed to mitigate ambient particulate matter with an aerodynamic diameter <2.5 μm (PM2.5), the major component of air pollutant contributing to adverse health outcomes [67]. The APPCAP comprises a series of regulatory mechanisms, including mandatory and fortified standards for enterprise air pollutant emission. It signifies a paradigm shift from total emission control to the enhancement of air quality. The policy also underscores the diversification of pollution control strategies and the optimization of pollution management approaches. A substantial investment of $270 billion was committed towards addressing the root cause of the pollution, which encompasses reducing coal dependency, regulating vehicle emissions, promoting the use of renewable energy, and upgrading emission standards enforcement [68]. Further, the APPCAP puts a strong emphasis on data transparency, advocating for the expansion of the air quality monitoring network and the enhancement of public data accessibility. Another significant feature of the policy is the transition from a singular territorial management approach to a combined territorial management and regional joint prevention and control strategy [69]. The implementation of the APPCAP has led to significant reductions in PM2.5 concentration and sulphur dioxide emissions, particularly in the pilot regions (e.g. Beijing-Tianjin-Hebei, Yangtze River Delta, Pearl River Delta, Central Liaoning, Shandong, and Wuhan).

12.4.2 Secondary and Tertiary CVD Prevention

To tackle the increasing prevalence of CVD, the management of CVD has advanced recently through introducing novel techniques for managing CVD. This section introduces the updated approach in managing CVD in China, highlighting recent advances in CVD management, the role of rehabilitation, and the potential contributions of traditional Chinese medicine. In response to the increased medical expenditure related to the advanced CVD management, the government's policies relating to reimbursement and health insurance are also discussed.

Coronary Artery Disease (CAD)

For managing stable CAD, the Chinese guidelines for percutaneous coronary intervention recommend patients who have prescribed optimal medical therapy but still present with ischemic symptoms to have revascularization therapy. Therefore, statistics from the annual report indicates that the number of cardiovascular interventional therapy is increasing steadily in China. With the increasing experience, the procedural mortality was low (i.e. 0.23% in 2017) and over 90% of the cases were adopted trans-radial approach. In addition, the experienced centres started to perform percutaneous coronary interventions on those patients with complicated lesions, such as patients with left main bifurcation disease, and chronic total occlusion [70, 71].

For managing patients with acute coronary syndrome, China has adopted a comprehensive approach to streamline the logistics of managing these patients in order to achieve timely diagnosis and initiation of reperfusion treatment. With the support of the National Health Commission, the first Chinese Chest Pain Centre was established in 2011, and the Chinese Society of Cardiology officially began to accredit chest pain centres in 2013 [72]. These centres compose healthcare professionals with different expertise, including the medial staff from the emergency medical system, emergency department, cardiology department, and the imaging department, which aims to optimize the diagnosis and treatment for patients with acute coronary syndrome and other acute cardiovascular diseases. The essential standard for accreditation is the centre should be equipped with the ability to perform emergency percutaneous coronary intervention around the clock. For patients with ST-segment elevation myocardial infarction (STEMI), the door-to-balloon time is expected to be 90 min for patients undergoing percutaneous coronary intervention [73]. Since then, many hospital-based chest pain centres were established throughout China. To standardize clinical practices and facilitate quality improvement, a nationwide quality improvement initiative named the National Chest Pain Centres Programme was launched in 2016, which aims to monitor and improve the quality of care for patients with acute chest pain. A large-scale study reviewed the data of patients with acute coronary syndrome from the Hospital Quality Monitoring System database of 746 hospitals, using propensity score matching to compare hospitals with and without chest pain centre accreditation during 2013 to 2016 and found that patients admitted to accredited chest pain centres had lower in-hospital mortality, shorter length of stay and more likely to receive percutaneous coronary intervention than those patients admitted to hospitals without accreditation [74].

Heart Failure

In recognizing the disparity in treatment of heart failure across hospitals in different regions of China, the China Heart Failure Registry was established to assess the management and outcomes of heart failure patients. The first stage of the results from 2012 to 2015 was published in 2017 [75], followed by the second stage from

2017 to 2020. According to the first stage registry data of 13,687 patients, the in-hospital mortality rate was 4.1%. The overall using rates of diuretics, angiotensin-converting enzyme inhibitors or angiotensin receptor blockers (ACEI/ARB), and β-blockers at admission ranged 25% to 30%, which was relatively low [75]. For those patients with heart failure with reduced ejection fraction (HFrEF), the use of ACEI/ARB, β-blocker, and mineralocorticoid receptor antagonist was 67.5%, 70.0%, and 74.1%, respectively [75]. The clinical outcomes of heart failure patients were improved according to the second stage of the registry data for 34,938 patients hospitalized during 2017–2020, the mortality rate was reduced to 2.8% [76]. Such an improvement should be related to the increased use of guideline-directed medical therapy. The second-stage registry data showed that 78.2% discharged alive patients were prescribed with diuretics, 78.7% patients with HFrEF were prescribed with renin-angiotensin system inhibitors, including ACEI, ARB, or ARNI [76], ARNI is the dual inhibitor of angiotensin II receptor and neprilysin, which has been approved by the China Food and Drug Administration in 2017 for the treatment of HFrEF. Moreover, device therapy with cardiac resynchronization therapy and implantable cardioverter defibrillator for heart failure patients is also increasing in China [71].

Arrhythmia

Bradycardia is a common heart rhythm disorder in China. According to the statistics of the online registration system of the National Heath Commission, a total of 99,306 pacemakers were implanted in 2021, a 15.2% increase as compared with 2020 [77]. The novel techniques of left bundle branch pacing and Hitchcock Purkinje system pacing are rapidly progressing in China. The technique of left bundle branch pacing was rapidly adopted in China. According to the database of the Chinese Society of Pacing and Electrophysiology, there were 5000 cases conduction system pacing performed in China, while 80% of these causes were left bundle branch pacing [78]. In addition, the implantable cardioverter defibrillator and cardiac resynchronization therapy have also been increasingly used in China for preventing sudden cardiac deaths in patients with CVD.

Atrial fibrillation affects 1.6% of Chinese aged 18 years or older [79], and it accounts for a quarter of the stroke in China. According to the Chinese atrial fibrillation Registration study included patients from 32 hospitals during 2011 to 2014, it showed that 36.5% and 28.5% of patients with CHA_2DS_2-VASc scores ≥2 and 1, respectively, were treated with oral anticoagulants, while 21.4% of the patients with 0 point were also prescribed with the anticoagulant [80]. Another study retrospectively reviewed 10,725 patients with AF at their first hospitalization during 2008 to 2018 in three large-scale hospitals and reported that 24.4% of patients were prescribed with anticoagulant at the time of admission [81]. Radiofrequency catheter ablation is extensively adopted as a treatment modality in China. The data from the National Arrhythmia Intervention Quality Control Centre indicated that the annual growth rates of this procedure increased from

13.2% to 17.5% from 2009 to 2021. The incidence of periprocedural ischemic stroke as low as 0.4% and that of intracranial haemorrhage stroke was 0.1% [82], which demonstrated the safety profile of the radiofrequency catheter ablation procedure performed in China.

Cardiac Rehabilitation

Cardiac rehabilitation has been well established in Western developed countries and being proved to be efficacious in reducing rehospitalization and mortality and improving health-related quality of life in patients with CAD. However, its development in China was until recent years. The number of cardiac rehabilitation centres was <10 in 2012, which increased to 500 in 2017 [71]. Despite such rapid growth in the number of cardiac rehabilitation centres in China, the service remains inadequate. A national survey involving 454 hospitals (51% of the largest level IIIA hospital) in China revealed that only 24% having an operational cardiac rehabilitation programme [83]. As a result, the density of cardiac rehabilitation programmes was found to be low, with only two programmes available per 100 million inhabitants [83]. Hospitals that had rehabilitation programmes were more likely to be university or government hospitals, have more inpatient cardiovascular beds, and provide secondary CVD prevention services [83]. Nevertheless, the participation rate of cardiac rehabilitation remains low, with approximately 5% of eligible for service enrolled [84]. The major barriers to participate in cardiac rehabilitation include regional disparities in availability, with rehabilitation programmes concentrated in urban areas while rural regions lack facilities and trained healthcare professionals, and patients' limited knowledge and awareness of the benefits of cardiac rehabilitation, leading to low referral and uptake rates [85]. In addition, patients face hurdles such as distance or transportation difficulties, high costs, time constraints, a preference for home-based exercise, and lack of social support [85].

Despite reforms, the concentration of health services in the public hospital and pharmaceutical sectors has hindered progress, leading to increased health and insurance costs [86]. The utilization of primary health facilities has decreased from 62% and 29% in 2009 to 54% and 18% in 2017 for outpatient and inpatient services, respectively [87], while hospitalization lengths have increased due to a shortage of long-term care facilities [88]. The high proportion of out-of-hospital deaths of CVD (e.g. 79% for coronary heart disease) suggests the need for improved out-of-hospital care, which might include community-based interventions to recognize and quickly respond to symptoms [11]. Consequently, urgent implementation of an integrated health and social care approach, particularly in community settings, is advocated to enhance affordability and quality of care for patients with CVD.

Efforts to mitigate these challenges are underway. Researchers in China are also exploring innovative models of cardiac rehabilitation to enhance accessibility. A home-based cardiac rehabilitation programme that utilizes telehealth services to deliver education, physical activity tracking, remote blood pressure and heart-rate monitoring, individualized exercise plans and lifestyle advice, and has proven to be effective, accessible, and easy to use [89]. Despite these promising developments, cardiac rehabilitation in China is still in its early stages, and much work is needed to improve its accessibility and utilization. Future research and policy should focus on addressing the barriers to cardiac rehabilitation, developing innovative delivery models, and educating patients and healthcare professionals about the importance and benefits of cardiac rehabilitation.

Traditional Chinese Medicine as CVD Treatment

While conventional medicine plays a crucial role in managing CVD, there is growing interest in the potential role of complementary and alternative medicine, especially traditional Chinese medicine (TCM), in the management of CVD [90]. TCM has evolved over 2000 years to be used in preventing and treating diseases in China. Substantial research has been conducted to examine the role of TCM in managing CVD risk factors [91]. Several TCM herbs (e.g. red sage root) have been investigated for their potential therapeutic benefits (e.g. angina symptoms) [92]. Some of these herbs and formulas have been found to have anti-inflammatory, anti-oxidant, and anti-atherosclerotic properties, and some may help in regulating blood pressure and lipid levels [91].

For the management of CVD, several TCM drugs have been tested in randomized controlled trials and reported favourable results regarding their efficacy and safety for CVD [92]. The Chinese clinical practice guidelines only recommend one TCM drug, which is Qiliqiangxin. It comprises extracts from 11 types of traditional Chinese herbs, is a patent drug approved by the China Food and Drug Administration for the treatment of heart failure. Basic research studies have shown that Qiliqiangxin is effective against cardiac remodelling and heart failure after ischemic and hypoxic injuries [93, 94]. Moreover, a multi-centre, randomized placebo-controlled study ($N = 512$) found that Qiliqiangxin is effective in reducing the plasma N-terminal pro-B-type natriuretic peptide (NT-proBNP) level during 12 weeks of treatment as compared with the placebo group. In addition, Qiliqiangxin demonstrated superior effects in New York Heart Association functional classification, left ventricular ejection fraction, 6-min walking distance, and quality of life in comparison with the heart failure patients in the placebo group [95]. However, the effects on long-term outcomes remain to be investigated.

For the management of acute myocardial infarction (AMI), the use of TCM is common in Western medicine hospitals. The data from a large representative sample of 162 Western medicine hospitals showed that nearly all of these hospitals used early intravenous TCM for management of AMI [96]. Salvia miltiorrhiza (danshen) was most commonly prescribed for one third (35.5%) of all patients admitted with AMI, despite no evidence of its benefit or harm being recorded [96]. There is an urgent need to conduct clinical studies to evaluate the efficacy and safety of TCM for treating CVD.

Health System Policies

The National Healthcare Security Administration (NHSA) of China was established in 2018 to oversee the country's health insurance system [97]. One of its responsibilities is managing the national formulary-the National Reimbursement Drug List (NRDL) [97]. This list illustrated the medications that are covered by the national health insurance system. These drugs have been evaluated and approved for reimbursement based on their effectiveness, safety, and cost-effectiveness. The list serves as a reference for healthcare providers for medication prescription and for patients' information on which medications are covered by their insurance. To ensure the NRDL remains relevant and up to date, the NHSA has implemented a dynamic adjustment mechanism.

In alignment with Healthy China 2030, the National Health Commission initiated two consecutive 3-year plans in 2015 to improve medical services, address healthcare bottlenecks, and enhance Internet-based medical services [98]. The Commission has issued a notice to further improve the appointment treatment system and strengthen the construction of smart hospitals, with three core aspects: (1) accelerate the establishment of an improved appointment treatment system to enhance the patient experience; (2) innovate and perfect the smart hospital system using technology for efficient, safer, and more personalized medical services; (3) promote the development of Internet diagnosis and treatment and Internet hospitals to relieve the pressure of offline diagnosis. These measures have been instrumental in managing the COVID-19 pandemic and meeting public medical needs [98].

12.5 Challenges and Opportunities in Tackling Cardiovascular Disease Burden

China's urbanization and lifestyle shifts have led to a surge in non-communicable diseases, notably CVD, driven by risk factors such as unhealthy diets, sedentariness, tobacco use, and harmful alcohol consumption. However, China's unique social and cultural practices offer an ample opportunity for promoting cardiovascular health.

Despite significant healthcare advancements, China still grapples with disparities in healthcare access and quality, particularly between urban and rural areas and among different socioeconomic groups. Enhancing primary healthcare services, especially in underserved regions, is vital for early CVD detection and management. Despite substantial investments in primary health care, gaps persist in quality and integrated service delivery. Addressing these challenges requires comprehensive strategies, including strengthening physician training, establishing performance accountability, integrating clinical care with basic public health services, and enhancing coordination between primary healthcare institutions and hospitals. Leveraging digital data and innovative technologies can modernize the primary healthcare system, improving disease surveillance and promoting patient self-management. Equipping primary healthcare workers with skills in CVD risk assessment and integrating CVD care into routine services can improve prevention and management.

The rising trend of integrating TCM with Western medicine for CVD management, driven by patient preferences, presents both challenges and opportunities. Developing suitable care models and ensuring safe practices require establishing guidelines for the combined use of TCM and Western therapies, training healthcare providers in both systems, and creating integrated clinics. Research into TCM mechanisms can uncover new therapeutic strategies. However, more high-quality research is needed on CVD prevention and management, including the efficacy of TCM and digital health rehabilitation programmes.

The widespread tradition of communal activities such as Tai Chi and dancing in parks not only encourages physical exercise but also fosters social engagement, which can be leveraged for further health promotion. These gatherings can serve as platforms for health education, screenings, and peer support initiatives. Moreover, the abundance of parks and public spaces presents prospects for organizing health events and facilitating outdoor exercises. Additionally, traditional dietary habits, rich in vegetables, grains, and lean proteins, can be promoted to encourage healthy eating, and the mind-body emphasis in practices like Tai Chi and Qigong contributes a holistic health approach to combining physical activity with stress reduction.

Patient education and empowerment is a key aspect of managing CVDs. Implementing educational programmes and providing resources can help patients make healthier lifestyle choices. Addressing the mental health-CVD connection is also essential, which involves screening for mental health conditions in CVD patients and integrating mental health care into primary health care. Investing in healthcare infrastructure in underserved areas can reduce access and quality disparities. Innovative solutions like mobile clinics or telemedicine can reach patients in remote areas. Public-private partnerships can also facilitate resource and knowledge exchange, leading to innovative local solutions.

The "Healthy China 2030" initiative emphasizes the significance of international cooperation in achieving its health objectives. Collaboration in disease surveillance and response, where partnerships with global organizations like the WHO can enhance China's capacity to handle disease prevention. In research and development, joint ventures with international counterparts can promote medical advances. Sharing knowledge and experiences in health policies and systems can lead to mutual growth and understanding. China is also expected to have an active presence in global health diplomacy, addressing worldwide health challenges and contributing to global health security. This can involve participation in international forums, contributing to international health funding mechanisms, and providing aid and assistance to other countries. The initiative also seeks to promote the understanding and use of TCM on a global scale. These forms of international cooperation can help China to achieve its health goals while also contributing to global health.

In summary, while the CVD burden in China is significant, there are considerable opportunities for innovation and improvement. By capitalizing on these opportunities, China can make substantial strides in preventing and managing CVDs, thereby enhancing population health and well-being.

References

1. Institute for Health Metrics and Evaluation. Global health data exchange, 2019. https://vizhub.healthdata.org/gbd-results/.
2. Disease, N. C. f. C. 中国心血管健康与疾病报告2022. 2022. https://www.nccd.org.cn/News/Columns/Index/1089.
3. Ma Q, et al. Temporal trend and attributable risk factors of stroke burden in China, 1990–2019: an analysis for the Global Burden of Disease Study 2019. Lancet Public Health. 2021;6:e897–906. https://doi.org/10.1016/S2468-2667(21)00228-0.
4. Yang G, et al. Rapid health transition in China, 1990–2010: findings from the Global Burden of Disease Study 2010. Lancet. 2013;381:1987–2015. https://doi.org/10.1016/S0140-6736(13)61097-1.
5. Roth GA, et al. Global burden of cardiovascular diseases and risk factors, 1990–2019: update from the GBD 2019 study. J Am Coll Cardiol. 2020;76:2982–3021. https://doi.org/10.1016/j.jacc.2020.11.010.
6. United Nations, D. o. E. a. S. A., Population division. World Population Prospects 2019, Volume II: demographic profiles; 2019. https://digitallibrary.un.org/record/3851011?ln=en.
7. United Nations. World population ageing 2019—highlights; 2019. https://www.un.org/en/development/desa/population/publications/pdf/ageing/WorldPopulationAgeing2019-Report.pdf.
8. Yan R, et al. Cardiovascular diseases and risk-factor burden in urban and rural communities in high-, middle-, and low-income regions of China: a large community-based epidemiological study. J Am Heart Assoc. 2017;6(2):e004445. https://doi.org/10.1161/JAHA.116.004445.
9. Chen H, et al. Geographic variations in in-hospital mortality and use of percutaneous coronary intervention following acute myocardial infarction in China: a nationwide cross-sectional analysis. J Am Heat Assoc. 2018;7:e008131. https://doi.org/10.1161/jaha.117.008131.
10. Wang W, et al. Prevalence, incidence, and mortality of stroke in China: results from a nationwide population-based survey of 480 687 adults. Circulation. 2017;135:759–71. https://doi.org/10.1161/CIRCULATIONAHA.116.025250.
11. Zhao D, Liu J, Wang M, Zhang X, Zhou M. Epidemiology of cardiovascular disease in China: current features and implications. Nat Rev Cardiol. 2019;16:203–12. https://doi.org/10.1038/s41569-018-0119-4.
12. Carney RM, Freedland KE. Depression and coronary heart disease. Nat Rev Cardiol. 2017;14:145–55. https://doi.org/10.1038/nrcardio.2016.181.
13. Chau JP, et al. Factors associated with post-stroke depression in Chinese stroke survivors. J Stroke Cerebrovasc Dis. 2021;30:106076.
14. Levine GN, et al. Psychological health, well-being, and the mind-heart-body connection: a scientific statement from the American Heart Association. Circulation. 2021;143:e763–83. https://doi.org/10.1161/CIR.0000000000000947.
15. Lichtman JH, et al. Depression as a risk factor for poor prognosis among patients with acute coronary syndrome: systematic review and recommendations. Circulation. 2014;129:1350–69. https://doi.org/10.1161/cir.0000000000000019.
16. Gheorghe A, et al. The economic burden of cardiovascular disease and hypertension in low- and middle-income countries: a systematic review. BMC Public Health. 2018;18:975. https://doi.org/10.1186/s12889-018-5806-x.
17. National Bureau of statistics of China. 2021.
18. Zhai F, et al. Dynamics of the Chinese diet and the role of urbanicity, 1991–2011. Obes Rev. 2014;15:16–26.
19. Shao Q, Tao R, Luca MM. The effect of urbanization on health care expenditure: evidence from China. Front Public Health. 2022;10:850872. https://doi.org/10.3389/fpubh.2022.850872.
20. Murray C. Health effects of dietary risks in 195 countries, 1990–2017: a systematic analysis for the Global Burden of Disease Study. Lancet. 2019;393:1958–72.

21. Chen Y, et al. The prevalence and increasing trends of overweight, general obesity, and abdominal obesity among Chinese adults: a repeated cross-sectional study. BMC Public Health. 2019;19:1293.
22. Popkin BM, Adair LS, Ng SW. Global nutrition transition and the pandemic of obesity in developing countries. Nutr Rev. 2012;70:3–21. https://doi.org/10.1111/j.1753-4887.2011.00456.x.
23. Min J, Xue H, Wang VHC, Li M, Wang Y. Are single children more likely to be overweight or obese than those with siblings? The influence of China's one-child policy on childhood obesity. Prev Med. 2017;103:8–13. https://doi.org/10.1016/j.ypmed.2017.07.018.
24. Hipgrave DB, Chang S, Li X, Wu Y. Salt and sodium intake in China. JAMA. 2016;315:703–5. https://doi.org/10.1001/jama.2015.15816.
25. Tian X, Wang H. Projecting national-level prevalence of general obesity and abdominal obesity among Chinese adults with aging effects. Front Endocrinol (Lausanne). 2022;13:849392. https://doi.org/10.3389/fendo.2022.849392.
26. Organization, W. H. Guideline: Sodium intake for adults and children. World Health Organization; 2012.
27. Ng SW, Howard AG, Wang H, Su C, Zhang B. The physical activity transition among adults in China: 1991–2011. Obes Rev. 2014;15:27–36.
28. Ng SW, Norton EC, Popkin BM. Why have physical activity levels declined among Chinese adults? Findings from the 1991–2006 China Health and Nutrition Surveys. Soc Sci Med. 2009;68(7):1305–14.
29. Zhang M, et al. Trends in insufficient physical activity among adults in China 2010–18: a population-based study. Int J Behav Nutr Phys Act. 2023;20:87. https://doi.org/10.1186/s12966-023-01470-w.
30. World Health Organization. The fatal link between tobacco and cardiovascular diseases in the WHO South-East Asia Region —May 2018. 2018. https://www.who.int/publications/i/item/the-fatal-link-between-tobacco-and-cardiovascular-diseases-in-the-who-south-east-asia-region%2D%2D-may-2018.
31. Wang X, et al. Regional differences in adults' smoking pattern: findings from China Kadoorie Biobank study in 10 areas in China. Zhonghua liu Xing Bing xue za zhi= Zhonghua Liuxingbingxue Zazhi. 2015;36:1200–4.
32. Yang G, Wang Y, Wu Y, Yang J, Wan X. The road to effective tobacco control in China. Lancet. 2015;385:1019–28. https://doi.org/10.1016/s0140-6736(15)60174-x.
33. Chen Z, et al. Contrasting male and female trends in tobacco-attributed mortality in China: evidence from successive nationwide prospective cohort studies. Lancet. 2015;386:1447–56. https://doi.org/10.1016/S0140-6736(15)00340-2.
34. Organization, W. H. Global status report on alcohol and health 2018. World Health Organization; 2019.
35. Manthey J, et al. Global alcohol exposure between 1990 and 2017 and forecasts until 2030: a modelling study. Lancet. 2019;393:2493–502. https://doi.org/10.1016/S0140-6736(18)32744-2.
36. Jiang H, Room R, Hao W. Alcohol and related health issues in China: action needed. Lancet Glob Health. 2015;3:e190–1. https://doi.org/10.1016/S2214-109X(15)70017-3.
37. Wu Y, Benjamin EJ, MacMahon S. Prevention and control of cardiovascular disease in the rapidly changing economy of China. Circulation. 2016;133:2545–60. https://doi.org/10.1161/CIRCULATIONAHA.115.008728.
38. Wu M, et al. Association of anxiety with cardiovascular disease in a Chinese cohort of 0.5 million adults. J Affect Disord. 2022;315:291–6. https://doi.org/10.1016/j.jad.2022.08.008.
39. Zhou L, Ma X, Wang W. Inflammation and coronary heart disease risk in patients with depression in China mainland: a cross-sectional study. Neuropsychiatr Dis Treat. 2020;16:81–6. https://doi.org/10.2147/NDT.S216389.
40. Wang Z, et al. Status of hypertension in China: results from the China hypertension survey, 2012–2015. Circulation. 2018;137:2344–56. https://doi.org/10.1161/CIRCULATIONAHA.117.032380.

41. Huang Y, et al. Prevalence of mental disorders in China: a cross-sectional epidemiological study. Lancet Psychiatry. 2019;6:211–24.
42. Liu Y, et al. Association between solid fuel use and nonfatal cardiovascular disease among middle-aged and older adults: findings from The China Health and Retirement Longitudinal Study (CHARLS). Sci Total Environ. 2023;856:159035. https://doi.org/10.1016/j.scitotenv.2022.159035.
43. Sun D, et al. Long-term exposure to ambient PM(2.5), active commuting, and farming activity and cardiovascular disease risk in adults in China: a prospective cohort study. Lancet Planet Health. 2023;7:e304–12. https://doi.org/10.1016/S2542-5196(23)00047-5.
44. Wei J, et al. Ground-level gaseous pollutants (NO2, SO2, and CO) in China: daily seamless mapping and spatiotemporal variations. Atmos Chem Phys. 2023;23(2):1511–32. https://doi.org/10.5194/acp-23-1511-2023.
45. Huang W, et al. Individual and joint associations of long-term exposure to air pollutants and cardiopulmonary mortality: a 22-year cohort study in Northern China. The Lancet Regional Health—Western Pacific. 2023;36 https://doi.org/10.1016/j.lanwpc.2023.100776.
46. Lv S, et al. Long-term effects of particulate matter on incident cardiovascular diseases in middle-aged and elder adults: the CHARLS cohort study. Ecotoxicol Environ Saf. 2023;262:115181. https://doi.org/10.1016/j.ecoenv.2023.115181.
47. Tan X, Zhang Y, Shao H. Healthy China 2030, a breakthrough for improving health. Glob Health Promot. 2019;26:96–9. https://doi.org/10.1177/1757975917743533.
48. The State Council, T. P. s. R. o. C. General Office of the State Council of the People's Republic of China on the issuance of China's Medium- and long-term plan for chronic diseases control and prevention (2017–2025); 2017. http://www.gov.cn/zhengce/content/2017–02/14/content_5167886.htm.
49. Yu D, et al. China nutrition and health surveys (1982–2017). China CDC Wkly. 2021;3:193–5. https://doi.org/10.46234/ccdcw2021.058.
50. Cai L, et al. China is implementing the national nutrition plan of action. Front Nutr. 2022;9:983484. https://doi.org/10.3389/fnut.2022.983484.
51. Gao C, Xu J, Liu Y, Yang Y. Nutrition Policy and Healthy China 2030 building. Eur J Clin Nutr. 2021;75:238–46. https://doi.org/10.1038/s41430-020-00765-6.
52. Wu F, et al. Evaluation of China healthy lifestyle for all interventions based on RE-AIM framework—China, 2007–2020. China CDC Wkly. 2022;4:403–6. https://doi.org/10.46234/ccdcw2022.091.
53. Zhang J, et al. Multilevel evaluation of 'China Healthy Lifestyles for All', a nationwide initiative to promote lower intakes of salt and edible oil. Prev Med. 2014;67:210–5. https://doi.org/10.1016/j.ypmed.2014.07.019.
54. China, G. A. o. S. o. 第一次全国体育场地普查历史回顾. 2004. https://www.sport.gov.cn/n4/n15291/n15294/c964610/content.html.
55. China, G. A. o. S. o. 第六次全国体育场地普查数据公报. 2014. https://www.sport.gov.cn/gdnps/content.jsp?id=567393.
56. Wang K, Wang X. Providing sports venues on mainland China: implications for promoting leisure-time physical activity and national fitness policies. Int J Env Res Public Health. 2020;17 https://doi.org/10.3390/ijerph17145136.
57. Lin H, et al. National survey of smoking cessation provision in China. Tob Induc Dis. 2019;17:25. https://doi.org/10.18332/tid/104726.
58. Ministry of Health of the People's Republic of China. Smoke-free healthcare facility standards, Ministry of Health of the People's Republic of China. Beijing, China; 2008. http://www.jsxyfy.com/_s2/2012/0815/c15a2088/page.psp [Chinese]
59. Tobacco use among youth. a cross country comparison. Tob Control. 2002;11:252–70. https://doi.org/10.1136/tc.11.3.252.
60. Warren CW, Jones NR, Asma S. Global youth tobacco surveillance, 2000–2007; 2008.
61. Mei X, Chen G, Zhong Q, Li YL, Li JL. Secondhand smoke exposure among never-smoking adolescents in Wuhan. China Sci Rep. 2022;12:14209. https://doi.org/10.1038/s41598-022-18612-y.

62. Song P, Jin C, Tang W. New medical education reform in China: towards healthy China 2030. Biosci Trends. 2017;11:366–9. https://doi.org/10.5582/bst.2017.01198.
63. Anon. A step change for tobacco control in China? Lancet. 2014;384:2000. https://doi.org/10.1016/S0140-6736(14)62319-9.
64. Lv J, et al. Implementation of the WHO framework convention on tobacco control in mainland China. Tob Control. 2011;20:309–14.
65. Ministry of Finance of the People's Republic of China. Notice of Ministry of Finance and State Administration of Taxation on adjusting and perfecting consumption tax policies (no. 33). Beijing: Ministry of Finance; 2006. (in Chinese)
66. The State Council, T. P. s. R. o. C. The Central Committee of the Communist Party of China and the State Council issued the "Healthy China 2030" Planning Outline; 2016. https://www.gov.cn/zhengce/2016-10/25/content_5124174.htm.
67. Yu Y, Dai C, Wei Y, Ren H, Zhou J. Air pollution prevention and control action plan substantially reduced PM2.5 concentration in China. Energy Econ. 2022;113:106206. https://doi.org/10.1016/j.eneco.2022.106206.
68. Greenstone M, Schwarz P. Is China winning its war on pollution? 2018. https://aqli.epic.uchicago.edu/wp-content/uploads/2018/08/China-Report.pdf.
69. Wang J, Lei Y, Ning M. Implementation of action plan for air pollution control: declaration of war on PM2.5. Environ Prot. 2014;42(6):28–31. (in Chinese)
70. Chinese Society of Cardiology, Chinese Medical Association. Chinese guideline for percutaneous coronary intervention in patients with left main bifurcation disease. Cardiol Discov. 2022;2:134–44.
71. Bei Y, Shi C, Zhang Z, Xiao J. Advance for cardiovascular health in China. J Cardiovasc Transl Res. 2019;12:165–70.
72. Zhang Y, Huo Y. Current status and future prospects of chest pain center accreditation in China. Chin J Fronts Med Sci. 2017;9:1–5.
73. Zhang Y, Huo Y. Early reperfusion strategy for acute myocardial infarction: a need for clinical implementation. J Zhejiang Univ Sci B. 2011;12:629–32.
74. Sun P, et al. Effectiveness of chest pain centre accreditation on the management of acute coronary syndrome: a retrospective study using a national database. BMJ Qual Safety. 2021;30:867–75.
75. Zhang Y, et al. Contemporary epidemiology, management, and outcomes of patients hospitalized for heart failure in China: results from the China heart failure (China-HF) registry. J Card Fail. 2017;23:868–75.
76. Zhang Y, et al. Clinical performance and quality measures for heart failure management in China: the China-Heart Failure registry study. ESC Heart Failure. 2023;10:342–52.
77. Report TW, Health OC, China DI, Hu SS. Report on Cardiovascular Health and Diseases in China 2022: an updated summary. Biomed Environ Sci. 2023;36:669–701.
78. Zhang S, Zhou X, Gold MR. Left bundle branch pacing: JACC review topic of the week. J Am Coll Cardiol. 2019;74:3039–49.
79. Shi S, et al. Prevalence and risk of atrial fibrillation in China: a national cross-sectional epidemiological study. Lancet Regional Health–Western Pacific. 2022;23
80. Chang S-S, et al. Current status and time trends of oral anticoagulation use among Chinese patients with nonvalvular atrial fibrillation: the Chinese atrial fibrillation registry study. Stroke. 2016;47:1803–10.
81. Bai Y, et al. Prevalence of recommended anticoagulation by guidelines preadmission and its impact on the incidence of acute myocardial infarction (AMI) and in-hospital outcomes after AMI in atrial fibrillation patients. J Thromb Thrombolysis. 2022;54:91–6.
82. Liu Y, et al. Incidence and outcomes of cerebrovascular events complicating catheter ablation for atrial fibrillation. EP Europace. 2015;18:1357–65.
83. Zhang Z, et al. Availability and characteristics of cardiac rehabilitation programmes in China. Heart Asia. 2016;8:9–12. https://doi.org/10.1136/heartasia-2016-010758.

84. Liu X, et al. Translation, cross-cultural adaptation, and psychometric validation of the Chinese/Mandarin Cardiac Rehabilitation Barriers Scale (CRBS-C/M). Rehabil Res Pract. 2021;2021:5511426. https://doi.org/10.1155/2021/5511426.
85. Xie X, Chen Q, Liu H. Barriers to hospital-based phase 2 cardiac rehabilitation among patients with coronary heart disease in China: a mixed-methods study. BMC Nurs. 2022;21:333. https://doi.org/10.1186/s12912-022-01115-6.
86. Fang EF, et al. A research agenda for ageing in China in the 21st century (2nd edition): focusing on basic and translational research, long-term care, policy and social networks. Ageing Res Rev. 2020;64:101174. https://doi.org/10.1016/j.arr.2020.101174.
87. Meng Q, Mills A, Wang L, Han Q. What can we learn from China's health system reform? BMJ. 2019;365:l2349. https://doi.org/10.1136/bmj.l2349.
88. Organization, W. H. China country assessment report on ageing and health; 2015.
89. Dorje T, et al. Smartphone and social media-based cardiac rehabilitation and secondary prevention in China (SMART-CR/SP): a parallel-group, single-blind, randomised controlled trial. Lancet Digit Health. 2019;1:e363–74. https://doi.org/10.1016/S2589-7500(19)30151-7.
90. Guo L, et al. A multi-center, randomized, double-blind, placebo-parallel controlled trial for the efficacy and safety of shenfuqiangxin pills in the treatment of chronic heart failure (Heart-Kidney yang deficiency syndrome). Medicine (Baltimore). 2020;99:e20271. https://doi.org/10.1097/MD.0000000000020271.
91. Jiang Y, et al. Effect of traditional Chinese medicine on the cardiovascular diseases. Front Pharmacol. 2022;13:806300. https://doi.org/10.3389/fphar.2022.806300.
92. Hao P, et al. Traditional Chinese medicine for cardiovascular disease: evidence and potential mechanisms. J Am Coll Cardiol. 2017;69:2952–66. https://doi.org/10.1016/j.jacc.2017.04.041.
93. Tao L, et al. Traditional Chinese Medication Qiliqiangxin attenuates cardiac remodeling after acute myocardial infarction in mice. Sci Rep. 2015;5:8374.
94. Li X, et al. Traditional Chinese medicine as a therapeutic option for cardiac fibrosis: pharmacology and mechanisms. Biomed Pharmacother. 2021;142:111979.
95. Li X, et al. A multicenter, randomized, double-blind, parallel-group, placebo-controlled study of the effects of qiliqiangxin capsules in patients with chronic heart failure. J Am Coll Cardiol. 2013;62:1065–72.
96. Spatz ES, et al. Traditional Chinese medicine for acute myocardial infarction in western medicine hospitals in China. Circ Cardiovasc Qual Outcomes. 2018;11:e004190.
97. Wang W, et al. Use of real world data to improve drug coverage decisions in China. BMJ. 2023;381:e068911. https://doi.org/10.1136/bmj-2021-068911.
98. Administration, C. M. Interpretation of the "Notice on further improving the system of appointment diagnosis and treatment and strengthening the construction of smart hospitals"; 2020. http://www.nhc.gov.cn/yzygj/s3594r/202005/4fede18997024bd28912aef7f68b370b.shtml.
99. National Bureau of Statistics of China. China Statistical Yearbook; 2023. https://www.stats.gov.cn/sj/ndsj/2023/indexeh.htm.
100. Li Y, et al. Prevalence of diabetes recorded in mainland China using 2018 diagnostic criteria from the American Diabetes Association: national cross sectional study. BMJ. 2020;369
101. Zhang L, et al. Prevalence of overweight and obesity in China: results from a cross-sectional study of 441 thousand adults, 2012–2015. Obes Res Clin Pract. 2020;14:119–26.
102. Wang M, et al. Trends in smoking prevalence and implication for chronic diseases in China: serial national cross-sectional surveys from 2003 to 2013. Lancet Respir Med. 2019;7:35–45.
103. Liu S, et al. Burden of cardiovascular diseases in China, 1990–2016: findings from the 2016 Global Burden of Disease Study. JAMA Cardiol. 2019;4:342–52. https://doi.org/10.1001/jamacardio.2019.0295.
104. Centre for Health Protection, Department of Health & the Government of the Hong Kong Special Administrative Region. Report of Population Health Survey 2020–22 (Part II); 2023. https://www.chp.gov.hk/en/features/37474.html.

105. Health Bureau & Hong Kong. Vibrant, healthy and tobacco-free Hong Kong; 2021. https://www.healthbureau.gov.hk/tobacco-free/assets/pdf/consultation_document_en.pdf.
106. Ke L, et al. Prevalence, awareness, treatment and control of hypertension in Macau: results from a cross-sectional epidemiological study in Macau, China. Am J Hypertens. 2015;28:159–65. https://doi.org/10.1093/ajh/hpu121.
107. International Diabetes Federation. Diabetes in Western Pacific—2021; 2021. https://diabetesatlas.org/idfawp/resource-files/2021/11/IDF-Atlas-Factsheet-2021_WP.pdf.
108. Yang Q, et al. The multimorbidity and lifestyle correlates in Chinese population residing in Macau: findings from a community-based needs assessment study. Healthcare (Basel). 2023;11 https://doi.org/10.3390/healthcare11131906.
109. Lisaon Office of the Cenral People's Government in the Macao S.A.R. Macao Has achieved remarkable results in controlling tobacco hazards. 2021. http://www.zlb.gov.cn/2021-06/07/c_1211190256.htm.
110. Cheng HM, Lin HJ, Wang TD, Chen CH. Asian management of hypertension: current status, home blood pressure, and specific concerns in Taiwan. J Clin Hypertens (Greenwich). 2020;22:511–4. https://doi.org/10.1111/jch.13747.

Further Reading

Cheng HM, Lin HJ, Wang TD, Chen CH. Asian management of hypertension: current status, home blood pressure, and specific concerns in Taiwan. J Clin Hypertens (Greenwich). 2020;22(3):511–4. https://doi.org/10.1111/jch.13747.

Centre for Health Protection, Department of Health, the Government of the Hong Kong Special Administrative Region. Report of Population Health Survey 2020–22 (Part II). 2023. Accessed January 7, 2024. https://www.chp.gov.hk/en/features/37474.html.

Health Bureau, Hong Kong. Vibrant, healthy and tobacco-free Hong Kong. 2021. January 7, 2014. https://www.healthbureau.gov.hk/tobacco-free/assets/pdf/consultation_document_en.pdf.

International Diabetes Federation. Diabetes in Western Pacific—2021. 2021. Accessed January 11, 2024. https://diabetesatlas.org/idfawp/resource-files/2021/11/IDF-Atlas-Factsheet-2021_WP.pdf.

Ke L, Ho J, Feng J, et al. Prevalence, awareness, treatment and control of hypertension in Macau: results from a cross-sectional epidemiological study in Macau, China. Am J Hypertens. 2015;28(2):159–65. https://doi.org/10.1093/ajh/hpu121.

Liu S, Li Y, Zeng X, et al. Burden of cardiovascular diseases in China, 1990–2016: findings from the 2016 global burden of disease study. JAMA Cardiol. 2019;4(4):342–52. https://doi.org/10.1001/jamacardio.2019.0295.

Li Y, Teng D, Shi X, et al. Prevalence of diabetes recorded in mainland China using 2018 diagnostic criteria from the American Diabetes Association: national cross sectional study. BMJ. 2020, 369:m997.

Lisaon Office of the Cenral People's Government in the Macao S.A.R. Macao Has achieved remarkable results in controlling tobacco hazards. 2021. Accessed January 11, 2024. http://www.zlb.gov.cn/2021-06/07/c_1211190256.htm

National Bureau of Statistics of China. China statistical yearbook. 2023. Jan 5, 2024. https://www.stats.gov.cn/sj/ndsj/2023/indexeh.htm.

Wang Z, Chen Z, Zhang L, et al. Status of hypertension in China: results from the China Hypertension Survey, 2012–2015. Circulation. 2018;137(22):2344–56. https://doi.org/10.1161/circulationaha.117.032380.

Wang M, Luo X, Xu S, et al. Trends in smoking prevalence and implication for chronic diseases in China: serial national cross-sectional surveys from 2003 to 2013. Lancet Respir Med. 2019;7(1):35–45.

Yang Q, Zhang Q, Ngai FW, et al. The multimorbidity and lifestyle correlates in Chinese population residing in Macau: findings from a community-based needs assessment study. Healthcare (Basel). 2023;11(13) https://doi.org/10.3390/healthcare11131906.
Zhang L, Wang Z, Wang X, et al. Prevalence of overweight and obesity in China: results from a cross-sectional study of 441 thousand adults, 2012–2015. Obes Res Clin Pract. 2020;14(2):119–26.

Chapter 13
WHO, UN, and Sustainable Development Goals: Effective Measures for Prevention of CVD in Developing Economies

Kathryn A. Taubert and Sidney C. Smith, Jr.

13.1 Introduction

Cardiovascular disease (CVD) is the number one cause of death globally. According to the World Health Organization (WHO), CVD is responsible for taking almost 18 million lives per year. Over 80% of these CVD deaths are attributed to myocardial infarction and stroke, with one-third of these deaths occurring prematurely (under 70 years of age) [1].

From the beginning of the twentieth century through 1970, there was a sharp rise in deaths attributable to heart disease in the United States and other similar high-income countries (HICs) [2, 3], as shown in Fig. 13.1 [3] CVD, especially heart attack, previously was referred to as a "disease of affluence" or "rich man's disease" because of its prevalence and mortality in higher income countries. In lower income countries, the leading causes of death in much of the twentieth century were still infectious diseases and malnutrition. However, CVD mortality began rising in low- and middle-income countries (LMICs) in the latter part of the twentieth century, and by the first decade of the twenty-first century, CVD was the largest cause of death in all the developing regions of the world with the exception of Sub-Saharan Africa where it is the leading cause of death in those over the age of 45 [4]. Although the mortality from CVD began to plateau and, in some instances, decline in HICs from the latter part of the twentieth century, it remains the number one cause of mortality globally [5].

K. A. Taubert (✉)
Department of Physiology, UT Southwestern Medical Center, Dallas, TX, USA
e-mail: kathryn.taubert@utsouthwestern.edu

S. C. Smith, Jr.
Division of Cardiology, Department of Medicine and Cardiology, School of Medicine, University of North Carolina, Chapel Hill, NC, USA
e-mail: scs@med.unc.edu

T. Romero et al. (eds.), *Global Challenges in Cardiovascular Prevention in Populations with Low Socioeconomic Status*,
https://doi.org/10.1007/978-3-031-79051-5_13

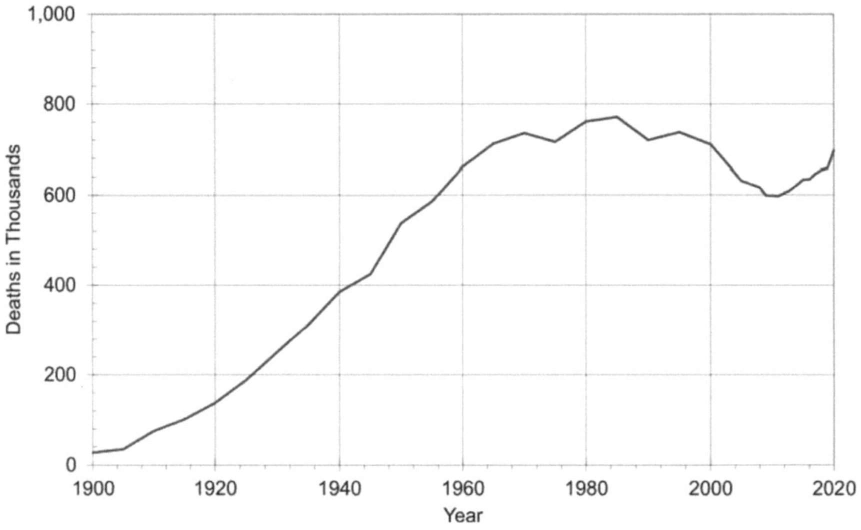

Fig. 13.1 Deaths attributable to CVD, United States, 1900–2020. CVD (*ICD-10* codes I00–I99) does not include congenital heart disease. Before 1933, data are for a death registration area, not the entire United States. Reprinted with permission Circulation.2023;147:e93–e621©2023 American Heart Association, Inc. (From Ref. [3])

Cardiovascular disease is in the category of noncommunicable diseases (NCDs; also referred to as chronic diseases). Other major NCDs include cancer, diabetes, and chronic lung disease, and these four are collectively responsible for 74% of all deaths worldwide. Over 75% of all NCD deaths, and 86% of the 17 million people who died prematurely (before reaching 70 years of age) *occur in low- and middle-income countries* [6]**.** The burden of NCDs, led by CVD, was the greatest in LMICs and many of those countries were ill-equipped to deal with this epidemic.

This chapter describes the initiatives from the World Health Organization (WHO) and the United Nations (UN) that have been designed to tackle this epidemic of noncommunicable diseases, especially CVD. The focus will be on the WHO plan for prevention and control of NCDs and the UN plan to "ensure healthy lives and promote well-being" which is a part of the UN Sustainable Development Goals. A helpful glossary of organizations, programs, and their targets/goals, is included in Table 13.1.

Table 13.1 Organizations and initiatives

United Nations (UN)—an intergovernmental organization whose stated central mission is the maintenance of international peace and security
World Health Organization (WHO)—the directing and coordinating authority on international health within the UN system. Their mission is to promote health, keep the world safe and serve the vulnerable, with measurable impact for people at country level
Member State—countries that are members of the UN or WHO are referred to as Member States
UN General Assembly (UNGA)—is the main policy-making body of the UN. It is made up of the 193 UN Member States
World Health Assembly (WHA)—is the main decision-making body of the WHO. It is made up of 194 WHO Member States
UN High-Level Meeting (UN HLM)—convened by the UN General Assembly (UNGA) ad attended by all Member States. the meeting is dedicated to a specialized topic and is taken in exceptional circumstances through a UN resolution and vote, with the purpose of reaching agreement on cooperation measures and solutions on important global issues
Global Action Plan (GAP)—the WHO Global Action Plan for the Prevention and Control of NCDs was endorsed by the WHA in 2013. The GAP provides Member States, international partners and WHO with a road map and menu of policy options which, when implemented collectively, will contribute to progress on 9 global NCD targets to be attained in 2025, including a 25% relative reduction in premature mortality from NCDs by 2025. It is often referred to as **"25 by 25" or "25 × 25". Note:** In 2019 the World Health Assembly extended the WHO Global Action Plan for the Prevention and Control of NCDs end date to 2030
NCD Global Monitoring Framework—allows monitoring of trends and assessment of progress made in the implementation of national strategies and plans on NCDs. The Global Monitoring Framework for the Prevention and Control of NCDs comprises 9 global targets and 25 indicators (adopted at the 2013 WHA meeting)
SDGs—Sustainable Development Goals—a product of the United Nations, the 17 goals are a call for action by all countries – richer and poorer—to promote prosperity while protecting the planet. They recognize that ending poverty must go hand-in-hand with strategies that build economic growth and address a range of social needs including education, health, social protection, and job opportunities, while tackling climate change and environmental protection

13.2 WHO and NCDs

The WHO is the directing and coordinating authority on international health within the United Nations (UN) system, and their mission is to promote health, keep the world safe and serve the vulnerable, with measurable impact for people at country level. Virtually every country in the world is a Member State of the WHO. The WHO collaborates closely with the UN system on certain public health issues.

As the implications of the rising global morbidity and mortality caused by CVD and other NCDs became more evident, WHO began having increased dialogue about what could be done. The World Health Assembly (WHA) is the decision-making body of the WHO. The WHA meets yearly, and a report from the WHO Director-General on NCD prevention and control [7] was an agenda item at the1998 WHA meeting [8]. After discussion concerning the growing impact of NCDs on the health of global populations, the WHA endorsed a plan for the integrated prevention and control of NCDs and urged Member States to collaborate with WHO in developing a global strategy for the prevention and control of NCDs, thus ensued several years of their meetings with Member States, nongovernmental organizations, and other relevant stakeholders. In 2000, the "Global Strategy for the Prevention and Control of Noncommunicable Diseases" report from the WHO Director-General was released to the WHA [9]. The report noted that the rapid rise of NCDs represented one of the major health challenges to global development in the coming twenty-first century. This challenge threatens economic and social development as well as the lives and health of millions of people. It was further noted that there was a vast body of knowledge and experience related to prevention of NCDs and immense opportunities for their control by global action [9]. Action plans were further revised in the WHO publication "2008–2013 Action Plan for the Global Strategy for the Prevention and Control of Noncommunicable Diseases" presented to the 2008 WHA meeting [10]. Mindful of the rapidly increasing burden of NCDs in LMICs and its serious implications for poverty reduction and economic development, it was agreed that the UN General Assembly would hold a dedicated High-Level Meeting (HLM) on the topic of NCDs in September 2011. A UN HLM is only convened through a UN resolution and vote, and the HLM on NCDs was only the second one on a health topic ever convened (the 2001 HLM on HIV/AIDS being the first).

The President of the UN General Assembly submitted a draft resolution titled "Political Declaration of the High-level Meeting of the General Assembly on the Prevention and Control of Non-communicable Diseases" and the resolution was adopted [11]. Following the Political Declaration adoption, WHO in consultation with other groups was tasked with developing a Global Monitoring Framework to enable global tracking of progress in preventing and controlling major NCDs, specifically calling out CVD, cancer, chronic lung diseases and diabetes, and key risk factors. The completed framework contains 9 global targets and 25 indicators. the nine areas that were selected to be targets (Fig. 13.2) include one mortality target, six risk factor targets (harmful use of alcohol, physical inactivity, dietary sodium intake, tobacco use, raised blood pressure, and diabetes and obesity), and two national systems targets (drug therapy to prevent heart attacks and strokes, and essential NCD medicines and technologies to treat major NCDs). The targets were stated to be both attainable and significant, and when achieved will represent major accomplishments in NCDs and risk factor reductions. The global NCD targets are intended to focus global attention on NCDs and would represent a major contribution to NCD prevention and control.

The overarching mortality target of "25% relative reduction in risk of premature mortality from cardiovascular diseases, cancer, diabetes, or chronic respiratory diseases" was adopted at the 2012 WHA meeting and the rest of the framework was adopted by Member States during the 2013 WHA meeting. As situations are not the same in all countries, Member States were encouraged to consider the development of national NCD targets and indicators building on the global framework. The nine voluntary global targets are aimed at combating global mortality from the four main NCDs, accelerating action against the leading risk factors for NCDs and

Fig. 13.2 Set of nine Global Noncommunicable Disease (NCD) goals targets for 2025. (From Ref. [12])

strengthening national health system responses. The targets are discussed in detail in the WHO document "Noncommunicable Diseases Global Monitoring Framework: Indicator Definitions and Specifications" [12]. As shown in the framework document, each target has one or more indicators. For example, for the target "A 25% relative reduction in the prevalence of raised blood pressure or contain the prevalence of raised blood pressure, according to national circumstances," the indicator is "Age-standardized prevalence of raised blood pressure among persons aged 18+ years (defined as systolic blood pressure 140 mmHg or greater and/or diastolic blood pressure 90 mmHg or greater) and mean systolic blood pressure." The purpose of the global monitoring framework is to provide detailed guidance to Member States so they can correctly measure each of the 25 indicators and monitor their progress over time. For each indicator, a complete definition is provided, appropriate data sources are identified and a detailed calculation, where applicable, is provided. All of the goals/targets have a "reach-by" date of 2025 with a baseline of

2010. The plan is often referred to as "25 by 25" or "25 × 25," reflecting a commitment to a 25 % reduction in NCD mortality by the year 2025. To monitor progress of the 25 by 25 targets and goals, follow-up HLMs on NCDs were scheduled for 2014, 2018, and 2025 (discussed later in this chapter).

13.3 UN and NCDs

As the WHO was finalizing the targets and indicators for the NCD framework, the UN had begun discussing the Sustainable Development Goals (SDGs), which would be the successor to the Millennium Development Goals. An Open Working Group was established to develop a set of Sustainable Development Goals for consideration and appropriate action by the General Assembly at its 68th session in 2013 [13]. Ultimately, the 2030 Agenda for Sustainable Development [14] was adopted by all UN Member States in 2015 and provides a shared blueprint for peace and prosperity for people and the planet, now and into the future.

At its heart are a group of goals which are an urgent call for action by all countries—developed and developing—in a global partnership. They recognize that ending poverty and other deprivations must go hand-in-hand with strategies that improve health and education, reduce inequality, and spur economic growth—and be sure no one is left behind. The 2030 Agenda went into effect in January 2016 with an "end-by" date of 2030. The agenda sets out 17 wide-ranging and ambitious goals (Table 13.2), and a total of 169 targets in support of these goals [15]. All of the goals have indicators by which progress can be measured. The 2030 Agenda for Sustainable Development recognized NCDs as a major challenge for sustainable development [16]. As part of the 2030 Agenda, Heads of State and governments committed to develop ambitious national responses to address NCDs, and this is reflected in Goal 3, which is to "ensure healthy lives and promote well-being for all at all ages." It is often referred to as the "health goal."

Thirteen targets are listed for Goal 3 [17] (Table 13.3), and target 3.4 states "By 2030, reduce by one-third premature mortality from noncommunicable diseases through prevention and treatment and promote mental health and well-being." This is an extrapolation of the WHO's reduction of premature mortality goal one-fourth (25%) in the 25 by 25 NCD framework but extended to 2030—hence the one-third (33%) reduction in premature mortality in the SDGs. After release of the NCD goals/targets, mental health was added, and this is reflected in the SDGs. Indicator 3.4.1 (for NCDs) is the "mortality rate attributed to cardiovascular disease, cancer, diabetes or chronic respiratory disease" in the UN SDG framework. This is defined as the percent of 30-year-old-people who would die before their 70th birthday from cardiovascular disease, cancer, diabetes, or chronic respiratory disease, assuming that they would experience current mortality rates at every age and would not die from any other cause of death (e.g., injuries or HIV/AIDS) [18].

There are other targets under Goal 3 that have implications for NCDs. These include:

Table 13.2 United Nations sustainable development goals to achieve by 2030. (From Ref. [15])

Goal 1.	End poverty in all its forms everywhere
Goal 2.	End hunger, achieve food security and improved nutrition and promote sustainable agriculture
Goal 3.	Ensure healthy lives and promote well-being for all at all ages
Goal 4.	Ensure inclusive and equitable quality education and promote lifelong learning opportunities for all
Goal 5.	Achieve gender equality and empower all women and girls
Goal 6.	Ensure availability and sustainable management of water and sanitation for all
Goal 7.	Ensure access to affordable, reliable, sustainable, and modern energy for all
Goal 8.	Promote sustained, inclusive, and sustainable economic growth, full and productive employment, and decent work for all
Goal 9.	Build resilient infrastructure, promote inclusive and sustainable industrialization and foster innovation
Goal 10.	Reduce inequality within and among countries
Goal 11.	Make cities and human settlements inclusive, safe, resilient, and sustainable
Goal 12.	Ensure sustainable consumption and production patterns
Goal 13.	Take urgent action to combat climate change and its impacts[a]
Goal 14.	Conserve and sustainably use the oceans, seas, and marine resources for sustainable development
Goal 15.	Protect, restore, and promote sustainable use of terrestrial ecosystems, sustainably manage forests, combat desertification, and halt and reverse land degradation and halt biodiversity loss
Goal 16.	Promote peaceful and inclusive societies for sustainable development, provide access to justice for all and build effective, accountable, and inclusive institutions at all levels
Goal 17.	Strengthen the means of implementation and revitalize the global partnership for sustainable development

[a]Acknowledging that the UN Framework Convention on Climate Change is the primary international, intergovernmental forum for negotiating the global response to climate change

- 3.5 (harmful use of alcohol)
- 3.8 (universal health coverage; UHC)
- 3.9 (air pollution)
- 3.a (tobacco)
- 3.b (support the research and development of vaccines and medicines)
- 3.c (health workforce)
- 3.d (early warning, risk reduction, and management of national and global health risks)

3.9 is called out here because although not included as one of the risk factors in 25 by 25, it is an established risk factor for CVD. 3.d is included because according to the political declaration of the third HLM on the prevention and control of NCDs, the COVID-19 pandemic poses further challenges for creating and maintaining healthy environments and people living with NCDs are at increased risk of severe illness and death due to COVID-19. NCDs need to be part of the national preparedness and response plans. The economic effects of the pandemic are likely to have a

Table 13.3 Targets for UN sustainable development goal 3. (From Ref. [17])

• 3.1 By 2030, reduce the global maternal mortality ratio to <70 per 100,000 live birth
• 3.2 By 2030, end preventable deaths of newborns and children under 5 years of age, with all countries aiming to reduce neonatal mortality to at least as low as 12 per 1000 live births and under-5 mortality to at least as low as 25 per 1000 live births
• 3.3 By 2030, end the epidemics of AIDS, tuberculosis, malaria and neglected tropical diseases and combat hepatitis, water-borne diseases, and other communicable diseases
• **3.4** By 2030, reduce by one third premature mortality from non-communicable diseases through prevention and treatment and promote mental health and well-being
• **3.5** Strengthen the prevention and treatment of substance abuse, including narcotic drug abuse and harmful use of alcohol
• 3.6 By 2020, halve the number of global deaths and injuries from road traffic accidents
• 3.7 By 2030, ensure universal access to sexual and reproductive health-care services, including for family planning, information and education, and the integration of reproductive health into national strategies and programs
• **3.8** Achieve universal health coverage, including financial risk protection, access to quality essential health-care services and access to safe, effective, quality, and affordable essential medicines and vaccines for all
• **3.9** By 2030, substantially reduce the number of deaths and illnesses from hazardous chemicals and air, water and soil pollution and contamination
• **3.a** Strengthen the implementation of the World Health Organization Framework Convention on Tobacco Control in all countries, as appropriate
• **3.b** Support the research and development of vaccines and medicines for the communicable and noncommunicable diseases that primarily affect developing countries, provide access to affordable essential medicines and vaccines, in accordance with the Doha Declaration on the TRIPS Agreement and Public Health, which affirms the right of developing countries to use to the full the provisions in the Agreement on Trade-Related Aspects of Intellectual Property Rights regarding flexibilities to protect public health, and, in particular, provide access to medicines for all
• **3.c** Substantially increase health financing and the recruitment, development, training, and retention of the health workforce in developing countries, especially in least developed countries and small island developing States
• **3.d** Strengthen the capacity of all countries, in particular developing countries, for early warning, risk reduction and management of national and global health risks

long-term impact on NCD prevention and control [17]. More information about SDG Goal 3 is available on the UN website [17].

13.4 On the Way to 2025 and 2030—Interim Program Reviews

In 2018, a report on the progress regarding NCDs was distributed to the UN General Assembly from Heads of State and Government and representatives of States and Governments [19]. Among many comments, it was recognized that action to realize the commitments made for the prevention and control of noncommunicable diseases is inadequate, that the level of progress and investment to date is insufficient to meet target 3.4 of the SDGs, and that the world has yet to fulfill its promise of implementing, at all levels, measures to reduce the risk of premature death and disability from noncommunicable diseases. It was acknowledged that the progress achieved by some countries in the implementation of their commitments made in 2011 and 2014 for the prevention and control of four major noncommunicable diseases, namely, CVD, diabetes, cancer, and chronic respiratory diseases, by reducing their main common risk factors, namely, tobacco use, harmful use of alcohol, unhealthy diets, and physical inactivity, and by addressing the underlying social, economic, and environmental determinants of noncommunicable diseases and the impact of economic, commercial, and market factors, as well as by improving disease management to reduce morbidity, disability, and mortality. Additionally, it was recognized that many countries still face significant challenges in the implementation of their commitments and remain deeply concerned that the burden of noncommunicable diseases continues to rise disproportionately in developing countries and that every year 15 million people between the ages of 30 and 69 die from noncommunicable diseases and that 86 % of these premature deaths occur in developing countries. The report included a commitment from these Heads of State and Government and representatives of States and Governments to increase their efforts and listed several actions that could be implemented [19].

Every year in July, governments join businesses, civil society, thought leaders and influencers at the UN High-Level Political Forum on Sustainable Development to review progress and accelerate global efforts to deliver meaningful progress on the 2030 Agenda for Sustainable Development and its 17 Sustainable Development Goals. Specific goals are reviewed at each meeting [20].

From the various follow-up meetings and other reports, it has become clear that the NCD goals were not on track to achieve their 2025 targets. Progress slowed down even more with the onset of COVID-19.

In 2019, the World Health Assembly extended the WHO Global Action Plan for the Prevention and Control of NCDs 2013–2020 to 2030 and called for the development of an Implementation Roadmap for 2023 to 2030 to accelerate progress on preventing and controlling NCDs. This was detailed in a 2021 WHO discussion paper "Development of an Implementation Roadmap 2023–2030 for the Global Action Plan for the Prevention and Control of NCDs 2013–2030" [21]. Considering the relatively slow progress in the achievement of the 9 NCD targets, the WHA has requested WHO to develop an implementation roadmap to support the implementation of the extended NCD GAP in countries. In line with the extension of the NCD GAP to 2030, the NCD Global Monitoring Framework targets are also extended to 2030. Changes have been made in several of the original 9 voluntary 25 by 25 NCD targets due to the end-date extension to 2030 (or other reasons). Specifically, there are changes in the mortality target as well as the alcohol, physical inactivity, sodium, tobacco, and blood pressure targets. These changes that were made are shown in Table 13.4 [21].

To assess national-level responses to NCDs, WHO has implemented NCD country capacity surveys periodically since 2001. Since the first survey round, the NCD Country Capacity Survey has been conducted a further seven times, most recently

Table 13.4 NCD global monitoring framework indicating target metric changes due to end-date extension from 2025 to 2030. (From Ref. [21])

Premature mortality from NCDs	A 25% relative reduction in the overall mortality from cardiovascular diseases (CVD), cancer, diabetes, or chronic respiratory diseases	Unconditional probability of dying between ages of 30 and 70 from CVD, cancer, diabetes or chronic respiratory diseases	Target extended to **a one third relative reduction in the overall mortality from CVD, cancer, diabetes, or chronic respiratory diseases. This** target **is adapted as per the SDG target** on NCDs and with **2015 as the baseline** and an extrapolation of the 25% relative reduction to 2030, making it 33.3%
Harmful use of alcohol	At least 10% relative reduction in the harmful use of alcohol, as appropriate, within the national context	Total (recorded and unrecorded) alcohol per capita (aged 15+ years old) consumption within a calendar year in liters of pure alcohol, as appropriate, within the national context	Target extended to a **20% relative reduction in harmful use of alcohol.** The proposed revision of the target is under the draft action plan on alcohol that will be considered by EB 150 and WHA75
Physical inactivity	A 10% relative reduction in prevalence of insufficient physical activity	Age-standardized prevalence of insufficiently physically active persons aged 18+ years (defined as <150 min of moderate-intensity activity per week, or equivalent)	Target extended to a **15% relative reduction in prevalence of insufficient physical activity** as part of the Global Action Plan on Physical Activity adopted by MS at WHA May 2018
Salt/sodium intake	A 30% relative reduction in mean population intake of salt/sodium	Age-standardized mean population intake of salt (sodium chloride) per day in grams in persons aged 18+ years	Target extended to a **40% relative reduction in mean population intake of salt/ sodium**
Tobacco use	A 30% relative reduction in prevalence of current tobacco use	Age-standardized prevalence of current tobacco use among persons aged 18+ years	Target extended to a **40% relative reduction in prevalence of current tobacco use**
Raised blood pressure (BP)	A 25% relative reduction in the prevalence of raised BP or contain the prevalence of raised BP, according to national circumstances	Age-standardized prevalence of raised BP among people aged 18+ years (defined as systolic BP140 mmHg or greater and/or diastolic BP 90 mmHg or greater) and mean systolic blood pressure	Target extended to a **33% relative reduction in the prevalence of raised blood pressure**

Note: No changes were made to the diabetes and obesity target or to the two national systems response targets in 2021. The surveys are completed by the NCD focal point within each country's ministry of health or similar agency, and the countries are asked to report on a number of topics relating to NCDs. The resulting report is titled "Assessing national capacity for the prevention and control of noncommunicable diseases: report of the 2021 global survey" [22]. Results are reported by WHO region and by the World Bank Income Group for the following topics:

- aspects of NCD infrastructure
- plans, policies, and strategies
- surveillance
- health systems capacity
- NCD-related disruptions during the COVID-19 pandemic

In April 2022, an International Strategic Dialogue on NCDs and the SDGs was held in Accra, Ghana, hosted by the Government of Ghana, Government of Norway, and the WHO [23]. It is now recognized that insufficient global action on NCDs, combined with the COVID-19 pandemic, are creating the very real possibility that SDG targets 3.4 and 3.8 will not be met. Just 14 countries are on track to achieve SDG target 3.4 to reduce by one-third the premature mortality of NCDs through prevention and treatment and promote mental health and well-being by 2030.

The International Strategic Dialogue seeks to:

- Raise the priority accorded to the prevention and control of NCDs within the national SDG response in low- and middle-income countries
- Bring together national and international actors and partners to share knowledge and ideas with key stakeholders on what would it take globally for low- and middle-income countries to achieve SDG 3 on health, with a particular focus on SDG 3.4 (NCDs) and SDG 3.8 (UHC) targets
- Raise the political visibility of Heads of State and Government who are providing a strategic leadership role in the prevention and control of NCDs to a global level

The dialogue will launch:

- An International NCD Compact 2022–2030 to accelerate the progress towards the NCD and SDG targets [24]
- An (informal) International Group of Heads of State and Government on the Prevention and Control of NCDs (NCD Presidential Group) that will meet annually during the high-level general debate of the UNGA from 2022 towards 2025

13.5 What Can Be Done to Reach the 25 by 25 NCD Goals and the SDG Goal 3?

It is clear that failing to meet the 25 by 25 NCD goals would jeopardize success for SDG 3.4. There is also the socioeconomic impact. As pointed out on the WHO website, "Poverty is closely linked with NCDs and the rapid rise in NCDs is predicted to impede poverty reduction initiatives in low-income countries, particularly by increasing household costs associated with health care. Vulnerable and socially disadvantaged people get sicker and die sooner than people of higher social positions, especially because they are at greater risk of being exposed to harmful products, such as tobacco, or unhealthy dietary practices, and have limited access to health services. In low-resource settings, healthcare costs for NCDs quickly drain household resources. The exorbitant costs of NCDs, including treatment, which is often lengthy and expensive, combined with loss of income, force millions of people into poverty annually and stifle development" [25].

There have been many suggestions and recommendations by WHO, UN, and associated agencies as well as from NGOs, global health experts, and others. Some groups weighed in on strategies before or shortly after the Global Monitoring Framework for NCD was being populated with constructing goals and targets. For instance, a study by Sacco and colleagues [26] titled "The Heart of 25 by 25: Achieving the Goal of Reducing Global and Regional Premature Deaths from Cardiovascular Diseases and Stroke—A Modeling Study from the American Heart Association and World Heart Federation concluded that "Aggressive strategies to achieve multiple WHO targets, especially for raised blood pressure and tobacco control, will be required to meet the 25 by 25 overall goal. Success is possible if the individual WHO targets are met, and healthcare systems are strengthened. Achieving these goals can be accomplished only if countries and regions set priorities, implement cost-effective population-wide strategies, and collaborate in public-private partnerships across multiple sectors."

In an article by Sridhar and colleagues, regarding the (then) upcoming HLM, they listed five critical elements Member States should address to hopefully make the new measurable goals and means of building accountability may be within reach [27]. These are briefly summarized as:

- meeting should spotlight the true scale of morbidity and mortality caused by NCDs and the economic consequences for households, health systems and national economies
- governments should commit to developing national NCD plans
- identify/create feasible financial avenues
- governments commit to strengthening national regulation of NCD risk factors
- incentives and mechanisms put in place to encourage cross-sectoral action and coordination

A publication by Thakur and colleagues covers the progress and challenges in achieving NCD targets for the sustainable development goals [28]. They give an overview of the status of the NCDs and SDGs, NCD targets within the SDGs, and progress and challenges affecting NCD targets of the SDGs. They conclude with key recommendations to achieve the NCD targets of the SDGs (summarized briefly here):

- Continue the dialogue from the three UN high-level meetings within global governing bodies

- Increase funding at national, regional, and international levels to invest in health systems, services, and workforce development. Funding should be guided by "best buy" interventions
- Design and scale-up solutions for high risk, resource-limited, and marginalized populations
- Create a unified national response to align and coordinate various stakeholders
- Strengthen early detection and monitoring for NCDs with consistent follow-up

A commentary written by a group of experts from the World Heart Federation titled "Accelerated reduction in global cardiovascular disease is essential to achieve the Sustainable Development Goals" stated that governments, with the support of all stakeholders, will need to do as follows [29]:

- Continue efforts to improve data on CVD and associated risk factors, particularly in low-income and middle-income countries, where information gaps exist.
- Ensure that their healthcare expenditure as a percentage of gross domestic product is at least 5%, in line with recommendations from the WHO.
- Implement policies to combat CVD, guided by the burden of disease and risk factors, and ensure that their implementation is adequately resourced and monitored for progress.

In 2022, the NCD Countdown 2030 collaborators published a health policy paper "NCD Countdown 2030: efficient pathways and strategic investments to accelerate progress towards the Sustainable Development Goal target 3.4 in low-income and middle-income countries" [30]. In this paper, the authors synthesized the evidence related to interventions that can reduce premature mortality from the major NCDs over the next decade and that are feasible to implement in countries at all levels of income. They stated that their recommendations are intended as generic guidance to help 123 low-income and middle-income countries meet SDG target 3.4. They concluded that "This Health Policy lays out an ambitious but pragmatic approach to helping LMICs get back on track towards achieving SDG target 3.4 in the wake of the COVID-19 pandemic. Focusing on a relatively small number of highly cost-effective NCD interventions to scale up fits with the progressive universalist approach to UHC."

Common barriers to success that are often mentioned at the national or subnational level include lack of money, lack of time, lack of champions at country level, healthcare provider inertia, patient inertia, government inertia—and, in the years we are living in, COVID-19.

13.6 Universal Health Coverage

Another issue vital to the success of the NCD Global Monitoring Framework and SDG 3.4 is UHC. According to the WHO, UHC means that all people have access to the full range of quality health services they need, when and where they need them, without financial hardship. It covers the full continuum of essential health services, from health promotion to prevention, treatment, rehabilitation, and palliative care. To deliver on this promise, countries need to have strong, efficient, and equitable health systems that are rooted in the communities they serve. Primary health care is the most effective and cost-efficient way to get there.

UHC is an issue discussed at both the WHO and the UN. In fact, the UN convened a High-Level Meeting on UHC which was held in September 2019 [31]. World leaders endorsed the most ambitious and comprehensive political declaration on health in history. However, post-meeting global monitoring reports on UHC indicate progress is not on track, and the COVID-19 pandemic has brought the world further away from the targets set by the political declaration, which included (1) progressively covering 1 billion additional people, with a view of covering all people by 2030; and (2) stopping the rise and reversing the trend of catastrophic out-of-pocket health expenditure and eliminate impoverishment due to health-related expenses by 2030.

In September 2023 at the second UN General Assembly High-Level Meeting on UHC, world leaders approved a new political declaration titled "Universal Health Coverage: expanding our ambition for health and well-being in a post-COVID world" [32]. The declaration contained 107 action points and is hailed as a vital catalyst for the international community to take big and bold actions and mobilize the necessary political commitments and financial investments to attain the UHC target of the SDGs by 2030. World leaders committed to redouble efforts towards UHC by 2030 [33].

Just ahead of this 2023 high-level meeting, the WHO and the World Bank released a jointly published comprehensive "Tracking Universal Health Coverage 2023 Global Monitoring Report," revealing an alarming stagnation in the progress towards providing people everywhere with quality, affordable, and accessible health care [34]. It is widely recognized that achieving universal health coverage by 2030 is crucial for fulfilling the promise of the 2030 Agenda for Sustainable Development and realizing the fundamental human right to health. Unfortunately, the report shows that based on the latest available evidence, more than half of the world's population is still not covered by essential health services. Additionally, two billion people face severe financial hardship when paying out-of-pocket for the services and products they needed. The report also found that, over the past two decades, less than a third of countries have improved health service coverage and reduced catastrophic out-of-pocket health spending. The UHC target measures the ability of countries to ensure that everyone receives the health care they need, when and where they need it, without facing financial hardship. It covers the full continuum of key services from health promotion to prevention, protection, treatment, rehabilitation, and palliative care. Alarmingly, global progress towards UHC has been largely stagnating since 2015, before stalling in 2019 [35]. Another high-level meeting on UHC is scheduled for 2027.

13.7 Available Resources

Many of the documents cited in this chapter can provide guidance to individuals or groups at the country level, whether they are policymakers, public health officials, advocates, or healthcare workers (especially those in primary healthcare clinics). For those working on the "frontline" of patient care (e.g., physicians, nurses, other trained healthcare professionals, and case managers), there are also tools available that can help. For example, the WHO HEARTS package can be quite useful [36]. The HEARTS technical package for CVD management in primary care provides a strategic approach to improving CV health in countries. It contains modules on healthy-lifestyle counseling, evidence-based treatment protocols, access to essential medicines and technology, risk-based CVD management, team-based care, and systems for monitoring. There is also an implementation guide as well as a tool for the development of a consensus protocol for the treatment of hypertension. The HEARTS package can be adapted for country or regional needs and supports ministries of health to strengthen CVD management in primary healthcare settings. The HEARTS modules are intended for use by policymakers and program managers at different levels within ministries of health, and within resource-limited settings, who can influence CVD primary care delivery. HEARTS is discussed in more detail in the hypertension chapter.

The WHO also maintains an essential medicines list which is intended as a guide for countries or regional authorities to adopt or adapt in accordance with local priorities and treatment guidelines [37]. Additionally, there is the list of WHO "NCD best buys" evidence-based, cost-effective treatments, and interventions to prevent and control NCDs. The list was most recently updated in 2023 [38].

The World Heart Federation (WHF) is another good source of materials. WHF is the organization representing the CVD community in Official Relations with the WHO. WHF addresses the determinants of CVD and mobilizes the global community through roadmaps, roundtables, and advocacy. Their global CVD roadmaps are particularly helpful. In 2014, the WHF launched an initiative to develop a series of Global Roadmaps, with the aim of identifying potential roadblocks on the pathway to effective prevention, detection, and management of CVD, along with evidence-based solutions to overcome them.

The CVD roadmaps have become the cornerstone of WHF activities as resources for implementation to guide initiatives to support heart health globally, translating science into policy and influencing agencies, governments, and policymakers alike. With this framework, countries can develop or update national NCD programs aligned with the WHO Global Action Plan for the Prevention and Control of NCDs. The overall aim is to drive efforts within national agendas to meet the ambitious target set out in the UN Sustainable Development Goals: a one-third reduction in premature mortality caused by NCDs (including CVD) by 2030.

There are roadmaps on the following topics:

- Atrial fibrillation
- Chagas disease

- Cholesterol
- CVD in people with diabetes
- Digital health in cardiology
- Heart failure
- Hypertension
- Rheumatic heart disease
- Secondary prevention of CVD
- Tobacco control

All of the roadmaps are published in a scientific journal and are also available through the WHF website at https://world-heart-federation.org/cvd-roadmaps/

13.8 Latest Snapshot of Where We Are

In 2023, the WHO Director-General presented a "Political declaration of the third high-level meeting of the General Assembly on the prevention and control of non-communicable diseases, and mental health" to the WHO Executive Board [39]. This report was submitted by the Director-General pursuant to the request in decision WHA72(11) (year 2019) "to consolidate reporting on the progress achieved in the prevention and control of noncommunicable diseases and the promotion of mental health with an annual report to be submitted to the Health Assembly through the Executive Board, from 2021 to 2031, annexing reports on implementation of relevant resolutions, action plans and strategies, in line with existing reporting mandates and timelines." The report presented an overview of the progress achieved in the prevention and control of NCDs, the promotion of mental health and well-being, and the treatment and care of mental health conditions.

The section of the report titled "Where we are today" says the following: "Global attention and national action on NCDs over the past two decades have been insufficient to reduce their burden against the nine voluntary targets of the global action plan and target 3.4 of the Sustainable Development Goals (by 2030 reduce by one-third premature mortality from NCDs through prevention and treatment and promote mental health and well-being). No country is on track to achieve all nine voluntary global targets for 2025 set by the Health Assembly in 2013 against a baseline of 2010. The failure of health system capacity to keep up with the needs for preventing and controlling NCDs is reflected in the lack of progress for NCDs of the universal health coverage service coverage index. The pandemic of coronavirus disease (COVID-19) has highlighted the urgent need to strengthen health systems through a radical reorientation towards primary health care as the foundation for progress towards universal health coverage, as well as to ensure health security and achieve health and well-being for all. The prevention and control of NCDs and the promotion, protection, and care of mental health are integral to this reorientation."

Another section says "The data broadly show that countries with policy, legislative and regulatory measures, including fiscal measures, for the prevention and control of NCDs, as well as strong and inclusive health systems, have had the best outcomes against NCDs. In those countries, people living with and affected by NCDs are more likely to have access to effective services, including protection against NCD risk factors, detection of hypertension and diabetes, treatment of NCDs, and consistent, high-quality follow-up and care."

The report goes on to say, however, that new data from WHO show that the NCD *targets are not just aspirational but achievable.* The data broadly show that countries with policy, legislative and regulatory measures, including fiscal measures, for the prevention and control of NCDs, as well as strong and inclusive health systems, have had the best outcomes against NCDs. In those countries, people living with and affected by NCDs are more likely to have access to effective services, including protection against NCD risk factors, detection of hypertension and diabetes, treatment of NCDs, and consistent, high-quality follow-up and care.

Glossary

Global action plan Provides Member States, international partners, and WHO with a road map and menu of policy options which, when implemented collectively, will contribute to progress on nine global NCD targets to be attained in 2025 (later extended to 2030).

Sustainable development Development that meets the needs of the present without compromising the ability of future generations to meet their own needs.

Universal health coverage This means that all people have access to the full range of quality health services they need, when and where they need them, without financial hardship.

References

1. World Health Organization. https://www.who.int/health-topics/cardiovascular-diseases#tab=tab_1 (accessed 26 January 2024).
2. Dalen JE, Alpert JS, Goldberg RJ, Weinstein RS. The epidemic of the 20th century: coronary heart disease. Am J Med. 2014;127:807–12.
3. Tsao CW, Aday AW, Almarzooq ZI, Anderson CAM, Arora P, Avery CL, et al. Heart Disease and Stroke Statistics—2023 Update: a report from the American Heart Association. Circulation. 2023;147:e93–e621. https://doi.org/10.1161/CIR.0000000000001123.
4. Gaziano TA, Bitton A, Anand S, Abrahams-Gessel S, Murphy A. Growing epidemic of coronary heart disease in low- and middle-income countries. Curr Probl Cardiol. 2010;35(2):72–115. https://doi.org/10.1016/j.cpcardiol.2009.10.002.
5. Roth GA, Forouzanfar MH, Moran AE, Barber R, Nguyen G, Feigin VL, et al. Demographic and epidemiologic drivers of global cardiovascular mortality. N Engl J Med. 2015;372:1333–41. https://doi.org/10.1056/NEJMoa1406656.
6. World Health Organization. https://www.who.int/news-room/fact-sheets/detail/noncommunicable-diseases (accessed 23 January 2024).

7. World Health Organization. https://apps.who.int/gb/ebwha/pdf_files/EB101/pdfangl/ang14.pdf (accessed 28 January 2024).
8. World Health Organization. https://iris.who.int/bitstream/handle/10665/258896/WHA51-1998-REC-1-eng.pdf#page=36 (accessed 3 January 2024).
9. World Health Organization. https://apps.who.int/gb/archive/pdf_files/WHA53/ea14.pdf?ua=1 (accessed 09 January 2024).
10. World Health Organization. https://www.who.int/publications/i/item/9789241597418 (accessed 09 January 2024).
11. United Nations. https://documents-dds-ny.un.org/doc/UNDOC/LTD/N11/497/77/PDF/N1149777.pdf?OpenElement (accessed 22 December 2023).
12. World Health Organization. Noncommunicable diseases global monitoring framework: indicator definitions and specifications. https://www.who.int/publications/m/item/noncommunicable-diseases-global-monitoring-framework-indicator-definitions-and-specifications (accessed 22 December 2023).
13. United Nations General Assembly. Outcome document–open working group on sustainable development goals, July 2014. https://sustainabledevelopment.un.org/focussdgs.html (accessed 03 January 2024).
14. Political declaration of the third high-level meeting of the General Assembly on the prevention and control of noncommunicable diseases. Presented to the EB Jan 2022. https://apps.who.int/gb/ebwha/pdf_files/EB152/B152_6-en.pdf (accessed 03 January 2024).
15. United Nations. Transforming our world: the 2030 Agenda for Sustainable Development. https://sdgs.un.org/2030agenda (accessed 08 January 2024).
16. United Nations. https://www.un.org/en/development/desa/population/migration/generalassembly/docs/globalcompact/A_RES_70_1_E.pdf (accessed 03 January 2024).
17. United Nations. https://www.un.org/sustainabledevelopment/health/ (accessed 26 January 2024).
18. Sustainable Development Goals (an official website of the US Government) https://sdg.data.gov/3-4-1/ (accessed 26 January 2024).
19. United Nations General Assembly. Resolution adopted by the General Assembly on 10 October 2018 A/res/73/2 downloaded from UN digital library https://digitallibrary.un.org/record/1648984?ln=en#record-files-collapse-header (accessed 26 January 2024).
20. United Nations. Monitoring and progress. https://www.un.org/sustainabledevelopment/monitoring-and-progress-hlpf/ (accessed 26 January 2024).
21. World Health Organization. https://cdn.who.int/media/docs/default-source/documents/health-topics/non-communicable-diseases/eb150%2D%2D-who-discussion-paper-on-ncd-roadmap-development-(20-aug-2021)%2D%2D-for-web.pdf?sfvrsn=58b8c366_17&download=true (accessed 12 January 2024).
22. World Health Organization. Assessing national capacity for the prevention and control of noncommunicable diseases: report of the 2021 global survey. Geneva: World Health Organization; 2023. Licence: CC BY-NC-SA 3.0 IGO
23. World Health Organization. https://www.who.int/news-room/events/detail/2022/04/12/default-calendar/international-strategic-dialogue-on-noncommunicable-diseases-and-the-sustainable-development-goals (accessed 26 January 2024).
24. World Health Organization. https://www.who.int/initiatives/global-noncommunicable-diseases-compact-2020-2030 (accessed 26 January 2024).
25. World Health Organization. Noncommunicable diseases fact sheet. https://www.who.int/news-room/fact-sheets/detail/noncommunicable-diseases (accessed 22 December 2023).
26. Sacco RL, Roth GA, Reddy KS, Arnett DK, Bonita R, Gaziano TA, et al. The heart of 25 by 25: achieving the goal of reducing global and regional premature deaths from cardiovascular diseases and stroke: a modeling study from the American Heart Association and World Heart Federation. Circulation. 2016;133(23):e674–90.
27. Sridhar D, Morrison JS, Piot P. Expectations for the United Nations high-level meeting on noncommunicable diseases. Bull World Health Organ. 2011;89(7):471. https://doi.org/10.2471/BLT.11.089292.

28. Thakur SJ, Nangia R, Singh S. Progress and challenges in achieving noncommunicable diseases targets for the sustainable development goals. FASEB BioAdv. 2021;3:563–8. https://doi.org/10.1096/fba.2020-00117.
29. Pineiro DJ, Codato E, Mwangi J, Eisele J-L, Narula J. Accelerated reduction in global cardiovascular disease is essential to achieve the sustainable development goals. Nat Rev Cardiol. 2023;20:577–87. https://doi.org/10.1038/s41569-023-00912-z.
30. NCD Countdown 2030 Collaborators. NCD Countdown 2030: efficient pathways and strategic investments to accelerate progress towards the Sustainable Development Goal target 3.4 in low-income and middle-income countries. Lancet. 2022;399:1266–78.
31. United Nations. https://www.uhc2030.org/un-hlm-2019/ (accessed 28 January 2024).
32. United Nations. https://www.un.org/pga/77/wp-content/uploads/sites/105/2023/09/UHC-Final-Text.pdf (accessed 28 January 2024).
33. https://www.who.int/news/item/21-09-2023-world-leaders-commit-to-redouble-efforts-towards-universal-health-coverage-by-2030 (accessed 28 January 2024).
34. World Health Organization. Tracking universal health coverage: 2023 global monitoring report. Geneva: World Health Organization and International Bank for Reconstruction and Development/The World Bank; 2023. Licence: CC BY-NC-SA 3.0 IGO. Available at https://iris.who.int/bitstream/handle/10665/374059/9789240080379-eng.pdf?sequence=1
35. World Health Organization. https://www.who.int/health-topics/universal-health-coverage#tab=tab_1 (accessed 26 January 2024).
36. World Health Organization. HEARTS. https://www.who.int/publications/i/item/9789240001367) (accessed 28 January 2024).
37. WHO model list of essential medicines 2023 https://www.who.int/publications/i/item/WHO-MHP-HPS-EML-2023.02 (accessed 28 January 2023).
38. World Health Organization. https://www.who.int/news/item/26-05-2023-more-ways%2D%2Dto-save-more-lives%2D%2Dfor-less-money%2D%2D%2D%2Dworld-health-assembly-adopts-more-best-buys%2D%2Dto-tackle-noncommunicable-diseases (accessed 26 January 2024).
39. World Health Organization. Political declaration of the third high-level meeting of the General Assembly on the prevention and control of non-communicable diseases, and mental health. https://apps.who.int/gb/ebwha/pdf_files/EB152/B152_6-en.pdf (accessed 26 January 2024).

Glossary

ABI The ratio of ankle systolic blood pressure to brachial systolic blood pressure.

Air pollution Gases and particles suspended in air that can be inhaled and produce health effects.

Artificial Intelligence Computer systems able to perform human tasks that require human intelligence (visual, speech recognition, translations between languages, decision-making).

Built environment The totality of the places and the infrastructure created, such as buildings, streets, and parks, and are the main settings where we live, work, study, and play.

CHIP Somatic mutations in leukocytes increase CHD risk.

Circadian Biological processes recurring naturally on a 24-h cycle even in the absence of light fluctuations.

Climate change It refers to long-term changes in temperatures and weather patterns.

DECIDE Diet Diet, ExerCIse, and CarDiovascular hEalth (DECIDE)-Diet is a multicenter randomized controlled feeding trial to evaluate Chinese heart healthy diets tailored to participants' own regional cuisine.

Doppler waveforms Waveforms of the ankle arteries are collected using a Doppler probe.

Duplex ultrasound Imaging modality to evaluate blood flow and vascular structure using high-frequency sound waves.

Environment Circumstances, objects, or conditions by which one is surrounded.

Environmental justice The fair treatment and meaningful involvement of all people regardless of race, color, national origin, or income, with respect to the development, implementation, and enforcement of environmental laws, regulations, and policies.

T. Romero et al. (eds.), *Global Challenges in Cardiovascular Prevention in Populations with Low Socioeconomic Status*,
https://doi.org/10.1007/978-3-031-79051-5

Environmental stressors Components of the natural or altered environment that could interact with organisms triggering a response that can lead to impaired health.

Free/Low-Cost Medical Care (FLCMC) Free and Low-Cost Medical Services "is a system that provides free or low-cost medical services so that people are not limited in their access to necessary medical care due to economic reasons."

Gender Male or female sex when considered with respect to cultural or social differences rather than biological ones.

Global Action Plan Provides Member States, international partners, and WHO with a road map and menu of policy options which, when implemented collectively, will contribute to progress on nine global NCD targets to be attained in 2025 (later extended to 2030).

Green spaces An area of grass, trees, or other vegetation set apart for recreational or aesthetic purposes in an otherwise urban environment.

Greenhouse gases (GHGs) The gases in the atmosphere that raise the surface temperature of planets such as the Earth.

HEARTS The WHO HEARTS technical package for CVD management in primary health care supports policymakers and program managers at different levels within the Ministry of Health, primarily in LMICs, who can influence CVD primary care delivery.

Living poorness person A person who is in actual economic distress and is at risk of becoming unable to maintain a minimum standard of living.

Long-term care insurance system The public assistance system is a public welfare program by the government that provides necessary protection to those in need and guarantees a minimum standard of living that is healthy and culturally acceptable.

Low- and middle-income countries (LMIC) LMIC is defined by the world bank as having a gross national income (GNI) per capita of US$ 1045 or less (low income), or between US$ 1046 and 12745 (middle income).

Non-communicable diseases Diseases that are not spread by infection or through other people but are typically caused by unhealthy behaviors.

PCSK It inhibits LDL cholesterol liver receptors increasing LDL blood levels and CHD risk. Drugs like Inclisiran inhibit PCSK synthesis.

PEN Package The WHO Package of Essential Noncommunicable (PEN) disease interventions for primary health care defines a minimum set of interventions to address major NCDs, including CVD, in primary care. The components are feasible even in low resource settings and can be delivered by primary care physicians and non-physician health workers.

Polygenic risk score (PRS) Genetic risk profiling and risk factor interaction to identify susceptible populations.

Post-exercise ABI Ratio of ankle and brachial systolic blood pressures after exercise (usually treadmill but can be heel raise)

Primordial prevention Risk factor reduction targeted towards an entire population through modifications on social and environmental conditions.

PVR Waveforms measured by cuffs inflated with a certain volume of air (usually ~60 mmHg)

SDOH (social determinants of health) The circumstances in which people are born, grow up, live, work, and age and the systems put in place to offer health care and services to a community.

SHAKE WHO technical package for salt reduction strategies to enable to achieve a reduction in population salt intake.

Social determinants of health The social, economic, and environmental conditions in which people are born, grow, live, work and age that impact health and well-being across the life course, and the inequities in access to power, decision-making, money, and resources that give rise to these conditions.

Sub-Saharan Africa (SSA) The region of Africa that lies south of the Sahara.

Sustainable development Development that meets the needs of the present without compromising the ability of future generations to meet their own needs.

TBI The ratio of great toe systolic blood pressure to brachial systolic blood pressure.

Universal Health Coverage This means that all people have access to the full range of quality health services they need, when and where they need them, without financial hardship.

Urban environment An area with an increased density of human-created structures in comparison to the areas surrounding it.

Index

T. Romero et al. (eds.), *Global Challenges in Cardiovascular Prevention in Populations with Low Socioeconomic Status*,
https://doi.org/10.1007/978-3-031-79051-5

MIX
Papier aus verantwortungsvollen Quellen
Paper from responsible sources
FSC® C105338

If you have any concerns about our products,
you can contact us on
ProductSafety@springernature.com

In case Publisher is established outside the EU,
the EU authorized representative is:
Springer Nature Customer Service Center GmbH
Europaplatz 3, 69115 Heidelberg, Germany

Printed by Libri Plureos GmbH
in Hamburg, Germany